MULTIPLE SCLEROSIS FOR DUMMIES®

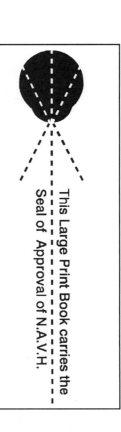

This Large Print Book carries the
Seal of Approval of N.A.V.H.

Multiple Sclerosis for Dummies®

Rosalind Kalb, PhD, Nancy Holland, EdD, RN, and Barbara Giesser, MD

Foreword by David L. Lander

Author of *Fall Down Laughing: How Squiggy Caught Multiple Sclerosis and Didn't Tell Nobody*

THORNDIKE PRESS

An imprint of Thomson Gale, a part of The Thomson Corporation

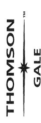

THOMSON

GALE™

Detroit • New York • San Francisco • New Haven, Conn. • Waterville, Maine • London

LIBRARY OF CONGRESS CATALOGING-IN-PUBLICATION DATA

Kalb, Rosalind.
Multiple sclerosis for dummies / by Rosalind Kalb, Nancy Holland, and Barbara Giesser ; foreword by David L. Lander. — Large print ed.
    p. cm.
Includes bibliographical references and index.
ISBN-13: 978-0-7862-9676-7 (hardcover : alk. paper)
ISBN-10: 0-7862-9676-3 (hardcover : alk. paper)
1. Multiple sclerosis — Popular works. I. Holland, Nancy. II. Giesser, Barbara S. III. Title.
RC377.K35 2007
616.8'34—dc22

2007012546

Thorndike Press® Large Print Health, Home, and Learning.

The text of this Large Print edition is unabridged.

Other aspects of the book may vary from the original edition.

Set in 16 pt. Plantin.

Published in 2007 by arrangement with John Wiley & Sons.

Printed in the United States of America on permanent paper

10 9 8 7 6 5 4 3 2 1

Dedication

We dedicate this book to our teachers—beginning with Labe Scheinberg, MD, who launched a generation of clinicians committed to the care of people with MS and their families and ending with our patients and colleagues who have taught us everything else we know about this disease.

Authors' Acknowledgments

Okay, it's time to admit that we didn't do this all by ourselves. We need to thank quite a few people for their assistance along the way:

Stephen Reingold, PhD, for his ongoing encouragement, wealth of knowledge, and willingness to share the initial brainstorm.

Dorothy Northrop, MSW, ACSW, Kimberly Calder, MPS, and Steven Nissen, MS, CRC, from the National MS Society for their time, expertise, and commitment to helping people with MS develop and maintain their vocational and financial safety nets.

Nancy Reitman, RN, MA, for her ideas, behind-the-scenes research, and willingness to pitch in whenever and wherever.

Joyce Nelson, CEO of the National MS Society, John Richert, MD, Executive Vice President of Research and Clinical Programs at the National MS Society, and Adrienne Glasgow, Chief Financial Officer of the National MS Society, for their dedication to people affected by MS and their enthusiastic support of this project and its authors.

And thank you to the amazing group at Wiley:

Lindsay Lefevere—the Acquisitions Editor who paved the way and got us all fired up.

7

Publisher's Acknowledgments

We're proud of this book; please send us your comments through our Dummies online registration form located at www .dummies.com/register/.

Some of the people who helped bring this book to market include the following:

Acquisitions, Editorial, and Media Development

Senior Project Editor: Alissa Schwipps

Acquisitions Editor: Lindsay Lefevere

Copy Editor: Jessica Smith

Technical Editor: David H. Mattson, MD, PhD

Senior Editorial Manager: Jennifer Ehrlich

Editorial Assistants: Erin Calligan Mooney, Joe Niesen, David Lutton, Leeann Harney

Cover Photo: © National Multiple Sclerosis Society

Cartoons: Rich Tennant (www.the5thwave.com)

Composition Services for Original Edition

Project Coordinator: Erin Smith

Layout and Graphics: Carl Byers, Carrie Foster, Shane Johnson, Stephanie D. Jumper, Laura Pence

Alissa Schwipps—our Senior Project Editor who patiently provided invaluable guidance and assistance every step of the way.

Jessica Smith—the Copy Editor who made sure you could read what we wrote.

The Composition team—this team turned our thoughts into the book you're holding.

We also want to thank David Mattson, MD, PhD, for his very thoughtful and valuable technical review of the material.

8

Special Art: Kathryn Born, Medical Illustrator
Proofreaders: John Greenough, Techbooks
Indexer: Techbooks
Anniversary Logo Design: Richard Pacifico

Publishing and Editorial for Consumer Dummies
Diane Graves Steele, Vice President and Publisher, Consumer Dummies
Joyce Pepple, Acquisitions Director, Consumer Dummies
Kristin A. Cocks, Product Development Director, Consumer Dummies
Michael Spring, Vice President and Publisher, Travel
Kelly Regan, Editorial Director, Travel
Publishing for Technology Dummies
Andy Cummings, Vice President and Publisher, Dummies Technology/General User
Composition Services
Gerry Fahey, Vice President of Production Services
Debbie Stailey, Director of Composition Services

9

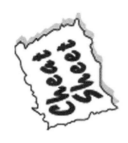

Multiple Sclerosis For Dummies®

Hints for Managing Your Energy Bank

✔ Set priorities to ensure the best use of your daily energy supply.

✔ Make deposits (naps are great!) in addition to your withdrawals.

✔ Use your energy supply efficiently by doing the following:

- Using the right tools/mobility devices
- Making your home/work spaces accessible and convenient
- Asking for help when you need it

✔ Do the most difficult tasks when you have the most energy.

✔ Pace yourself instead of pushing yourself to the point of exhaustion.

✔ Talk to your doctor about symptoms that disrupt your sleep.

✔ Stay cool—literally and figuratively.

✔ Review your medications with your doctor (some have sleepiness or fatigue as a side effect while others are prescribed to relieve it).

Strategies for Feeling Your Best

✔ Talk with your neurologist about treatment with one of the approved disease-modifying therapies to slow disease activity and progression and reduce further nerve damage as much as possible.

✔ Work with your MS team to manage your symptoms, avoid complications, and maintain your quality of life.

✔ Make time for rest, exercise, and healthy, balanced meals.

✔ See your general medical doctor routinely for physical exams and screening tests.

✔ Use the following effective cooling strategies:

- Avoid hot showers, hot tubs, and saunas.

- Limit your time in the hot sun.
- Exercise in a cool environment.
- Drink iced fluids.
- Check out cooling vests and scarves.

➤ Call a friend—there's no need to go it alone.

➤ Don't wait for a crisis—tap the resources that are out there to help you.

➤ Stay focused on your goals—you don't need to make a career out of MS.

Quick Tips to Boost Your Memory

➤ Substitute organization for memory whenever possible:

- Use an organizer or PDA to track dates, names, numbers, and tasks.
- Create reminder systems for yourself (a beeping watch for medication, a reminder in your computer about important meetings or due dates, a birthday/anniversary list).
- Keep important items (glasses, keys, medication) in a consistent place.
- Use a family calendar to track everyone's activities.
- Keep a file of clear, large-print directions in your car.
- Create a master grocery list and check off the items you need before each trip to the store.
- Use step-by-step templates for multi-step tasks (paying bills, balancing the checkbook, preparing a meal, packing a suitcase).

➤ Use all of your senses for learning—read it, say it, and write it down.

➤ Remember that smaller is better—organized (chunked) information, such as phone numbers and social security numbers, is easier to remember than long lists, so organize the stuff you need to remember into bite-size pieces.

➤ If you can't remember something, don't panic because the panicky feeling only makes it harder for your memory to work. Try a little patience and deep breathing to let your memory do its thing.

Partnering with Your Neurologist

✔ Call the National MS Society (800-FIGHT-MS or 800-344-4867) for a list of MS specialists in your area.

✔ For each visit to the neurologist, do the following:

• Be prepared to describe and prioritize problems and symptoms.

• Bring a list of questions.

• To catch everything the doc says, bring your partner or a friend or a tape recorder.

✔ Make sure your doctor has an up-to-date list of all the medications (prescription and over-the-counter) and supplements you're taking.

✔ If you don't understand something, ask (the goal is to know more rather than less when you leave the doctor's office).

✔ If you need a long consultation (to discuss family planning decisions, employment decisions, sexual dysfunction, and so on), schedule a separate appointment or phone call.

✔ Don't wait for a crisis—see your MS doctor on a regular basis.

✔ If you feel you need or want a second opinion, don't hesitate to get one.

A Snapshot of Your Healthcare Team

✔ **Neurologist:** Diagnoses and treats MS and other neurologic diseases.

✔ **Nurse:** Provides education and support for all treatment issues.

✔ **Rehabilitation specialists:** Promote independence, safety, and quality of life. For example, consider the following:

• **Physiatrist:** A physician specializing in rehabilitation medicine.

• **Physical therapist:** Promotes strength, mobility, and balance through exercise and training in the use of mobility aids.

• **Occupational therapist:** Promotes function in activities of daily living via energy management, assistive technology, and environmental modifications (may also treat cognitive symptoms).

• **Speech/language pathologist:** Diagnoses and treats problems with voice quality, speech, and swallowing (may also treat cognitive symptoms).

- **Vocational rehabilitation counselor:** Assists with career planning and retraining.

✓ **Mental health professionals:** Provide diagnosis, treatment, and support for a wide range of emotional issues, as well as education for stress management, goal-setting, and problem-solving strategies.

- **Psychiatrist:** A physician specializing in the diagnosis and treatment of mental health problems.

- **Psychotherapist (psychologist, social worker, counselor):** Provides counseling, information, and support for individuals and families.

- **Neuropsychologist:** Diagnoses and treats cognitive symptoms.

✓ Additional medical specialists: Provide specialized expertise in medical areas that may be impacted by MS or are of particular interest to folks with MS.

- **Neuroophthalmologist:** A physician specializing in neurologically-related visual symptoms.

- **Urologist:** A physician specializing in urinary problems and male sexual function.

- **Obstetrician/gynecologist:** A physician specializing in women's reproductive care.

For Dummies: Bestselling Book Series for Beginners

Contents at a Glance

15

16

Table of Contents

17

20

21

22

23

27

Foreword

It was twenty-some years ago when I first realized that my body was trying to tell me that there was something wrong. I had no idea what was happening nor would I know what to do about it if I did.

First there were the problems with my legs, then my arms, then my balance. With all the changing symptoms and the doctors not knowing what I had, I thought I had contracted hypochondria. I knew I had something, but what? I asked myself, "What is this? Does it have a name?"

When I found out I had multiple sclerosis, other than finally having a label for my problem, I still had no idea what to do with it. It was complicated. It was unpredictable. And there was no cure!

I was lost and had no idea which way to go.

Had I had a wonderful book as simple to navigate, yet as comprehensive as *Multiple Sclerosis For Dummies*, my family and I would have saved a lot of time and aggravation.

It took me years to realize that the most constructive way to deal with my MS was by playing an active role as part of my health care team. While you won't be able to be a doctor after reading *Multiple Sclerosis For Dummies*, you will be much more capable of asking your doctor the right ques-

31

tions, and that makes you an effective component of your own treatment.

While getting MS is no joke, *Multiple Sclerosis For Dummies* offers humor as another essential element for understanding and facing your MS. MS can take a lot of things away from you, but it cannot take away your sense of humor.

Multiple Sclerosis For Dummies is like a global positioning system for your condition; it'll keep you from feeling lost.

David L. Lander ("Squiggy")
Proud Member of the MS Community

32

Introduction

Being diagnosed with multiple sclerosis (MS) is definitely a bummer, but living with it doesn't have to be. This book is all about how to live your life with MS without making a full-time job of it. After diving in, you'll be more informed and more prepared no matter how your MS behaves.

If you've never heard of MS before and you want to know what may be in store, this book is definitely for you. You also want to take a gander through this book if all you've ever heard about MS is the bad stuff. We suggest this because the fact is, you've probably met several people at work, at the gym, or in your neighborhood, who have MS and you didn't even know it. And, even if the people you happen to know with MS don't seem to have a symptom or care in the world, you now have another good reason to keep reading: Everyone's MS is different and no one can predict exactly what yours will be like.

The three of us—a neurologist, a nurse, and a psychologist—have worked with, and learned from, people with MS for over 30 years (actually it's 82 years if you add our careers together end to end!). We wrote this book as a team effort so we could send a loud and clear message that you're not alone. Health professionals trained in neurology,

33

nursing, psychology, rehabilitation medicine, and a variety of other disciplines, as well as voluntary organizations, such as the National Multiple Sclerosis Society, are ready to help you every step of the way.

About This Book

Don't worry: In this book, we're not going to try and tell you everything there is to know about MS. Instead, we only give you what you need in order to make educated choices and comfortable decisions. We provide lots of information that's easy to access and easy to swallow regarding what happens in MS—what kinds of symptoms it can cause, how it can affect your life at home and at work, what you can do to feel and function up to snuff, and how you can protect yourself and your family against the long-term unpredictability of the disease. We also throw in useful tips, introduce you to the members of your healthcare team, and point you in the direction of other useful resources. And we even promise to make you chuckle once or twice along the way.

Feel free to pick and choose what you want to read—you don't have to take a cover-to-cover approach if you're more comfortable with a hop, skip, and jump style. Each chapter tackles a different aspect of living with MS so that you can zero in on the stuff that's most relevant to you.

Conventions Used in This Book

We used the following conventions throughout the text to make things consistent and easy to understand:

- ✔ All Web addresses appear in monofont.
- ✔ New terms appear in *italics* and are closely followed

34

by an easy-to-understand definition.

✔ **Bold** is used to highlight the action parts of numbered steps.

✔ Because most people with MS receive their MS-related care from a neurologist (a physician who specializes in the diagnosis and treatment of diseases of the nervous system), we use the terms *neurologist*, *doctor*, and *physician* interchangeably whenever we're referring to the person who's treating your MS. When we're talking about other medical specialists—such as internists, family practice doctors, urologists, gynecologists, physiatrists, psychiatrists—we refer to them by their specialty titles.

✔ We talk about a lot of medications in this book, which you may or may not ever need. In case you do, we always give the brand name first, because that's the one you're most likely to see in advertisements or hear other people talk about, followed by the chemical name in parentheses.

What You're Not to Read

Even though we poured heart and soul into every page of this book, we know that you won't want to read it all—and most likely you won't need to. So, we make it easy for you to identify "skippable" material by sticking it into sidebars. This is the stuff in the gray boxes that's interesting and related to the topic at hand, but not essential for your health and well-being.

Foolish Assumptions

Even though no two people have MS in exactly the same

way, we assume that you—our readers—still have quite a few things in common. We've written this book with these thoughts about you in mind:

- You have MS or care about someone who does.

- However much you already know about MS, you want to know more—in language that's easy to access and easy to understand.

- You're looking for ways to manage your MS and the symptoms it can cause.

- You want to be healthy, active, and productive in spite of whatever challenges MS is throwing your way.

- You wish you had a crystal ball, but you're willing to settle for some helpful suggestions on how to deal with the unpredictability of MS.

How This Book Is Organized

This book is divided into seven parts to help you gather all the information you need about MS. However, every part can stand alone, so you don't have to read one before another. In fact, if you're looking for only a few things in particular, just check out the table of contents or the index and skip directly to those topics. The following is a rundown of the seven parts.

Part 1: When MS Becomes Part of Your Life

Whether MS has entered your life with a bang or a whimper, you need to know what it's all about. So, in this part, we fill you in on the basic facts as well as the big mysteries that remain to be solved. We show you the usual steps in-

36

volved in getting a diagnosis and suggest ways to handle any reactions that you may have during those early days (as well as those that may crop up as the realities of the disease begin to sink in). This part also gives you good ideas on how to begin making room in your life for a chronic, unpredictable illness—without giving it more of your attention than it needs.

It's always good to know that you don't have to deal with tough stuff on your own—so, in this part, we also spend some time introducing you to the healthcare professionals who are going to help you manage your MS.

Part II: Taking Charge of Your MS

The best way to feel more confident in the face of any new challenge is to come up with a game plan. And you're in luck because this part of the book is designed to do just that. It helps you get started with the planning process and gives you tips on how to work with your healthcare team to make the treatment choices that best meet your needs.

Each chapter describes a part of the MS treatment package—including all the immediate and longer-term strategies for slowing disease activity, dealing with pesky relapses, and managing symptoms. We talk about the importance of early treatment and describe the available options. And, we zero in on ways to manage the physical symptoms that can pop up along the way, as well as the ones that can mess with your head, such as mood changes and problems with memory and thinking.

Alternative medicine is a hot topic for people with MS, so in this part, we also give you pointers on how to sift through the available products and services to find those that are safe and effective for people with MS.

Part III: Staying Healthy and Feeling Well

You can be healthy with MS—in fact, the healthier you are the better you're going to feel. So, this part is all about how to take care of yourself with a healthy, balanced diet, the right kind of exercise, restful sleep, and some good stress management strategies.

Throughout the chapters of this part, we emphasize the importance of looking beyond your MS (or your family member's MS) to develop an overall wellness plan involving regular checkups by your family doctor and dentist and the preventive health screens recommended for your age group.

In this part, we also give you an idea of what to do when your MS isn't behaving very nicely. When the disease progresses in spite of available treatments, it's important to know how to manage your symptoms, avoid messy complications, and keep your life on track.

Part IV: Managing Lifestyle Issues

The key to coping well with your MS is finding ways to fit it into your life. So, in this part, we begin with a reminder that people's responses to your MS are going to depend in large part on how you present it to them. We then go on to give you lots of strategies for helping others understand what your MS is all about.

We also include a chapter that shows how to make MS part of the family. This chapter describes the ways in which families are affected when someone they love gets MS, and it also shares tips to help family members communicate and problem-solve more comfortably.

Because MS is diagnosed most often during early adulthood, when people are busy starting or adding to their families, this part fills you in on all the good news for prospective parents (yes, people with MS can have happy, healthy kids!). It gives you lots of parenting tips to help you deal with those bundles of joy that quickly grow into toddlers and teens.

Part V: Creating Your Safety Nets

The hallmark of MS is its unpredictability. Because everyone's MS is different and no one has a crystal ball, anxiety about the future is pretty common. To reduce that anxiety as much as possible, this part is all about making sure that you're armed and ready to deal with whatever comes along.

We give you tips on how to stay in the work force as long as you're interested and able, strategies for getting and maintaining insurance coverage, and recommendations for how to plan effectively for the unpredictable future. When you're living with MS, developing these kinds of safety nets can help you feel less vulnerable and more in control.

Part VI: The Part of Tens

In this part, we give you some key suggestions in a handy top-ten format. One chapter lists ten tips to live by when you have MS and another lists the mistaken notions about MS that you can finally put to rest. We round out this part with ten strategies to make traveling with MS as trouble-free as possible.

Part VII: Appendixes

This is the last-but-definitely-not-least part. We start with a glossary so you can look up any of those technical words that trip you up when you're reading about MS, attending an educational meeting, or even talking to your doctor. Then we point you toward some important resources that you may want to tap along the way—including other books

39

that zero in on some of the issues covered here, Web sites with accurate, up-to-date information, and community agencies and organizations that you can tap for information or assistance if the need arises.

Icons Used in This Book

To make this book easier to read and simpler to use, we include some icons that can help you pick out the key ideas and points of information throughout the book.

This icon highlights shortcuts that help you conserve valuable resources, such as energy, time, and money.

When you see this icon, it tells you that the information that follows is essential and that you should keep it in mind as you deal with your MS.

This icon flags dangers to your health, safety, or general well-being.

This icon reminds you when it's time to check in with your neurologist or another specialist on your healthcare team.

Where to Go from Here

This book is organized so that all you need to do is shut your eyes and point in order to find complete information about one aspect of MS or another. If you prefer the eyes-open method but aren't sure where you want to start, we recommend Part I. It gives you basic info about MS and how it's diagnosed, as well as some tips for sorting out all of the feelings that an MS diagnosis can stir up. If you've already been there and done that, you may want to check out specific treatment strategies in Part II, or discover ways to feel more bright-eyed and bushy-tailed in Part III. If you're wondering how MS may affect your relationships with the important people in your life, you can focus on Part IV. And if you're someone who likes to get all your ducks in a row from the get-go (and even if you're not), you can check out Part V for suggestions on how to feel securely prepared in spite of the unpredictability of MS.

No matter where you choose to begin, begin now. Make it your priority to educate yourself about MS and the strategies you and your family members can use to live well in spite of it.

41

Part I

When MS Becomes Part of Your Life

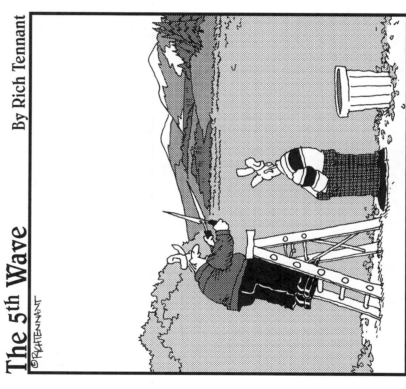

The 5th Wave   By Rich Tennant

"Living with MS is like owning a large hedge. The more you manage it, the better the outlook."

In this part . . .

We're guessing that multiple sclerosis (MS) has become part of your life recently. Either you or someone you care about has been diagnosed with MS and you're wondering what it's all about. This part gives you the big picture, starting with an overview of what doctors know—and don't know—about this chronic, unpredictable disease and what you can do to live comfortably and productively in spite of it. The good news is that you aren't ever alone in your efforts to overcome the challenges of MS—your healthcare team, which we introduce to you in this part, will always be right beside you.

Chapter 1

Meeting MS Face to Face

Because you've picked up this book, we're assuming that your doctor has delivered the news that you have multiple sclerosis (MS). Or, perhaps he or she said that you *may* have this disease, or that you *probably* have this disease (which makes you wonder why you can't get a clear answer). Whether you got the news yesterday or several months ago, you're probably trying to figure out what it means for you, for your future, and for your family. In other words, you have about a zillion questions about what's in store.

Chances are, the answers you've received so far haven't

Introducing the Roles Your Immune and Nervous Systems Play in MS

Surprise! Even though MS is described as the most common *neurologic* disorder diagnosed in young adults, the problem doesn't appear to originate with the nervous system. Instead, decades of research have pointed to the body's immune system as the culprit. Some kind of malfunction in the immune system interferes with the functioning of the body's nervous system, resulting in the symptoms commonly associated with MS. The current thinking is that the glitch is an *autoimmune* problem, which basically means that your body is mistakenly destroying some of its own healthy tissues and cells. But, this thinking has yet to be proven. We explain the autoimmune process in the section "What happens in MS" later in the chapter, but for

been all that satisfying—mostly because MS still can't be cured, no one knows what causes it, and no doctor can predict with any certainty how your MS is going to behave in the future. However, the good news is that the treatment options are expanding, and people with MS are busy getting on with their lives—and you will too.

In this chapter, which is an introduction to MS and an overview of what we cover in the rest of the book, we fill you in on the available MS info—including what scientists have been able to discover about the workings of this disease and what questions remain to be answered. We explain why your MS is different from everyone else's, and we introduce you to the treatment strategies that can help you manage your MS. Finally, we glance at the ways that MS can affect life at home and at work, and we show you what you can do to ensure the best possible quality of life for you and the people you love.

46

now, it's important to understand how the immune system is supposed to work when it's healthy.

The immune system: Your body's frontline defender

The *immune system*—which is a complex network of glands, tissues, and circulating cells—is your body's frontline defense in the fight against infection by viruses, bacteria, and other bad guys. When confronted with an infection, the immune system gears up to neutralize the foreign invader and make you healthy again.

In order for your immune system to do its job properly, it has to be able to distinguish between the good guys (the cells, tissues, and organs that make up your body) and the bad guys (any foreign invader, such as a virus or bacteria that doesn't share your genes). And get this: The immune system is so powerful that it would reject a pregnant woman's developing fetus (which shares only some of her genes) if the hormones of pregnancy didn't suppress her immune system. (Check out Chapter 16 to read more about how pregnancy hormones appear to affect MS.)

The nervous system: Your body's CEO

The *nervous system*, which controls all bodily functions, is made up of *neurons*, each of which consists of a cell body and its long extension—the *axon*. And each axon is covered by a protective or insulating coating called *myelin*. The neurons are gathered into small- and large-sized bundles called *nerves*.

The system is basically divided into two parts: The *central nervous system* (CNS), which consists of the brain, spinal cord, and optic nerves, is the target of the damage done in MS. The *peripheral nervous system* (PNS) includes the branching network of nerves and axons that connects the CNS to muscles, sensory organs, and glands in the rest of the body.

The nervous system conducts three basic kinds of electrical signals throughout the body:

- ✔ **Motor signals:** These signals, which move from the CNS, through the PNS, and to muscles and other organs, control movement, strength, and other bodily functions.

- ✔ **Sensory signals:** These signals go back to the CNS from the eyes, ears, skin, and other sensory organs, and they provide information about the environment from those organs.

- ✔ **Integrative signals:** These signals travel from nerve cell to nerve cell within the nervous system and are thought to be responsible for many cognitive functions, such as thinking and memory (check out Chapter 9 for information about cognitive changes in MS).

These electrical signals are like the current in an electrical wire: When everything is working fine, they travel long distances along the myelin-covered axons in the CNS, jumping from one axon to another as needed. The myelin (like the rubber or plastic insulation around an electrical wire), is what helps speed the electrical signals on their journey and smoothes out any bumps along the way.

What happens in MS

After you understand the role of the immune system and the nervous system, you can begin to understand how MS affects them. In autoimmune diseases like MS (and rheumatoid arthritis, myasthenia gravis, and Type I diabetes, among others), the immune system loses the ability to distinguish the good guys from the bad guys, and so it starts attacking the normal tissues in the body. In MS, this autoimmune response targets the myelin coating around the axons in the CNS as well as the axons themselves.

The autoimmune attack happens because of a breakdown in the *blood-brain barrier* (BBB), which allows immune cells that have been living harmlessly in your blood to travel into your CNS to attack the myelin and axons, resulting in the symptoms associated with MS. The autoimmune process in MS follows these steps (see Figure 1-1):

1. The inflammation that occurs during an MS *relapse* (also called an attack or exacerbation) damages the BBB, allowing the movement of immune cells into the CNS. (Skip to Chapter 6 for more info about MS relapses.)

2. Toxic substances are released into the CNS, which can increase inflammation and result in the breakdown of myelin (in a process called *demyelination*) and the axons.

3. Nervous system cells called *astrocytes* move into the locations where the damage has occurred and they form scar tissue (giving rise to the name *multiple sclerosis*, which means multiple scars).

49

The results of the autoimmune process aren't all that pretty: The inflammation can cause swelling, which interferes with the conduction of signals in the nervous system. The demyelination results in a loss of insulation around the neurons' axons, which slows or interrupts nervous system conduction. And finally, the axons can be broken (a process referred to as *axonal loss*), which breaks the connections between the nervous system and parts of the body. (Figure 1-2 shows the steps involved in demyelination and axonal loss.) This whole process results in the symptoms that we describe in Chapters 7, 8, and 9. (Flip to Chapter 6 to read about the treatments that can reduce the inflammation and slow the destructive process.)

REMEMBER

Figure 1-1:
A view of the autoimmune process.

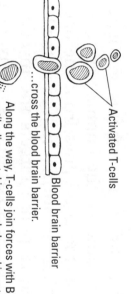

Activated T-cells

Blood brain barrier

...cross the blood brain barrier.

Along the way, T-cells join forces with B-cells, antibodies, cytokines, and chemokines to launch attacks on myelin and nerve fibers.

Demyelination disrupts transmission of impulses along the nerve fiber....

AND...

Direction of nerve impulse

Myelinated nerve fiber

Large, reactive astrocyte

Nerve cell body

Severely demyelinated axon

Scar tissue

Astrocytes are attracted to demyelinated areas on nerve fibers where they form scar tissue. Multiple scars means "multiple sclerosis."

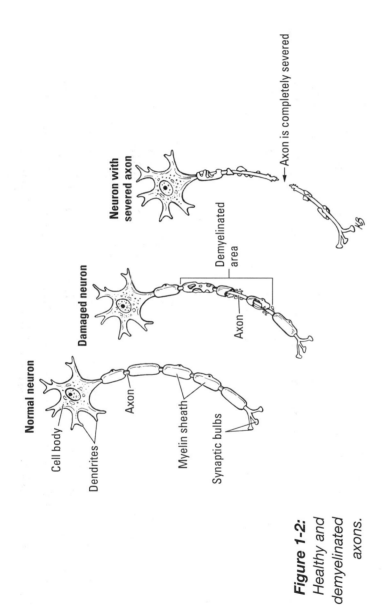

Figure 1-2:
Healthy and demyelinated axons.

Normal neuron

Cell body

Dendrites

Axon

Myelin sheath

Synaptic bulbs

Damaged neuron

Axon

Demyelinated area

Neuron with severed axon

Axon is completely severed

Taking advantage of the body's natural healing process

The body has a natural capacity to heal some of the damage caused by MS. For example, partial healing occurs following each MS relapse. Here's how it works: The inflammation that occurs during an MS relapse causes *edema*—the accumulation of fluids at the site of the damaged myelin (picture what happens when you sprain your ankle). Edema results in swelling that compresses the myelin-coated axons and interferes with the transmission of nerve signals. As the inflammation and swelling disappear, and the relapse comes to an end, some of the axons begin to decompress and are able to function normally again. The reduction of inflammation can happen through a natural healing process, or can sometimes be prodded along with steroid medications (which you can read about in Chapter 6).

51

In addition, the myelin coating that has been damaged by the inflammation has some ability—but not a whole lot—to heal or regenerate. As long as the axon itself remains intact, the natural regeneration of myelin can smooth out the conduction of nerve impulses and result in some amount of improvement of symptoms over time. Check out the National MS Society Web site at www.nationalmssociety.org/myelin for more information on myelin and current research efforts to stimulate this natural healing process.

After the nerve fiber itself has been damaged or severed, and scar tissue has formed, healing is much more difficult. Unfortunately, doctors haven't yet found a way to repair damaged axons or to remove the scars. Researchers are focusing a lot of attention on how to promote this kind of repair—and this is precisely where stem cell research may be most relevant in MS. To read about stems cells and their potential value in the treatment of MS, go to www.nationalmssociety.org/stemcell.

Exploring Possible MS Triggers

Assuming that MS is, in fact, an autoimmune disease, it's important to figure out what actually triggers the immune system's attack on the nervous system. Most scientists agree that no single virus or bacterium causes MS all by itself. They have also concluded that no single thing in the environment or in a person's diet is directly responsible for the disease.

Currently, scientists believe that the disease is caused by a combination of several factors—including gender, racial or ethnic, geographic, genetic, and lifestyle factors that interact with an infectious trigger of some kind (for example, one or more viruses or bacteria) to stimulate the autoimmune process. This means that when a person with a genetic susceptibility to MS meets up with the environmental trigger or triggers, his or her immune system overreacts in a way that sets off the abnormal autoimmune process.

This sounds simple enough, but the question of why some people get MS and others don't remains one of the great mysteries of this disease. Solving this mystery is important because identifying the factors that make some people susceptible to MS and others not would help scientists figure out the cause of MS. And, identifying the cause would make it a whole lot easier to find more effective treatment and, eventually, a cure.

Gender clues

The fact that MS doesn't occur equally in women and men has long piqued the curiosity of scientists and physicians. It turns out that some interesting differences exist between the sexes (in regard to MS, that is) that may provide important clues to the cause of MS:

- MS is two to three times more common in women than in men. However, prior to the onset of puberty, boys are as likely to get MS as girls (check out Chapter 15 for more info about MS in kids).

- Men tend to develop MS at a later age than women do, and they're more likely than women to be diagnosed with primary-progressive MS. (You can read more about the disease courses in the section "Distinguishing the four disease types" later in the chapter.)

Ethnic or racial clues

MS isn't unique to one racial or ethnic group, but certain groups are much more susceptible than others. Scientists are using the following clues to help themselves understand the genetic and environmental factors that may be causing these group differences:

➤ MS is most common among Caucasians of northern European ancestry.

➤ African-Americans and Hispanics develop MS half as often as Caucasians.

➤ Asians develop MS less frequently than Caucasians and generally have different types of symptoms.

➤ MS is rare (or unheard of) in pure Africans, Inuits, and some isolated populations around the world that have never mingled with other groups.

Geographical clues

The geographical distribution of MS has been known for a long time: In general, the further you live from the equator, the greater your chances are of developing MS. Like a lot of other aspects of MS, no one knows why this is true, but here are some possible explanations:

➤ **Genetic/ethnic:** Residents in the temperate areas of the world (except certain groups like the Inuits) tend to be of northern European descent.

➤ **Climatic/meteorologic:** Residents of the tropics have greater exposure to the sun and vitamin D, which may offer some protection against MS.

➤ **Infectious:** Certain types of infectious agents may be more common in temperate areas of the world.

Each of these possible explanations is the subject of intensive study in the MS research community.

An interesting wrinkle in the geographical data—which no one can yet explain—suggests that timing may be the key. Data, particularly from Israel and South Africa, suggest that people who migrate from their birthplace *before* puberty take on the MS risk factor of their new home, whereas people who migrate *after* puberty maintain the risk level associated with their birthplace. Just remember that these are statistical statements that characterize large groups of people, not single people within that group. This means that these statements provide no kind of guarantee for you or your children. So, there's no need to pack your bags and relocate to the tropics.

Genetic clues

MS isn't an inherited disease. However, the evidence is quite strong that a genetic factor contributes to a person's risk of developing MS. The following facts point to a genetic component:

✔ Approximately 20 percent of people with MS have a close or distant relative with MS.

✔ The risk for someone who has one close relative with MS is 3 to 5 percent (compared to less than 1 percent in people without a relative with MS). For a person in a *multiplex family*—which has several members with MS—the risk of developing MS is even higher. Keep in mind, however, that even within the same family, close relatives can experience very different disease courses, symptoms, and levels of disability.

✔ If one identical twin develops MS, the risk for the other twin is about 30 percent—proving that the disease isn't directly inherited. Because identical twins share identical genetic traits, the risk would be would be 100 percent if genetics told the whole story.

Lifestyle clues

You've probably asked yourself (and your doctor) a hundred times what you did—or didn't do—to cause your MS. Just remember that it's clear from the study of geography, ethnicity, and genetics that the cause of MS—whatever it turns out to be—isn't anything simple or direct. You didn't *do* anything to cause MS to happen.

However, here are some intriguing findings related to lifestyle:

➤ Even though exposure to sunlight and vitamin D is primarily determined by how close to the equator a person lives, it may also be related to time spent outdoors. One study also found that people who got extra vitamin D from a daily multivitamin were at a lower risk for MS.

➤ Some studies have suggested that dietary factors may play a role in determining a person's susceptibility to MS. For example, it has been suggested that Inuits don't get MS because of their fish-heavy diet.

➤ A few studies have suggested that smoking may increase a person's risk of developing MS as well as the risk for disease progression, but no one has a clue why this may be true. So, if you're looking for yet another reason to quit smoking, its possible relationship to MS is a good one.

It's difficult to separate out these lifestyle findings from other factors because none of them happen in isolation. Genetics and geography are also operating regardless of one's smoking, sunning, or eating habits. So, in the meantime, flip to Chapter 11 for more info about diet and general wellness.

Understanding Why Your MS Is as Unique as Your Fingerprint

Here's something to think about: If you went to a large gathering of people with MS, chances are high that you wouldn't meet anyone whose MS was just like yours. MS is so variable from one person to the next that your experience with MS will be totally unique.

Even though the cause of this variability isn't clear, it probably has to do with the genetic and geographic factors we talk about in the section "Exploring Possible MS Triggers" earlier in the chapter. In addition, the inflammatory process that damages myelin and axons can happen just about anywhere in the central nervous system, with the random targets resulting in different kinds of symptoms (check out the section "Scanning the possible symptoms" later in the chapter).

Distinguishing the four disease types

A little over a decade ago, a group of MS specialists—researchers and clinicians—got together to develop a common language for talking about MS. The group identified the following four disease types or courses:

✔ **Relapsing-remitting MS (RRMS):** MS begins as a relapsing-remitting disease about 85 percent of the time. RRMS is characterized by unpredictable periods of worsening (called *relapses, exacerbations,* or *attacks*) followed by remissions. A *remission* may be complete, meaning that the person returns to his or her pre-relapse level of functioning, or partial, meaning that some of the symptoms are likely to be permanent.

✔ **Secondary-progressive MS (SPMS):** Within about 10 years, approximately 50 percent of those who are diagnosed with RRMS transition to SPMS, which is characterized by a steady (but not necessarily rapid) progression of disability without any remissions. These folks generally have fewer or no relapses as time goes on.

✔ **Primary-progressive MS (PPMS):** For about 10 percent of people, MS progresses right from the beginning, without any relapses or remissions. PPMS seems to differ from RRMS and SPMS in terms of its underlying disease process—it has less inflammatory action going on in the brain and spinal cord and more tissue degeneration and destruction early on. These differences may be the reason that the current treatments for MS (check them out in Chapter 6)— which mainly target the inflammation—work much better in relapsing forms of MS than they do in PPMS.

✔ **Progressive-relapsing MS (PRMS):** A very small number of people (less than 5 percent) are diagnosed initially with a progressive form of the disease, but then experience some relapses down the road.

Check out Figure 1-3 for a quick glance at the four disease types.

58

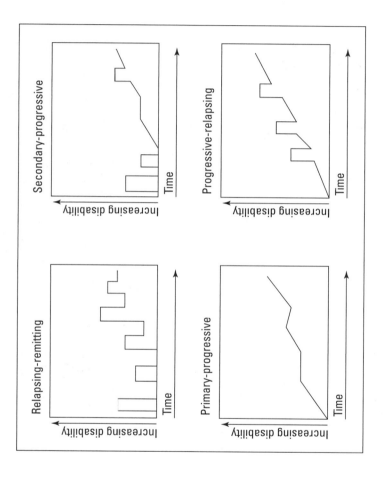

Figure 1-3:
The four disease types in MS.

Even though these categories may seem nice and neat, they really aren't. Within each of the groups is a tremendous variability, so don't be surprised if your MS doesn't quite fit any of the descriptions outlined here.

For example, regardless of their disease type, some folks may experience a course that's mild and relatively stable for many years, while others (more often those with PPMS or severe SPMS) may have a rapidly disabling course (see Chapter 13 for more on dealing with advanced disease). Unfortunately, no one can predict with any certainty whose MS is going to do what, which has led most MS specialists to conclude that early treatment with one of the available medications (refer to Chapter 6) is the best way to hedge your bets.

Scanning the possible symptoms

MS symptoms can involve virtually any sensory or motor

function that's controlled by the central nervous system. This means that the list of possible symptoms is long—including fatigue (by far the most common), visual changes, walking problems, and tremor (Chapter 7); bladder and bowel problems, sexual difficulties, sensory changes, and speech and swallowing problems (Chapter 8); and mood changes and problems with thinking and memory (Chapter 9).

Most symptoms tend to come and go, but some may come and stay. And they can range from mild to quite severe. The good news is that most people don't develop *all* of these symptoms, and most of the symptoms are treatable.

MS symptoms don't show up in any particular order. Often, however, visual changes are what bring someone to the doctor. Then, once in the doctor's office, it's pretty common for someone to remember an episode of one or more of these symptoms during high school or college that came and went without anyone paying much mind. That's why your doctor asks you so many questions and takes such a careful medical history when trying to arrive at a diagnosis. (Flip to Chapter 2 for information about the diagnostic process.)

Perusing the MS Treatment Menu

Reading about all the MS symptoms can definitely be an eye-opening experience. In fact, both your eyes and your mouth may be hanging wide open when you do. But try not to panic. With the help of your treatment team (flip to Chapter 4 for details), you can figure out how to manage your symptoms and take the necessary steps to control the disease as much as possible.

Because MS is so complex, treatment involves several different strategies, all of which are discussed in detail in Part II. However, for now, here are snapshots of several steps you can take to feel and function up to snuff:

✔ **Use disease-modifying therapy.** Your doctor will discuss with you whether you're a candidate for treatment with one of the disease-modifying therapies (flip to Chapter 6 for details). For example, if you have relapsing-remitting MS or secondary-progressive MS and are having periodic relapses, you're probably a candidate. These medications don't cure MS, but they do reduce the frequency and severity of relapses. And, they probably slow the progression of the disease to some degree.

✔ **Manage your relapses.** Relapses (also called attacks or exacerbations) can be treated with corticosteroids if necessary. Even though the corticosteroids don't have any long-term impact on the disease, they're often effective in reducing the inflammation and bringing the relapse to an end more quickly. When you have a relapse, you and your doctor will decide whether the symptoms are interfering enough with your everyday activities to warrant treatment. (Check out Chapter 6 for more on managing your relapses.)

✔ **Manage your symptoms.** You and your healthcare team will work together to manage your symptoms effectively (see Chapters 7, 8, and 9). Successful symptom management relies on effective teamwork—with you being a key player on your team. Your job is to report symptoms promptly, follow through with the treatment plan, and provide feedback on what treatments do and don't work for you. And, remember, as your symptoms change, so will the strategies you use to manage them.

✔ **Work with the rehabilitation team:** Like the mechanics that keep your car finely tuned and road-

61

ready, the rehab team helps you get in gear (check out Chapter 4 for more on this team). Physical and occupational therapists can help you do what you want to do, comfortably and safely, and prevent yucky complications. They're the experts when it comes to finding the right tools to solve problems with walking, seeing, holding on to stuff, or anything else you're having trouble with.

- **Promote your overall health and wellness.** Feeling your best involves more than just managing your MS. So, it's important that you not focus on your MS to the exclusion of your general health. Unfortunately, being diagnosed with MS doesn't protect you from the health problems that plague all mortals. This means that you have to get the proper nutrition, exercise, and preventive healthcare (Chapter 11) and you have to manage the stresses of your everyday life (Chapter 12).

- **Seek out emotional support.** Living with MS isn't a piece of cake. Even for those whose symptoms remain mild and manageable, the unpredictability alone is enough to stress people out. So, Chapter 3 shows you how to deal with your new diagnosis and come to grips with a chronic illness. The fact is that adjusting to this intrusion in your life—and your family's life—is an ongoing process that begins with your first symptoms and continues through all the changes that MS can bring.

Fortunately, you don't have to cope with this alone. Throughout this book, we suggest ways to get the support you need—from your healthcare team, from the National MS Society and other organizations, and from those close to you. Check out Part IV for suggestions on how to communicate with others about your MS and about how to deal with the emotional stresses that MS can cause for you and the people you love.

Recognizing How Your MS Affects Your Loved Ones

When you throw a pebble into a lake or stream, there's always a ripple effect. Getting diagnosed with MS is similar because when one person in a family is diagnosed with MS, the entire family is affected by it. To help you adjust, we devote Chapter 15 to making MS a part of your family. Even though the symptoms are yours, your loved ones share everything from the impact of those symptoms on daily life to the financial pressures caused by MS. And like you, each family member is going to react to all of these challenges.

Talking about the tough stuff

One of the first hurdles for family members is figuring out how to talk comfortably—and honestly—with one another about the intrusion of MS in their lives. No one asked for MS, and no one likes it, so all of you are likely to feel sad, anxious, and maybe even a little resentful about the whole thing. Talking about these heavy-duty feelings can be difficult, particularly when you're all worried about creating more upset or worry for people you love.

Family members also tend to have different ways of dealing with tough stuff. For example, you may be a talker while your partner is the strong, silent type. These different—and sometimes conflicting—coping styles are another barrier to communication. So Chapter 15 offers you strategies for starting—and continuing—the tough conversations.

63

Keeping daily life on track

As you may have noticed, MS symptoms can disrupt the rhythms of daily life. You may find that you can't do some things as well or as fast as you used to do them, and that you need to swap some chores and responsibilities with other family members. If you and your family members are finding that plans—especially outings and trips—are disrupted by pesky symptoms or unexpected relapses, check out Chapter 15 for ideas on how to keep the good times rolling, and Chapter 23 for ten traveling tips to keep in mind.

Because MS symptoms are so unpredictable, you may all need to be a lot more flexible and creative than you have ever been before. Your goal as a family is to make sure that MS doesn't interfere with your plans and priorities any more than absolutely necessary.

Maintaining healthy partnerships

Couples generally don't know what they're getting into with that "in sickness and in health" line. So chances are, you're probably learning from scratch how to adapt your partnership to the challenges of MS. In Chapter 15, we provide strategies to help you keep your partnership feeling comfortable and balanced. And in Chapter 8, we tell you how to manage the symptoms that can interfere with your sexual relationship. Regardless of the path your MS takes, the goal is to maintain a healthy, mutually satisfying partnership.

If you aren't already in a committed relationship, you're probably in the dating scene, which is challenging enough without MS symptoms getting in the way. If this sounds like your situation, turn to Chapter 14 for tips on how to talk about your MS with a prospective partner.

Becoming confident parents

When young adults are diagnosed with MS, some of the first questions they ask are about having kids. Young women want to know how a pregnancy will affect their MS and whether their MS will harm the baby. Men and women both have questions about how MS will affect their ability to be good parents.

Although Chapter 16 gives you all the details about conception, pregnancy, childbirth, and breastfeeding, here's a sneak preview: Women and men with MS can be terrific parents of healthy, happy children. We suggest some important stuff to keep in mind when making your family plans—such as the unpredictability of MS, the depth of your financial resources, and the strength of your support system. And, we recommend some strategies to help you and your partner come to the decisions that are right for both of you.

But, we don't stop with childbirth, because that's over in a jiffy. Chapter 17 is full of parenting tips, including how to talk to your kids about MS, how to keep your MS symptoms from getting in the way of quality time with your kids, and how to keep MS from being the center of everyone's attention.

Minimizing the Impact of MS on Work and Play

MS is generally a relapsing-remitting disease, which means that symptoms come and go in an unpredictable way. So, don't make big decisions about any major life activities in the middle of a relapse or a particularly stressful week. Too many people end up leaving the workforce when they're first diagnosed or during a subsequent relapse, only to discover a few weeks or months down the road that they're feeling fine—but now they're unemployed. (If stress is getting you down, flip to Chapter 12 for ways to manage it.)

If you're considering leaving your job because of your MS, be sure to take advantage of all the legal protections that are available to you before thinking about disability retirement. The Americans with Disabilities Act (ADA) and other statutes are in place to help you stay employed as long as you want and are able to. Chapter 18 describes the provisions of the ADA, gives you pointers on how and when to disclose your MS at the workplace, and walks you through the steps for requesting accommodations from your employer.

Fun and recreation are just as important as work. Too often, people begin to give up activities they can no longer do easily or well. Before they know it, they've given up a lot of the things that make their life fun, full, and interesting. We talk a lot in this book about getting comfortable with doing things differently. After you decide that it's okay to be creative, you'll find a way to do just about everything that's important to you. People with MS swim, ski, sail, play golf, go camping, and travel all over the world. Chapter 7 describes the tools and strategies that can help you get around some of your symptoms, and Chapter 23 gives you ten tips for travel.

Taking Steps to Protect Your Quality of Life

Given the unpredictability of MS, you're probably wondering what you can do to safeguard your quality of life. The short answer is: You have to be a master at thoughtful planning and decision-making. We know that most folks don't enjoy second-guessing the future, but the best way to enjoy your comfort and security down the road is to get all your ducks in a row now. So, check out Chapter 19 for info on how to ensure that your insurance coverage is the best that it can be, and Chapter 20, which gives you tips on how to plan for an unpredictable future. In the meantime, here's the shorthand prescription for protecting your quality of life: *Hope for the best, but plan for the worst.*

You aren't alone. Lots of people are with you on your MS path, including the scientists who continue to look for answers, the health professionals who want to partner with you in your care, and the voluntary health organizations, such as the National MS Society, that offer information and support. We offer this book as a friendly guide through the process.

Chapter 2

So, What Is It, Doc?
Getting a Diagnosis

In This Chapter

▼ Sorting out the diagnostic criteria

▼ Discovering the tools used to diagnose MS

▼ Realizing why an MS diagnosis takes so long

*D*iagnosing multiple sclerosis (MS) is a bit like going on a treasure hunt—you need to collect a lot of stuff in order to get the prize—or in this case, the booby prize.

To make your treasure hunt just a bit easier, in this chapter, we discuss the diagnostic criteria of MS, and we describe the various kinds of tests your doctor may do to make the diagnosis and find the cause for whatever symptoms or problems you're having. We also explain why the diagnostic process can sometimes take a long time. You can believe us when we tell you that physicians today are as eager as you are to find the right answer. Unlike the old days when little help was available to a person with MS, now several safe and effective treatments are available to help slow the disease and reduce the risk of permanent neurologic damage. So, a prompt, accurate diagnosis is a goal that you and your doctor share.

Clarifying the Diagnostic Criteria

One of the reasons that MS can be so difficult to diagnose is that *neurologists* (physicians who specialize in the diagnosis and treatment of nervous system disorders) have not yet found any specific tests that can be used to identify it. For example, you can't culture it like you do with strep throat, or see it on a chest X-ray like you can with pneumonia. Instead, an MS diagnosis is a *clinical* one, which means that the doctor pieces it together from a variety of sources, including your past history, the symptoms you report, the results of the neurologic examination, and whatever other tests may be needed.

So, if you go to your primary care physician with problems or symptoms that sound like MS, he or she may recommend that you see a neurologist to help sort out the evidence. Chapter 4 gives you tips on how to find the right neurologist and other MS specialists for your healthcare team.

Before we describe exactly what's involved in the diagnostic process, you first have to understand what the neurologist is trying to find. In order to make a diagnosis of MS, he or she must find evidence of *dissemination in time and space*. Yes, it's truly a mouthful, but it's a good term to know because it's the basis for the long-established diagnostic criteria for multiple sclerosis. In a nutshell, what this term means is:

➧ The diagnosis requires objective evidence of two *relapses* (in other words, two episodes of *demyelination* in the central nervous system (CNS), which includes the brain, spinal cord, and optic nerves). Demyelina-

69

tion is the term used to describe the damage caused to the myelin coating surrounding the nerve fibers. A relapse (also known as an attack, exacerbation, episode, or flare) is defined as the sudden appearance or worsening of an MS symptom (or symptoms) that lasts at least 24 hours (although in reality, most attacks last several days or weeks).

Take a look at Chapter 1 for a description of the disease process. Also, see the section "Identifying a clinically isolated syndrome (CIS)" later in this chapter if your doctor says that you may have MS because you've experienced a single clinical episode or event caused by demyelination in your CNS.

- The two relapses must be separated in *time* (by at least one month) and in *space* (as evidenced by areas of inflammation or damage in different areas of the CNS).

- There must be no other explanation for these relapses or for the symptoms that the person is experiencing. In other words, the physician must rule out all other possible diseases or conditions that may be causing the problems.

In the early days, neurologists had to rely exclusively on a person's medical history, current symptoms, and the results of the neurologic exam (which we describe in the upcoming section "Getting Familiar with the Neurologist's Diagnostic Tools") to see if these criteria for an MS diagnosis had been met. However, in 2001, the International Panel on the Diagnosis of Multiple Sclerosis, under the leadership of W.I. McDonald, FRCP, issued a refinement of the criteria (referred to in the MS world as the *McDonald criteria*) that described how certain kinds of laboratory tests could be used to provide additional evidence of dissemination in time and space.

In other words, the diagnosis of MS still requires evidence of at least two relapses that have occurred in different parts of the CNS and different points in time, but there are now more tools at the neurologist's disposal for collecting that evidence.

In 2005, the International Panel met again to review data collected since 2001 and to tweak the criteria. These revisions, conveniently called the "2005 Revisions to the McDonald Diagnostic Criteria for MS," help enhance the speed and accuracy of an MS diagnosis. You can take a peek at the specifics on the National Multiple Sclerosis Society Web site at www.nationalmssociety.org/clinician resources.

Getting Familiar with the Neurologist's Diagnostic Tools

Fortunately, the MS world has moved beyond the days of the *hot bath test*—when physicians used to put people in a hot bath to try and bring out MS symptoms. They used this quick-and-dirty—okay, quick-and-clean—method because they knew that heat tends to slow nerve conduction in someone with MS and cause their symptoms to flare up (check out Chapter 6 for info about the effects of heat on MS).

Today, neurologists rely on a person's medical history, the neurologic exam, and a variety of laboratory tests to help confirm the diagnosis and rule out other conditions. Here are some other conditions that your doctor needs to rule out before confirming a diagnosis:

✔ Infections such as Lyme disease, syphilis, and HIV/AIDS

- Inflammatory diseases such as systemic lupus erythematosus or other causes of vasculitis

- Metabolic problems such as vitamin B12 deficiency or certain genetic disorders

- Diseases of the spine

All these conditions and more are running through your doctor's mind as he or she tries to find an explanation for your symptoms.

To access the National MS Society's handy publication about the diagnostic process, go to www.nationalmssociety.org/diagnose.

Medical history

The neurologist's ability to piece together the evidence of a diagnosis is only as good as the information that he or she is given. So, come to the appointment with all your medical records and test results, and be prepared to answer a lot of questions about past and present complaints, relevant family history, the places you've traveled, your use of alcohol or drugs, and any medications you take. This information is valuable in three ways:

- It helps the neurologist rule out other problems (for example, a virus contracted while visiting another part of the world, neurologic problems resulting from substance abuse, and side effects from medications).

- It lets the neurologist know whether you have any history in your family of MS or other autoimmune diseases.

- It can indicate whether you have ever experienced

any symptoms—no matter how mild or fleeting—that may be indicative of MS. Examining your history is one of the primary ways the neurologist has for identifying past MS relapses.

For example, suppose Susie goes to her neurologist complaining of numbness and tingling down her right side that began about a week ago. When taking her history, the neurologist finds that Susie experienced an episode of blurred vision when she was a teenager. The blurred vision passed after a few days and no one gave it another thought. However, for the doctor, these separate events point to a diagnosis of MS.

The point is, don't show up empty-handed for your appointment with the neurologist. He or she can take your history and examine you, but can't give you any definitive information or even know what tests to recommend without reviewing your records, including previous test results and other doctors' findings.

Neurologic exam

The neurologic exam is an important tool both for diagnosing MS and for assessing disease progression over time. It's important to understand the components of this examination because you're likely to experience it many times over the course of the disease.

During the neurologic exam, the doctor will evaluate both your symptoms and signs of MS. *Symptoms* are the problems or changes you're reporting. Because every person experiences and describes symptoms differently, they're always very subjective. However, this subjectivity doesn't make the symptoms less important, it just means that the neurologist has to rely on your experience of them to try and get a handle on what the problems may be and how severe they are. Examples of symptoms include problems with vision, walking, fatigue, bladder or bowel control, and so on.

On the other hand, *signs* are more measurable and objective pieces of evidence that you may have never even noticed, including involuntary eye movements, altered reflexes, or evidence of *spasticity* (tightness) in your legs (check out Chapter 7 for more information about this common symptom).

The neurologic exam usually evaluates the following:

✔ **Functioning of the cranial nerves:** The neurologist will evaluate the 12 individual nerves in your head that control the senses, such as vision and touch, and activities related to talking and swallowing.

The neurologist can check for damage in your optic nerve by testing your visual acuity using an eye chart, and by looking through an ophthalmoscope to examine the head of the optic nerve (the optic disc). A pale optic disc may indicate earlier damage to the nerve even if you don't remember ever experiencing any problem with your vision. The doctor also checks for double or blurred vision (by evaluating your eye movements), abnormal responses of the pupils, and other signs of neurologic damage.

The neurologist also assesses the movements of your tongue and throat, evaluates the strength of your facial muscles, and checks for reduced or altered sensations in your face.

✔ **Strength and coordination:** The neurologist may evaluate your strength by pushing on your arms and legs and asking you to resist the pressure. You may also be asked to squeeze his or her hand as hard as you can to determine your level of strength.

To evaluate your coordination, the neurologist may ask you to do the following:

- Walk down the hall so he or she can assess your speed and stability.
- Stand and move the heel of one foot up and down the opposite leg (which is often called the *heel-knee-shin test*).
- Walk on your heels and then on your toes.
- Walk a *tandem gait* by placing the heel of one foot directly against the toe of the other foot in alternating fashion.
- Touch his or her finger and then your nose many times rapidly (called the *finger-to-nose test*), first with the eyes open and then with them closed.

✔ **Sensation:** The neurologist may evaluate your *position sense* by asking you to close your eyes and describe where your hands and feet are in space. He or she may test your *vibration sense* by placing a tuning fork against various parts of your body. The doctor may also touch you softly or use very gentle pinpricks or a cotton ball at various points on your arms or legs to check for changes in sensitivity to touch.

✔ **Reflexes:** The neurologist may check your reflexes (at the ankle, knee, and elbow) to see if they're equal on both sides of your body.

Testing for the *Babinski reflex* (named after the French neurologist Josef Babinski) is also important because this abnormal sign in anyone more than one year old is always an indication of damage in the central nervous system. To do this test, the doctor runs a blunt instrument down the side of your foot from the heel to the little toe. The normal plantar reflex to this stimulus is to curl your toes (as generally happens whenever a person's foot is tickled). The abnormal (Babinski reflex) response, which is common in MS, is for your toes to fan upward and outward.

✓ **The presence of Lhermitte's sign** (named after Jean Lhermitte, another French neurologist): The neurologist may ask you whether you ever experienced a sudden, fleeting, electric-like shock down your body when you bend your head forward. The presence of this neurologic sign can be used to confirm damage in your CNS. Even though Lhermitte's sign can occasionally occur for other reasons, it's generally attributable to MS.

The neurologist probably will do this kind of in-depth exam only during your initial visit. Unless you've experienced a major change in your symptoms or you're participating in a *clinical trial* (research study) of some kind, he or she will most likely do an abbreviated version of the exam during subsequent check-ups, focusing primarily on any new problems you may have.

Various medical tests

When a patient's medical history and neurologic exam provide evidence of two episodes of demyelination that are separated in time and space, no other tests are technically needed to make the MS diagnosis. However, other tests are used to confirm the diagnosis or to help the neurologist identify a second episode of demyelination (if it wasn't apparent from the history or exam), and to rule out other diseases that could be masquerading as MS. We explain these tests in the following sections. Read on for details.

Magnetic resonance imaging (MRI)

Figure 2-1 shows a conventional MRI scanner. The *MRI scan* is a highly-sensitive, non-invasive way to view areas of damage in the CNS.

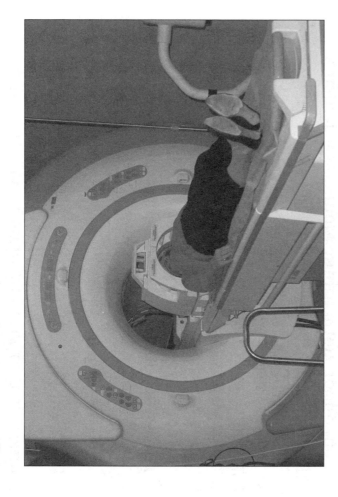

Figure 2-1: A conventional MRI scanning machine.

A contrast material called *gadolinium*, delivered by intravenous infusion during the scan, is often used to highlight new or active areas of inflammation in the CNS caused by a breakdown in the *blood-brain barrier* (BBB), which is the barrier that generally works to keep bad stuff from passing from your bloodstream into your CNS. (Check out Chapter 1 for more information about what happens in the immune system when you have MS.)

As part of the diagnostic process, most neurologists want to see an MRI scan of your brain and spinal cord. Even though an MRI scan is a valuable tool in the diagnostic process, it can't, by itself, determine if a patient has MS.

Normal aging and other diseases besides MS can cause *plaques* (also called lesions or, more informally, spots or scars) in the brain that look like MS. So, your doctor has to use other tools to ensure an accurate diagnosis. Also, neurologists know that about 5 percent of people with definite MS can have a normal-appearing brain MRI scan, at least for awhile, which means that scanning may need to be repeated in a few months in order to help confirm the diagnosis or rule it out. However, the longer the brain scan remains normal, the more the MS diagnosis would have to be called into question.

Current MRI technology allows doctors to view the CNS in different ways, and they've discovered that different types of scans yield different kinds of information. When studying your MRI images, the neurologist is looking for evidence of new disease activity as well as signs of more chronic damage to the *axons*, which are the parts of nerve cells that carry messages from one cell to another (these damaged axons are called *black holes*). He or she is also looking to find the total amount of damage that has occurred, which is referred to as *lesion load.* (Flip to Chapter 1 for more information about the damage that MS can cause to the myelin and the axons in the CNS.)

Be sure to ask your neurologist to review your MRI images with you so that he or she can explain what kinds of changes have occurred in your brain or spinal cord and what these changes indicate about your MS. Because docs tend to use a lot of technical jargon when they talk about MRI scans, be sure to ask questions if you don't understand the information you're being given.

A conventional MRI scanner is an enclosed cylindrical magnet. The scanning procedure requires that you lie perfectly still for several seconds to several minutes at a time, for a minimum of 45 minutes or so. So, if you have difficulty in enclosed spaces (for example, if you suffer from claustrophobia), the physician making the referral can give you a sedating medication prior to the scan. Alternatively, some MRI facilities offer machines with openings on the sides. To date, however, the scans taken in open-sided machines don't provide the same degree of clarity.

Because an MRI scanner uses strong magnets to obtain images of the body, it can't be used by patients who have cardiac pacemakers or certain kinds of metal implants. So, when scheduling the scan, the MRI office staff member will ask whether you have any prosthetic joints, a pacemaker, any implanted ports or infusion catheters, an intrauterine device (IUD), or any metal plates, pins, or screws from prior surgeries. Not all metal causes a problem, so don't assume that you can't have an MRI just because you've had a pin or screw implanted some time in the past. The staff member will also ask if you have any body tattoos or tattooed eyeliner (some people with tattoos have reported swelling or burning in the tattooed areas, and some tattoos contain metallic components that can interfere with image quality).

At the time of the scan, the MRI technician will ask you to remove anything that may interfere with the quality of the images of your head, such as hairpins, jewelry, eyeglasses, hearing aids, and removable dental work. Because of the loud banging noise made by the scanner, the technician will offer you ear plugs or earphones to wear during the procedure. If the gadolinium enhancement we mentioned earlier in this section is required, he or she will insert an intravenous needle into your vein. You'll then be positioned comfortably (sort of) on a sliding table that rolls into the cylindrical tube. You'll be able to communicate with the technician at all times in the event that you need assistance.

Other than the discomfort you feel from having to lie perfectly still in a confined space with loud noises banging in your ears (sounds fun, huh?), the MRI procedure is painless.

Evoked potential testing

Evoked potential tests, or EP tests, are recordings of the central nervous system's electrical response to the stimulation of specific nerve pathways that are commonly affected in MS (for example, visual, auditory, and sensory pathways).

These electrical responses are recorded from brain waves by using electrodes taped to your head. Because demyelination results in a slowing of response time, EPs can sometimes provide evidence of demyelination along nerve pathways that isn't otherwise apparent to the neurologist from the medical history or neurologic exam.

For example, if Susie goes to her neurologist with one symptom that's characteristic of MS, such as numbness and tingling or extreme fatigue, but she has no evidence in her history of a prior neurologic event, the neurologist may request EP testing to look for another area of demyelination that never caused Susie to experience any symptoms.

Of the three types of EP tests that neurologists use (visual, auditory, and sensory), the visual evoked potential test is the most useful in diagnosing MS because 80 percent of people with the disease have slowed responses on this test. The Revised McDonald Criteria include specifications for its use in reaching a confirmed diagnosis of MS. So, if Susie's visual EP is abnormal, her neurologist has evidence of two separate areas of demyelination, helping to confirm the MS diagnosis. But, if Susie's EPs are all normal, the doctor needs to continue looking for additional evidence of demyelination.

When you're undergoing an EP test, a gel (to promote electrical conduction) and electrodes are applied to your head and body at certain locations that are determined by the type of response being recorded. For example, when visual evoked responses are recorded, the electrodes are placed at the back of your scalp over the brain areas that register visual stimuli. For other EP tests, the electrodes are placed at different points on the head and body.

Different stimuli are delivered for each test. For example, a strobe light or screen with a checkerboard pattern is flashed for the visual test; clicking noises or a tone are delivered through headphones for the auditory test; and a mild electrical pulse is delivered at the wrist or knee for the general sensory test. The procedure, which takes approximately 45 minutes per test, is non-invasive and completely painless except for the slight (and we mean slight) discomfort caused by the mild shock given for the sensory evoked potential test.

Lumbar puncture

The *lumbar puncture*, or LP (also known as the spinal tap), allows your neurologist to examine the *cerebrospinal fluid* (CSF) that bathes your spinal cord. The doctor obtains the CSF by inserting a spinal needle into your lower spine (see Figure 2-2).

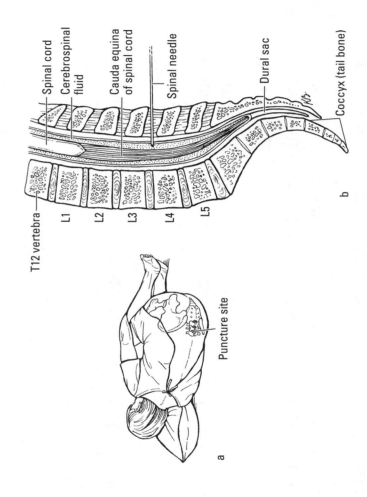

Spinal cord
Cerebrospinal fluid
Cauda equina of spinal cord
Spinal needle
Dural sac
Coccyx (tail bone)

T12 vertebra
L1
L2
L3
L4
L5

b

Puncture site

a

Figure 2-2: *How the lumbar puncture is administered.*

The CSF is then analyzed for evidence of an abnormal immune response in the CNS. Specifically, the neurologist is looking for increased production of certain immune proteins (IgG). Using a method called *protein electrophoresis*, some of this IgG may show up as stripes or bands (called *oligoclonal bands*). Approximately 79 to 90 percent of patients with MS have these bands, making them an important piece of evidence in the diagnostic process.

Because other conditions can also produce oligoclonal bands and because 10 to 21 percent of people with MS can actually have normal cerebrospinal fluid findings, the LP by itself can't make the diagnosis. However, the findings can help the neurologist confirm other evidence of MS. The Revised McDonald Criteria also include specifications for the use of oligoclonal bands and elevated IgG in arriving at a confirmed diagnosis of MS.

The LP, which generally isn't high on anyone's list of fun things to do, can be performed in about 20 minutes in your neurologist's office. The doctor will inject a local anesthetic into your back. He or she will then insert a spinal needle into the fluid-filled space that surrounds the nerves below the bottom end of your spinal cord, withdraw a small amount of CSF (we promise that it's really not as awful as it sounds), and then ask you to straighten your legs. Immediately after removing the needle, the doctor will apply pressure to the puncture site and then ask you to lie still for about 45 minutes. This waiting period helps minimize the risk of severe headache caused by the leakage of CSF, which occurs following approximately 20 percent of LP procedures.

Blood tests

Even though no definite blood tests exist for MS, blood tests can positively rule out other causes for neurologic symptoms, such as Lyme disease, collagen-vascular diseases, certain hereditary disorders, and HIV/AIDS.

Identifying a clinically isolated syndrome

A *clinically isolated syndrome* (CIS) is a first clinical episode lasting at least 24 hours that is caused by demyelination in one or more sites in the CNS. It can't be diagnosed as MS because one episode doesn't meet the criterion for dissemination in time (described in the "Clarifying the Diagnostic Criteria" section earlier in this chapter). A person with CIS can have a single neurologic sign or symptom (for example, an attack of optic neuritis) that's caused by a single lesion, or more than one sign or symptom (for example, an attack of optic neuritis accompanied by weakness on one side) that results from lesions in more than one site. A person who experiences a clinically isolated syndrome may or may not go on to develop multiple sclerosis.

So, if Susie goes to the neurologist with a single attack of optic neuritis, the doctor's challenge is to determine what the chances are that she's going to experience a second demyelinating event in the future (which would fulfill the diagnostic criteria for MS). Neurologists know from CIS studies that when a person with CIS also has brain lesions on an MRI scan that are similar to the those seen in MS, the patient has a high risk of a second demyelinating event, and therefore a diagnosis of MS, within several years. They also know that the more lesions there are, the higher the risk. However, individuals who experience CIS with no brain lesions on an MRI scan, and normal spinal fluid, are at relatively low risk for developing MS over the same time period. This means that the neurologist is going to look carefully at Susie's brain MRI—and repeat it over time—to help figure out the next steps to take.

To date, three large studies have been carried out (and a fourth is underway) to determine whether early treatment of CIS actually delays the second demyelinating event, and therefore the diagnosis of MS. So far, each of the *interferon medications*—Avonex (interferon beta-1a), Betaseron (interferon beta-1b), and Rebif (interferon beta-1a)—has been shown to delay the second demyelinating event (see Chapter 6 for more on these medications), and Avonex and Betaseron have been FDA-approved for this use. The study with Copaxone (glatiramer acetate) will be ongoing for some time.

As with many other situations in MS, there are no right or wrong answers when it comes to treatment of CIS. Some people are ready to begin an injectable medication this early in the game—before the diagnosis has been confirmed—while others aren't. The best strategy is to review your options thoroughly with your neurologist. (Flip to Chapter 6 for more information about the importance of early treatment.)

Understanding Why the Road to Diagnosis Can Be Full of Twists and Turns

Given all the tests available to help confirm or rule out a diagnosis of MS, you're probably wondering why it sometimes takes so long for the diagnosis to be confirmed. In the old days, before MRI technology and EP testing, a diagnosis could sometimes take years if a person's second relapse didn't occur for a long time. Fortunately, neurologists today usually arrive at answers more quickly because the available tests are used to identify other areas of demyelination that never caused recognizable symptoms.

But—and this is a big but—the diagnosis still can't be made until evidence of a second relapse is found, separated in time and space from the first. So, if a person has a neurologic episode of some kind, but then doesn't have another one for several years, doctors have no way to make a definitive diagnosis (flip to the section, "Identifying a clinically isolated syndrome" earlier in the chapter for details about this situation). Living with the possibility of MS hanging over their heads is difficult for people. However, it's also difficult being told they have MS when it turns out later that they really don't.

 For this reason, getting a second opinion—preferably from an MS specialist neurologist—is generally a good idea (see Chapter 4). Don't worry about offending your doctor by seeking a second opinion—a good doctor won't mind at all. In fact, the best docs encourage it.

You've Been Diagnosed—
So What's Next?

*N*ow that you have a diagnosis of multiple sclerosis (MS), you're probably trying to figure out what happens next. That's a good question, because one of the major challenges we talk about in this chapter is how unpredictable MS can be. At this point, you may be experiencing one or more uncomfortable or annoying symptoms, or the symptoms that led to your diagnosis may have all but disappeared. Either way, you now have to deal with the fact that MS is part of your life—and no two people deal with it exactly the same way.

So, in this chapter, we describe the most common reactions people have to receiving an MS diagnosis, as well the longer-term feelings that can come into play as time goes on. We also recommend some initial steps for your MS journey and propose strategies for dealing with the changes, challenges, and choices that a chronic illness like MS can bring to your life.

First Things First: Sorting Out Your Feelings

Everyone's initial reaction to getting an MS diagnosis is going to be different. Whatever you're experiencing, whether it's shock, denial, anxiety, anger, or even relief (or some combination of all of these), keep in mind that these reactions are normal, and that you—and those who care about you—are going to reexperience some variation of them whenever MS brings new symptoms and challenges into your life.

As tempting as it may seem, trying to ignore these feelings or keep them under wraps will just make it more difficult for you to begin taking care of yourself and your MS. The following sections help you recognize and deal with these common reactions to an MS diagnosis.

Shock: "This can't be happening"

Shock is a pretty typical first reaction. But, it generally doesn't last all that long because the day-to-day realities of symptoms, doctor visits, tests, treatment decisions, and insurance companies tend to drive the diagnosis home pretty quickly. If you experience this reaction, cut yourself a little slack and recognize that you're going through a stressful time. Take a little breathing time. After you've relaxed a bit, start the process of finding out what you need to know about MS, and then mobilize your support team (flip to Chapter 4 for details).

Denial: "This isn't happening"

Denial, that uncanny ability humans have to avoid feelings and thoughts that feel too stressful and difficult to handle, can feel wonderful. It's what allows people to plow ahead and live their lives in spite of whatever awful problem is confronting them. Without some healthy denial, a person newly diagnosed with a chronic disease like MS may just feel like giving up and giving in to whatever the disease has in store. So, as you can imagine, we're in favor of a reasonable dose of denial. If you're curious what a reasonable dose is, think of it this way: It's simply the amount that allows you to think about your MS without jumping to the conclusion that all will be doom and gloom.

On the other hand, we also know that denial can get in the way. It can stop people from educating themselves about the disease, from making thoughtful treatment decisions, from planning effectively for a future characterized by unpredictability, and from talking openly with loved ones about ways to support one another.

Because 75 to 85 percent of people are diagnosed with a relapsing-remitting course (see Chapter 1 for a description of this course), denial can be particularly tempting. For example, following an episode of heightened disease activity and uncomfortable symptoms, a remission comes along. You feel fine—just like your old self—and you desperately want to believe that the doctor was wrong and that nothing is wrong with you. But, you have to remember this: The medications currently available are most effective early in the disease. You may not be feeling any symptoms, but the disease is active nonetheless, and permanent damage to nerve cells can occur even in the earliest stages of the disease.

In fact, recent magnetic resonance imaging (MRI) studies have shown that even the *white matter* in the brain that appears normal (called, appropriately enough, *normal-appearing white matter*) on brain scans isn't really normal—the disease has begun to alter it (flip to Chapter 1 to see how MS affects the central nervous system (which includes the brain, spinal cord, and optic nerves). So, the point at which you're tempted to try and forget the whole thing is the very time when medications can begin reducing disease activity and the risk of permanent disability. In other words, act now; don't bury your head in the sand.

Confusion: "Why me?"

When bad things happen to you, it's natural to want to know why. Particularly because the cause of MS remains a mystery, people are quick to wonder if something they did—or didn't do—made them get MS. So, we want to emphasize here (and again when we talk about progressive disease in Chapter 13) that *there's nothing you or anyone else did to make you get MS, and there's nothing you or anyone else could have done to prevent it.* Unfortunately, MS is just one of those unfair and painful things that can happen to anyone—and for no good reason at all.

Anxiety: "What's going to happen to me?"

The fact of the matter is that for the rest of your life you'll be wondering what your MS has in store for you. You'll ask yourself and your doc: "What's going on with me today—and what's likely to go on tomorrow, next month, or next year?" The anxiety that surrounds the unpredictability of MS typically begins long before the diagnosis—when a person begins experiencing strange symptoms—and continues until that person develops a strategy or mindset to deal with the unknown.

The trick seems to lie in finding a balance between taking each day as it comes and taking steps to protect your quality of life regardless of what the future brings. (Check out Part V for several chapters on how to strike this balance.)

Anger: "Why can't you fix what's happening to me?"

While anger is a pretty normal reaction to a life-changing disease, the challenge lies in figuring out where to direct that anger. Initially, you may find yourself angry at the doctor for giving you this news, at the medical community for not being able to cure it, or at some higher power for letting it happen. Over time, you may also find yourself angry at the pharmaceutical companies for the prices of their products, the insurance company for their high co-pays or limited formularies, or your town or workplace for not being more accessible for someone with a disability. The list can get pretty long.

When all that anger doesn't make your MS go away, it can begin to spill over into other areas of your life—for instance, with your partner, your kids, your colleagues, or even your most loyal friends. So, right from the get-go, it's a good idea to begin figuring out how to put that anger to work. Using anger positively allows you to focus and fuel your coping strategies; it can energize your efforts to find answers, solve problems, and overcome obstacles that get in your way.

Relief: "Thank goodness—I thought it was something worse!"

For anyone not experiencing relief following an MS diagnosis, this reaction probably seems impossible. But, for those people who thought they might have a brain tumor,

90

Other important resources for people with a recent diagnosis

If you or someone you love has recently been diagnosed with MS, you may be wondering "So what do I do now?" Because emotions can kick in quickly, whatever words the doctor said after giving you the diagnosis may be lost in a blur. Obviously, you'll have opportunities to talk about it further in follow-up visits, but it may reassure you to know that many helpful resources are available to help you navigate the next few days, weeks, and months.

The National MS Society offers a variety of publications and programs:

✔ The best place to start is with a learn-at-home program called *Knowledge Is Power* (www.nationalmssociety.org/knowledge), which is available by mail or online.

✔ The Society's resource page for those with a recent diagnosis is www.nationalmssociety.org/newlydiagnosed.

✔ Webcasts are available at www.nationalmssociety.org/webcasts.

The Multiple Sclerosis Association of America (MSAA) is another good resource to tap:

✔ Information for people who are newly diagnosed is available at www.msaa.com/newly.html.

✔ MSAA programs and resources are described at www.msaa.com/programs/programs.html.

The Multiple Sclerosis International Federation provides information about MS in English, German, French, Spanish, Italian, and

Russian at www.msif.org.

Multiple Sclerosis For Dummies should give you all you need, but if you're itching to read more, you may find the following books particularly useful as well:

✔ *Multiple Sclerosis: A Guide for the Newly Diagnosed*, 2nd edition, by Nancy Holland, T. Jock Murray, and Stephen Reingold (Demos Medical Publishing); a third edition is due out in early 2007.

✔ *Multiple Sclerosis: The First Year* by Margaret Blackstone (Marlowe & Company).

Alzheimer's disease, ALS (Lou Gehrig's disease), or any number of other frightening things, MS is greeted as a much better option. An MS diagnosis may also be a relief for people who were told to consult a mental health specialist because their mysterious symptoms were "all in their head." For them, the diagnosis comes as a welcome validation of the symptoms—either physical or cognitive—that they have been living with. Finally they can get the support and treatment they need.

Even though a feeling of relief is comfortable in the short term, it's important not to let that feeling get in the way of doing what you need to do to—like making important treatment decisions and beginning to figure out how to fit MS into your life. (Check out Chapter 5 for ideas on how to start managing your MS.)

Deciding on the Next Steps

Following a major change in your life, trying to figure out what to do next can be tricky. Some people get so caught up in wanting to make the *right* choices that they find it difficult to make any at all. So, here are our suggestions for getting started.

Catch your breath before making any major changes or decisions

People diagnosed with MS may do a surprising number of things during their first moments of shock—quit jobs, leave relationships, take to their beds, tell the world about the diagnosis, decide never to have children, and so on. Consider yourself forewarned: You need to give yourself time to explore the disease and live with its ups and downs before deciding to change your life. You may be surprised to discover that you really don't have to change much at all.

We have known too many people who resign from their jobs ("I'll never be able to do this kind of work any more") or break off engagements ("I could never saddle the person I love with my MS") in the throes of an early exacerbation, only to find themselves jobless and bored to tears—not to mention lonely—when the MS goes into remission. So, give yourself a chance to get to know your MS a bit before taking any drastic steps.

Have a heart-to-heart conversation with your neurologist about treatment

We can't emphasize enough how important it is to consider early treatment with one of the approved disease-modifying therapies—before significant, irreparable damage can occur. So, broach the subject with your neurologist as soon as possible. Your doctor can help you figure out if you're a good candidate for this kind of treatment, if now is the right time to start, and which one of the medications may be best for you (you can review all the options in Chapter 6).

To find out more about the importance of early treatment and the role of the disease-modifying therapies in managing your MS, check out the *Disease Management Consensus Statement* from the MS specialist physicians on the National MS Society's Medical Advisory Board (www.nationalmssociety.org/consensus).

Begin talking about MS with the people in your life

The quickest way to feel less alone with your new diagnosis is to begin talking about it with others. However, figuring out whom to tell, and when to tell them, isn't always easy. Some people—particularly those who have been waiting for some time to get a diagnosis—want to rush out and tell everyone they know that the mystery has finally been solved. Other people, however, tend to want to keep it a secret, telling no one or as few people as possible. The most reasonable approach is probably somewhere in the middle.

Try picturing yourself surrounded by circles of gradually increasing size. Your best bet is to start by talking first with those in your "inner circle," and then gradually working your way outward on a need-to-know basis. (Chapter 14 is filled with ideas about how to talk comfortably with various people in your life about your MS.)

Telling the most important folks first

In general, sharing information with your partner, your best friend, your parents—whomever you feel closest to—is the place to start. Those closest to you—the people who know you well enough to sense when something is wrong even without you telling them—can help you begin the process of living with MS. In turn, you can help them understand what the disease is all about.

There are no hard-and-fast rules about how to share this

information with others, but it's helpful to keep in mind that each person's reaction will be different. You need to be prepared to deal with their feelings (as well as your own) and to provide some basic information about the disease.

Figuring out who else needs to know

Deciding who else to clue in can be tricky—mostly because spur-of-the-moment decisions about disclosing your MS can have long-term implications, particularly in relation to your current job and future career options (flip to Chapter 18 for more information about disclosure on the job).

The point is that once the information is public, you can't take it back. You may, for example, want people to know that MS is responsible for all of the symptoms you're currently experiencing. But, if the disease goes into remission and your symptoms get better, you may wish you hadn't told quite so many people—particularly your boss or colleagues at work whose attitudes about chronic illness or disability are likely to impact their interactions with you over the long-term.

For more help with your disclosure decisions, we recommend the publication "Disclosure: The Basic Facts," which is available on the National MS Society Web site at www .nationalmssociety.org/disclosure or by calling (800) FIGHT-MS (800-344-4867). In the meantime, here are some pointers:

✔ Give yourself and those closest to you some time to get used to the idea before trying to figure out who else needs to know.

✔ Before making any decisions about disclosing your MS at your workplace, check out Chapter 18. Even though you may decide that you want your co-

95

workers to know what's going on, it's worthwhile to spend a little time thinking about what you want them to know and why you want them to know it.

- If you have children, be sure to keep them in the loop. Not only does this help them understand what's going on, it also ensures that they hear this important information from you rather than from a well-meaning relative or friend who accidentally spills the beans. (See Chapter 17 to find out when and how to share this information with your kids.)

- If you're currently dating, you don't have to disclose your diagnosis the first time you meet someone. But, don't wait until you're walking down the aisle either. (Flip to Chapter 14 for tips on knowing when and how to broach the topic with someone you're interested in.)

Make a commitment to your health

Sometimes people get so bogged down thinking about, or dealing with, their MS, that they forget that MS is only one aspect of their overall health and well-being. Like filling your pantry before a snowstorm or your gas tank before a long trip, getting and staying healthy and fit is the best possible preparation for your MS journey.

MS doesn't provide any magical protection against other common health problems, so it's just as important for you as it is for everyone else to take good care of yourself by getting regular checkups and pursuing a healthy lifestyle. For some ideas on how to feel your best now and into the future, refer to Chapter 11, which is all about strategies for maintaining your health and wellness in spite of MS, starting with getting sufficient rest and exercise, eating a healthy diet, and managing your stress.

Facing the Longer-Term Challenges of a Chronic Illness

Living with MS differs from most people's prior experiences with illness. The first and foremost difference is that MS doesn't go away. Most people are used to temporary inconveniences, such as the flu, a strep throat, or a sinus infection—all of which are pretty awful while they're around, but mercifully gone after a short course of treatment (or the patience to wait them out).

Until a cure is found, however, MS is here to stay. It may be quiet and well-behaved much of the time, but it's always there. And it's this fact that you may find difficult to get a handle on. Suddenly nothing is quite the same, but you can't tell how different it's going to be from one day or week to the next. This unpredictability challenges people's efforts to make decisions and plans. In this section, we describe some of the most common reactions to these longer-term challenges, and we suggest strategies for how to deal with them.

The how-to of healthy grieving

You may be asking "What's grieving got to do with it? I'm still here. MS isn't going to kill me. What's to grieve?" But, believe it or not, grieving is an important—and healthy—part of living with MS. It's what prepares and empowers you (and those who care about you) to identify satisfying and creative ways to deal with whatever changes MS brings to your life.

Even though the process of grieving is different for different people, certain aspects of it are the same for everyone—starting with a feeling of loss.

Recognizing feelings of loss

For many people, an MS diagnosis is life's first big kick in the teeth. Because people are most often diagnosed in their 20s or 30s, MS may represent the first significant threat to those powerful feelings of strength and invincibility that motivate young adults to take on the world. This first chink in their armor can feel like a loss of control over their destiny, and grieving over that loss is the first important step to managing it.

As if being diagnosed with MS isn't hard enough on your self-esteem, the symptoms of the illness can also lead to significant feelings of loss. Symptoms that appear and disappear without warning can threaten a person's feelings of confidence and control (see the upcoming section "Living with Unpredictability"). The best way to sum up the losses is to say that the road ahead, which once looked and felt pretty smooth and straight, now has some unpredictable bumps and turns in it. Just remember that it's okay to feel sad about that.

To help them feel as if they aren't losing control, many of our patients talk about starting each day with what they call the "MS body check." It's a little bit like taking morning roll call to see who has shown up for the day. The roll call may sound a bit like this: "How's my left leg doing today? Hmmm, are those fingers still a little numb? How's the right eye—am I still seeing two of everything when one would be quite sufficient?" The body check is their way of sorting out what's going on with their MS from the get-go so that they can make their plans for the day accordingly.

A word to the wise: People express grief differently. While crying is probably the most obvious way to express feelings of loss and sadness, anger, irritability, and withdrawal are pretty common too. (Flip to Chapter 9, where we talk

98

about how to distinguish some of these normal expressions of distress and sadness from more serious mood changes and depression.)

Answering the "Who am I now?" question

You spend a lifetime assembling an image of who you are. A helpful way to think about this is to visualize one of those jigsaw puzzles made from a favorite photograph. Since birth, you've gradually added pieces to your puzzle—your personality style, sense of humor, special strengths and weaknesses, and tastes for this and that. But, then, when MS comes along, you suddenly have an oddly-shaped piece that needs to be added, and it takes some time to figure out how to make that piece fit into the whole picture. The first step is to deal with the loss of the puzzle as you knew it. The picture you had of yourself—your self-image—suddenly re-quires some tweaking. In a sense, you need to get to know yourself all over again.

People react in a variety of ways to the task of redefining themselves. Some people "go to pieces" initially—express-ing their grief by throwing up their hands in despair and temporarily losing sight of who they are. Others muster their emotional defenses and try to avoid adding the new piece to their puzzle for as long as possible. Then there are those people who gently nudge the pieces of their puzzle this way and that in an effort to figure out just how MS is going to fit in without jumbling the puzzle too much. All of these are part of the grieving process.

The most comfortable outcome of this grieving process is to find that your puzzle is still intact—to recognize that you're still you, with all the things that make you unique, in-teresting, lovable, and strong, in spite of the new piece that you have to add. In fact, healthy grieving allows you to put the other pieces in your puzzle to work. For example, you can use your coping skills, creativity, and determination to

99

figure out how to manage any changes that MS brings to your life.

Don't forget that the process is a continuous one: Each time a new symptom appears or the disease alters the way you do things, the grieving happens all over again. You'll be fiddling with those puzzle pieces forever. Of course, every-one (with MS or without) goes through exactly the same process as time, life events, and aging bring about changes. You'll have the advantage, however, because you'll already know how to make the adaptive process work for you.

In case you're thinking that every new piece in the puzzle is going to be unwelcome and uncomfortable, here's the good news: When going through the grieving process, you'll discover strengths and talents you never knew you had. Solving problems, meeting challenges, and figuring out cre-ative workarounds all add to feelings of pride, mastery, and self-esteem.

Letting go of the past and grabbing hold of the future

Healthy grieving involves letting go of the past so you can get on with the future. From one day, month, or year to the next, your MS may alter none, some, or many of your daily activities. When it does get in your way, you need to be ready to go after your goals in spite of it, and the only way you'll be able to do that is to be ready to do things differ-ently.

If, for whatever reason, your original goals aren't possible any more, don't assume that you have no goals in your fu-ture. Instead, allow yourself to think about different goals or perhaps a new direction. It's natural to be sad and angry when things don't go as smoothly as they used to or when goals have to be changed—that's what grieving is all about. The next step, however, is to put that emotional energy to use in order to map a new plan for yourself.

100

Living with unpredictability

Most people spend their childhood years waiting eagerly to become adults. They're convinced that as adults, they too will be in charge and have control over what happens in their day-to-day lives. Of course, the average, healthy person is never in control of as much as he or she would like to be, but add in MS and you get a harsh reminder that life can be pretty unpredictable. In this section, we show you how to grapple with the extra dose of unpredictability that MS can bring to everyday life.

Addressing the "Why can't they tell me what's going to happen next?" question

Among people with MS, one of the most frequently heard questions is about what's going to happen next. We have had many patients say to us, "I can handle the way things are today—if someone could just tell me that nothing else is going to go wrong, I know that I could manage." This same sentiment is expressed by those with one or two mild symptoms as well as those with many severely disabling symptoms. The point is that people generally cope pretty well with the changes that MS brings—after a period of upset, they figure out how to adapt and change the way they do things. The bigger challenge, however, is never knowing when they may have to adapt all over again.

The hard truth about MS is this: It may be difficult to predict from morning to night (let alone from one week, month, or year to the next) how you're likely to feel. Similarly, no one can tell you with any certainty just how your MS is likely to behave over the long term. Statistically speaking, the following factors seem to predict a better outcome:

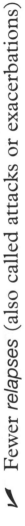

✔ Fewer *relapses* (also called attacks or exacerbations)

in the initial years following the diagnosis (Check out Chapter 1 for more information about MS relapses.)

✔ Longer interval between relapses

✔ More complete recovery from relapses

✔ Relapses that are primarily sensory in nature (for example, numbness, tingling, visual changes)

✔ Fewer findings on the neurologic exam after five years

Unfortunately, however, no matter what predictions you receive, you have no guarantees. So, your optimal strategy will always be to hope for the best while being prepared for whatever else comes along (check out Chapter 20 for strategies to help you feel prepared).

Taking control of the uncontrollable

We understand that controlling the uncontrollable sounds a bit like trying to organize the raindrops, but the fact is that there is a lot you can do to live more comfortably with a chronic, unpredictable disease. For example, do the following:

✔ **Educate yourself:** The more you know about MS, the better prepared you'll be to deal with whatever comes your way. Even though keeping your head in the sand may feel like a comfortable strategy, it leaves you uninformed and off-guard. By becoming familiar with the kinds of symptoms and changes that MS can cause, you're primed to recognize and deal with them if they happen to occur.

✔ **Create your support network:** The starting point

for dealing with an unpredictable disease like MS is to recognize that you don't have to do it alone.

From the get-go, your best strategy is to identify your resources (for example, voluntary health organizations, such as the National MS Society and the Multiple Sclerosis Association of American, Internet sites, and community resources) and recruit your team (family members, friends, colleagues, other people with MS, health professionals, and anyone else whose input you value). Over time, this network will be crucial to your coping efforts.

✔ **Start treatment early:** Even though doctors still don't have a cure for MS, several medications have been shown to slow disease progression and reduce the number and severity of attacks (flip to Chapter 6 for details). Early treatment can help prevent some of the irreversible damage that's known to occur even in the earliest stages of the disease.

✔ **Get to know your body:** Because no one else's MS is quite like yours, your own body's behavior will be your very best source of information and guidance. For example, pay attention to important cues: Does heat make your symptoms feel worse? Or are you more sensitive to cold? When is your energy at its peak? How do you react to stress? Are you better able to concentrate and remember things earlier in the day or later? Do you have side effects from any of the medications you're taking? Does it take you longer to do things than it used to?

And while you're busy trying to figure out all this important information for yourself, remember to share it with the key people in your life. No one can read your mind, and being clued in to how your MS behaves makes it easier for people to provide help and support when you need it (Chapter 14 has tips for how talk with others about your MS).

- **Plan activities for the "best" part of your day:** You may start the morning feeling ready to take on the world and end the day ready to take a long vacation. After you have a pretty good idea of how your body reacts over the course of a day, try to plan accordingly.

  If you have more energy in the morning, plan to get the big stuff done early. If a nap in the afternoon gives you an energy boost, figure out how best to make use of that bonus. If thinking and concentrating become more difficult as the day wears on, be sure to tackle the mind-bending tasks first thing. (Check out Chapter 7 for strategies to manage some of the various symptoms that can occur with MS).

- **Always have a back-up plan:** One day you're loaded for bear and the next you just feel loaded down. The best way to deal with the demon of unpredictability is to be prepared for it: Every big plan should have a back-up. Even though this extra planning may seem tiresome and impractical, our patients tell us that it gradually becomes second nature. For example, people get into the habit of thinking about alternatives just in case their fatigue kicks in, their symptoms flare, or a relapse happens. This is a particularly important strategy for parents (see Chapter 16).

- **Put all that emotional energy to the best possible use:** No, it isn't fair that you got MS. Yes, you resent that you can't do all the things you want to do the way you used to do them. And, yes, you're angry about having to deal with challenges and uncertain-

104

ties that others don't have to face. But, remember, anger that isn't put to good use is just a wasteful drain of precious energy. You'll feel better and function better if you direct all that energy toward your goals, taking on the challenge of MS by meeting it one day at a time.

Tap that anger to do something good for yourself: Rearrange the stuff in your kitchen to make it more accessible; call your National MS Society chapter to find out how to advocate for the rights of people with disabilities; join a self-help group in your community or start one of your own; or talk to your boss about some accommodations that would allow you to be more comfortable and productive on the job (see Chapter 18). In other words, doing is better than stewing.

Making Treatment and Lifestyle Choices That Work for You

When we started our careers in MS more than 25 years ago, the major issue confronting people with MS was that all of their choices were being taken away. People were told that no treatment was available for their MS, and that they should quit their jobs, go to bed, and give up on any ideas of having children. And besides all that, they were told that exercise was bad for them. Fortunately, those days are gone.

Today, your choices are unlimited. MS specialists are telling people with MS to continue pursuing their dreams and doing whatever works for them. It's true that those of you diagnosed with MS in your teens, twenties, or thirties will be living with this disease for decades. But, there's no need to make a career of MS. You have the opportunity to carve out your own path, making the choices along the way that make the most sense for you. The goal is to figure out how to accommodate the unpredictability of MS into the life you want to live.

You may encounter some unexpected roadblocks along the way, and you may have to take an unexpected detour every now and then, but you're still the one in the driver's seat. The more flexible and creative you're willing to be, the more options you'll have available to you.

Minimizing the stress of decision-making

Considering that options used to be sparse, having more of them is definitely a step in the right direction. But, in our professional roles as physician, nurse, and psychologist, we have also heard from people with MS (and their families) how stressful choices can be. In other words, having no choices felt awful, but having lots of choices brings its own set of challenges—particularly when the "right" and "wrong" answers aren't clearly marked. What's "right" for one person may be way off the mark for someone else.

Getting comfortable with the decision-making process and with the decisions you end up making, is important to living comfortably with a chronic illness like MS. So, each chapter of this book gives you the information you need to make educated choices that feel right for you.

Here are just some of the areas in which the options for people with MS have increased dramatically in recent years: Choosing among treatment options (Chapter 6); managing symptoms (Chapters 7, 8, and 9); making family planning decisions (Chapter 16); and making employment decisions (Chapter 18).

Don't be surprised when the people who care about you

106

most—your partner, parents, extended family members, friends, and colleagues—have lots of opinions about what you should and shouldn't do and about what's best for you. In fact, get used to the idea that you'll likely get a lot more advice than you actually want. As if hearing all this unwanted advice weren't challenging enough, the kicker is that much of that advice is likely to be conflicting or even contradictory. Your challenge, together with your partner, is to sift through the various opinions to find what works for you. Above all, realize that you aren't going to please everyone.

Getting the professional help and personal support you need

In addition to your loves ones, several key players can help you identify your options and support your decision-making efforts along the way. First and foremost on this list are MS professionals. Referrals to professionals who are knowledgeable about MS are available from the National MS Society (800-FIGHT-MS) or from the Consortium of MS Centers (see a listing of member centers at www .mscare.org/cmsc/index.php?option=com_peoplebook&Ite mid=500). Your personal physician may also be familiar with specialists in the area.

Consider the following professionals:

✔ **MS specialist neurologists and nurses:** These professionals are the best sources of information about treatment (take a look at Chapter 4 for suggestions on how to put together your treatment team). It's their job to get to know you and your MS, and to recommend the treatment options that will be most beneficial for you.

MS specialists can also offer helpful information about the course of your MS and any indicators about how your MS may progress down the road. Even though they can't make definitive predictions, they can certainly tell you the factors that you need to be thinking about as you consider your treatment and lifestyle options. If the health professionals with whom you're dealing aren't willing or able to have this kind of conversation with you, it may be time to look around.

✔ **Rehabilitation professionals (including physical and occupational therapists):** Rehabilitation professionals can help you function at your best by doing the following:

- Evaluating your needs and making recommendations for home and office modifications to increase accessibility and conserve energy.
- Identifying tools and adaptive devices to enhance your comfort, productivity, and safety.
- Designing exercise programs to enhance your health, safety, and mobility.

✔ **Vocational counselors:** These counselors are trained to help you think through your employment options. Depending on your career path and the kinds of MS symptoms you're experiencing, you may want to discuss with an employment specialist how best to safeguard your future earning power.

✔ **Financial consultants:** Financial consultants can help you plan for the financial uncertainties of the future, such as reduced income due to disability-related retirement, treatment costs, and the possible need for long-term care of some kind.

108

✔ **Mental health professionals:** These professionals are a great resource for anyone who values an objective third ear. Clinicians who are experienced with chronic illness, and with MS in particular, can appreciate the complexities of the plans and decisions you're trying to make. Having thoughtful and supportive input as you try to sort through your options can be invaluable.

You can also get support from others with MS. However, *self-help groups*—also called support groups—sometimes get a bad rap (one group may be all doom-and-gloom, another has someone who monopolizes the conversation without contributing very much, and another hangs its hat on miracle cures). The fact is that, like everything else, some are wonderful and some aren't. But, when you find the right one for you, it can be the perfect place to share ideas with other people who "get it," brainstorm some problem-solving ideas, learn from others' successes, and get helpful feedback.

Every support group is different: Some are professionally led and others are peer led; some are more social and others have a more lecture and discussion format; some meet every week and others meet monthly; and some have a fixed membership targeting a particular group (for example, people with MS, partners, couples, the newly diagnosed, those people with more advanced disability, and so on) and others are open to anyone who wants to attend. It may take some trial and error to find a group that's just right for you, but it's truly worth the effort, particularly if you're trying to sort through important decisions in your life. You can call the National MS Society at (800) FIGHT-MS or the Multiple Sclerosis Association of America at (800) 532-7667 for information about groups in your area.

Chapter 4

Creating Your Healthcare Team

*J*ust about anyone would admit that today's healthcare system is complex (to say the least) and less than user-friendly—for example, figuring out which managed care plan would actually cover your medical costs is almost an impossible feat. You're in an age of specialization that requires all consumers to be knowledgeable, assertive, and organized about their own care. The average, mostly healthy person, at one point or another, comes across a healthcare challenge, but those faced with a chronic, unpredictable illness like multiple sclerosis (MS) may find the challenge even more daunting.

To help you avoid as many healthcare challenges as possible, in this chapter, we show you how to find and coordinate the care and support you need. A growing commu-

110

nity of healthcare professionals who have the expertise and experience to help you manage your MS is readily available. Unfortunately, a bunch of not-so-good ones (who have the best of intentions but little knowledge about MS) are also ready to "help" you out. So that you don't settle with the latter group, we'll show you how to scout out the best talent.

Working with Your Physician

Even though you are and will continue to be the center of your healthcare team, your neurologist is the glue that holds the team together. Most people, whether they're initially diagnosed by their general practitioner or referred to a neurologist for the assessment and diagnosis, receive their subsequent MS care from a neurologist. Because neurologists are trained in diseases of the nervous system, they're the physicians best qualified to diagnose and treat MS. Under ideal circumstances, your neurologist coordinates your care by identifying your treatment needs and referring you to the specialists who can best address your needs.

Finding a neurologist with the qualities you value

Because your relationship with your MS doctor will be a long and personal one (you may be discussing oh-so-comfortable subjects like leaky bladders and flagging sex lives), it's important to find someone you feel comfortable with. Comfort means different things to different people, but some key elements are trust, good communication, and mutual respect. The following sections discuss these elements and the other factors you want to look for.

Training and expertise

Keep in mind that not all neurologists are the same. Most general neurologists see patients with a variety of conditions, including stroke, Parkinson's disease, epilepsy, migraines, and perhaps MS. In other words, throughout his or her career, a neurologist may have seen many patients with MS, or very few. So, the fact that a physician is a board-certified neurologist doesn't guarantee any particular expertise in the treatment of MS.

If you have the luxury of choosing among neurologists in your healthcare plan and in your geographic area, one of the key bits of information you need to obtain before making a decision is the neurologist's experience and training in MS. As a starting point, you can contact the National MS Society at (800) FIGHT-MS (800-344-4867) for a list of MS specialists in your area. You can also ask your insurance company if your plan covers any MS specialists.

If you don't have the luxury of choosing among a number of neurologists, you may want to create a tag team—a local doctor who handles your routine care and an MS specialist with whom you and your doctor confer periodically. The specialist, who's likely to be more up-to-date on the latest treatments and symptom management strategies, can provide recommendations for you and your own doctor to follow. You may need to travel or pay out-of-pocket to go to a specialist, but the peace of mind you get knowing that you're receiving the best care and guidance possible is well worth it. (See the section "Knowing when to call in the MS specialist" later in the chapter for more details.)

If your current doctor says that nothing can be done for your MS, you're putting your care in the wrong person's hands. So, search out the specialists in your area through your insurance company or the National MS Society.

Bedside manner

You know yourself best, so be honest with yourself and decide what qualities are most important to you in a doctor. For some people, warm and fuzzy is the key qualification—if they don't feel comfortable and cozy in the doctor's office, they don't want to be there no matter how knowledgeable the doc is. For others, MS expertise trumps everything else, even if the doctor has the charm of a toad. Most people try to find some combination of both. Whether or not the neurologist is chatty or charming, you probably need to find someone whose personal style meshes well with your own.

Accessibility and convenience

In addition to knowledge and personality, it's important to consider how accessible the doctor is—in person or by telephone:

✔ **Access to the office:** Find out how accessible the neurologist's office is. Even if you aren't having any mobility problems at the moment, some time down the road, particularly during a relapse, you may need to see a physician whose office is easy to get to and easy to get into.

It's amazing how many doctor's office aren't accessible to people in wheelchairs or scooters. Check out the accessibility ahead of time—nothing is more frustrating than making your way to a doctor's office only to find that you have to park six blocks away and you can't maneuver your wheelchair over the curb.

✔ **Communication:** Find out whether the doctor is available for phone calls. Most neurologists don't take calls during office hours, but you should be able

113

to leave a message and get a return call from the doctor or nurse within a reasonable period of time (a day or two is not unreasonable). Having this kind of communication with the doctor's office is important because questions about symptoms and medication side effects are common. You'll find it comforting to know that you can count on getting a call back when you have a question or concern.

TIP

Ability to deal with the tough stuff

It's important to have a doctor who doesn't shy away from difficult topics and who works comfortably with other MS specialist clinicians. You need a doc who is

⌐ **Ready to answer the hard-to-answer questions:** As you probably know, MS is unpredictable and knowing exactly what lies in store for you is difficult. Nevertheless, you need to be able to talk with your MS physician about the treatment and lifestyle decisions you're trying to make with the expectation that he or she will take the time to respond honestly and thoughtfully. Your decisions need to be based on the best information your doctor can give you about your disease course. If your neurologist doesn't seem willing or comfortable having these kinds of conversations with you, it's probably time to look for another doctor.

Don't stick with someone who's a bit too glib with false assurances that you have nothing to worry about. For example, many doctors, particularly those without much experience in MS, find it difficult to deliver painful news. They're very quick to reassure people that their disease is mild or that their prognosis is good, without taking the time to explain how complex and unpredictable the disease can be. When

114

doctors aren't realistic, their patients can feel betrayed if the disease suddenly worsens down the road. So, look for a doctor you can trust to be forthright and realistic with you about your MS.

✔ **Comfortable with teamwork:** Try to determine whether your doctor knows when to call in the troops. The most experienced MS physicians know that MS care involves a lot of teamwork. They recognize the invaluable contributions made by all healthcare professionals. Some doctors work in MS centers where the other disciplines, such as nursing, rehabilitation, social work, and psychology, are available at a single site. Others collaborate with these specialists around the community.

The important point is that your doctors see themselves as working collaboratively in an interdisciplinary framework that assures you the kind of care you need. The doctor who feels that he or she is the only provider you need to handle your MS care is probably not your best bet.

Establishing a pattern of routine care

After the diagnosis has been confirmed, and you and your neurologist have decided on a course of treatment, the next step is to establish a pattern for your routine care. Most MS specialists like to see their patients about twice a year—more often if the MS has been active, and less often if things are pretty quiet or the patient is being monitored by a local neurologist closer to home. The purpose of these visits is to monitor disease progression and make sure that their symptoms are being adequately managed (see Chapters 7, 8, and 9 for details on managing symptoms). During these visits, the neurologist performs a neurologic exam to pick up on important information about your MS that you may not be aware of (see Chapter 2). Increasingly, MS specialists are also recommending periodic magnetic resonance imaging (MRI) scans to help them with their treatment decisions.

If your doctor indicates that there's no need to see you on a regular basis, or simply leaves it up to you call if there's a problem, he or she isn't monitoring your MS closely enough.

Making the most of your doctor visits

Your neurologist, of course, is trying to keep you as healthy as you can be, but don't forget that you have an equally important role to play. The best neurologists often say that they're only as good as the information they get from their patients.

Here are some tips for making your doctor visits count:

✔ **Bring your medical records to your first visit.** Any time you're seeing a neurologist for the first time, it's important to bring as much of your medical history as possible, including MRI films, test results, and records from your previous doctors.

✔ **Be on time.** Everyone gets frustrated when forced to wait hours on end in a doctor's office, but the fact is that people arriving late for appointments is one reason that doctors fall behind. They're also trying to give each patient the attention he or she needs, and one day it may be your appointment that runs over the scheduled time.

✔ **Keep track of your symptoms.** There's no need to make a career out of this, but brief notes on your calendar about your latest ups and downs can help you remember problems or changes that you want to mention during your office visit.

116

✔ **If you have a lot of stuff going on with your MS, prioritize the problems.** Chances are that your doctor won't want to tackle every symptom at once because it's generally recommended to start only one new medication at a time in order to check for side effects. So, if your bladder problems are making you crazy, don't wait until the last minute of your visit to mention them to your doc.

✔ **Come prepared with a list of your questions and make sure the most important ones are at the top of the list.** Most regular visits last from 15 to 20 minutes, and a majority of the time is usually taken up with the neurologic exam and a review of your symptoms, medications, and any problems you're having with side effects.

 If you need to talk in depth about a particular issue, such as sexual or cognitive issues or anything else that may take time, you may want to consider scheduling an extra appointment or a phone call so that neither you nor the doctor feels rushed.

✔ **Make sure to keep your doctor informed about all the medications (over-the-counter as well as prescription, including their dosages) and treatment strategies you're using for your MS or other conditions.** In fact, keeping a complete list in your wallet for easy reference is a good idea.

 It's important to keep your doctor informed because over-the-counter products can contain ingredients that interact with your prescription drugs, worsen symptoms, and affect your immune system in negative ways. And any of the medications you take may have side effects that individually or collectively make your MS symptoms worse. (See Chapter 10 for more about the pros and cons of complementary and alternative therapies.)

✔ **Don't expect your neurologist to have time to review a fistful of articles you've printed from the Internet.** But, if you see something of particular interest or concern, it's reasonable to ask about it. Most doctors are happy to take a look, particularly if it's something they've not heard about before.

You can also call the National MS Society for this kind of information. The Society's information and referral specialists are trained to handle your questions. You can call (800) FIGHT-MS or e-mail generalmailbox@nmss.org with your questions.

✔ **Don't hold back—speak up when you're concerned.** The doctor can't read your mind any more than anyone else can, so don't hesitate to talk to your doctor about your symptoms and concerns.

✔ **Bring an extra pair of ears (or a tape recorder).** Most people aren't at their most relaxed state when they're in a doctor's office. You may be so focused on what your next question is going to be that you forget to listen to what the doctor is saying. You may be so worried about what the doctor is going to say that you don't remember the answer all that accurately. Or, you may have some memory issues that make it difficult to remember what the doctor says.

To head off any forgetfulness or worry, you may want to bring a tape recorder to the appointment so that you can listen to it again later. Some people also like bringing a relative or friend along to listen. If neither of these options is possible for you, it's also okay to ask your neurologist to write down the key points, particularly relating to a new prescription or other treatment issues. In many MS centers, you'll

118

find that information is routinely given in written form as well as oral.

Knowing when to call in the MS specialist

If no MS specialist is available in your insurance plan or in your geographic area, you may be relying on your family doctor or a general neurologist for your routine care. However, sometimes you do need to contact a specialist.

Here are some of the times when you may want to connect with a specialist:

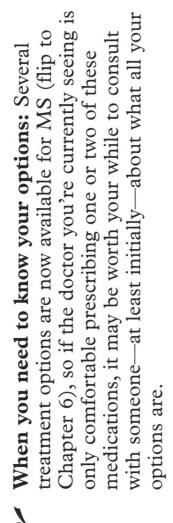

✔ **When you need to know your options:** Several treatment options are now available for MS (flip to Chapter 6), so if the doctor you're currently seeing is only comfortable prescribing one or two of these medications, it may be worth your while to consult with someone—at least initially—about what all your options are.

✔ **When your doctor doesn't have MS experience:** If the doctor you're currently seeing has had limited experience with MS, it's a good idea to schedule a yearly appointment with a specialist—even if you have to travel or pay out-of-pocket to do so. This yearly appointment ensures that you're getting the most up-to-date information.

MS specialists are used to providing these kinds of consultations to people from all over the world, and they'll happily write a letter to your own doctor to convey findings and recommendations. Many family doctors and general neurologists welcome this kind of input, particularly if their experience with MS is limited. If you're seeing a physician who makes you feel uncomfortable about going to see a specialist, you may want to consider working with another physician.

✔ **When your MS escalates and interferes with your life:** Because everyone's MS is so different, very little about MS care is "routine." If your MS progresses significantly in spite of treatment, your symptoms begin interfering in a major way with your everyday activities, or you're having troublesome side effects with your medications, a consultation with a specialist may be well worth your while. They've seen so many people with MS that they're more likely to have seen a patient whose situation is similar to yours than a doctor who has seen very few MS patients.

✔ **When your doctor doesn't routinely involve other specialties in your care:** In this case, a consultation with a specialist will help you identify ways in which nursing, rehabilitation, social work, mental health professionals, and many others may be of assistance to you.

Getting a second opinion

Even those people who are seeing an MS specialist sometimes feel the need to get a second opinion. And MS specialists would be the first to acknowledge how much of MS care is a combination of art and science. Given how many unanswered questions there are about MS, and the fact that none of the available treatments is completely effective in controlling the disease, doctors have differing opinions on how to handle just about every aspect of care.

Second opinions are particularly valuable in complex situations where the standard care or initial plan of attack isn't working as well as you expect. For example, if your MS hasn't responded adequately to any of the approved disease-modifying therapies, you may need to be given a combination of medications. Or, if your symptoms haven't

120

MD to MD: Sharing valuable resources

Your doctor has an important MS resource that he or she may not even know about. The National MS Society offers a program called MD-on-Call, which allows any physician to obtain a free consultation from an MS specialist on the Society's Medical Advisory Board. All your physician needs to do is call (866) MS-TREAT (866-678-7328) or send an e-mail to MD_info@nmss.org. Your physician can also request a literature search, articles from the Society's medical library, information about insurance, and guidance on how to set up an MS specialty center. If you think it may be difficult or uncomfortable to suggest this resource to your doctor, you can get a brochure describing the service for your doc by calling (800) FIGHT-MS (800-344-4867). You can then offer it to your doctor in case he or she hasn't heard about it.

been well-controlled with the first-line strategies, you may need to try something different. The second opinion may offer some useful insights or new ideas.

So, if you decide to go after another opinion, you can ask your neurologist for the names of colleagues he or she respects highly, or you can contact the National MS Society (800-FIGHT-MS) for additional recommendations.

The challenge for you, of course, is what to do with two different opinions. Ultimately, you need to rely on someone's expertise. You may take the second opinion back to your own doctor and let him or her decide whether it's a reasonable one to pursue. Or you may decide that you want to stay with the second doctor. Some people have pursued third opinions to decide which option is best (think game-winning tie-breaker).

Rounding Up Other Key Players

In this section, we talk about the other professionals who may become involved in helping you manage life with MS. If you're fortunate to have access to a comprehensive MS center, you may find many of these specialists all in one place. Otherwise, you'll need to round them up on your own.

As you read the following sections, you may wonder how you could ever possibly need all of these people on your healthcare team. Chances are you won't. Most people with MS experience only a few of the possible symptoms. But, some people face a lot more, so it's important for them to know who's out there and ready to help. The professionals described here have the expertise to handle whatever gets thrown your way.

The nurse for education, guidance, and support

Over the past several years, nurses have taken on a key role in MS care, and you'll find that many MS doctors are fortunate enough to have a nurse on staff. Nurses are involved in:

➤ Providing education to MS patients and their families

➤ Helping patients implement the doctor's treatment recommendations—particularly in relation to disease-modifying therapies and symptom management

➤ Responding to patients' questions and concerns

➤ Coordinating clinical trials for new drug treatments

Given the limited amount of time that most doctors have to spend with their patients these days, the nurse's role is particularly important in ensuring the comprehensiveness of your care. The nurse may be the one who responds to your phone calls, renews your prescriptions, trains you in self-injection techniques, helps you manage your side effects, and connects you with the specialists involved in your care. The nurse can be a tremendous ally and support person—in other words, he or she is your new best friend.

The rehabilitation specialists to help you keep on truckin'

Rehabilitation promotes a person's independence, safety, and overall quality of life. It's a personalized, interactive process designed to help each person maintain the highest possible level of function, given whatever impairments the MS may have caused. Each of the rehab specialists described in this section contributes something unique to MS care. Unfortunately, insurance coverage for these services varies greatly from one insurance plan to another, so you'll have to look carefully into your coverage to determine which services may be covered for you, and for how many visits.

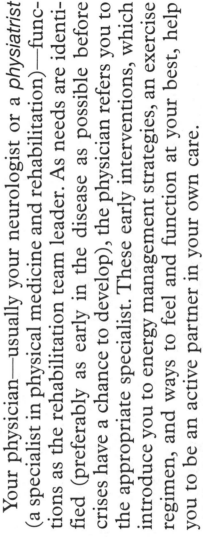

Your physician—usually your neurologist or a *physiatrist* (a specialist in physical medicine and rehabilitation)—functions as the rehabilitation team leader. As needs are identified (preferably as early in the disease as possible before crises have a chance to develop), the physician refers you to the appropriate specialist. These early interventions, which introduce you to energy management strategies, an exercise regimen, and ways to feel and function at your best, help you to be an active partner in your own care.

All of the following professionals work with you to ensure that your needs are met.

123

Rehabilitation recommendations for people with MS

The National MS Society's Medical Advisory Board recently developed a consensus statement concerning the role of rehabilitation in MS care. The paper, which is called "Rehabilitation: Recommendations for Persons with Multiple Sclerosis," is available online at www.nationalmssociety.org/expertopinionpapers. It was written to provide guidance to physicians, nurses, therapists, insurers, policy makers, as well as people with MS, concerning the optimal use of physical rehabilitation strategies in MS care. This document is important to read and share with your healthcare providers because it can be used to guide treatment and demonstrate the importance of rehabilitation to your insurance company.

Urologist

A *urologist* takes care of your urinary system, and if you're male, he or she takes care of your sexual organs as well. Because urinary symptoms are so common in MS, you may get to know your urologist pretty well over the years. (Check out Chapter 8 for info about bladder and sexual symptoms.)

Physical therapist

The *physical therapist's* (PT's) role is to evaluate and improve your strength, mobility, balance, and posture, and to provide fatigue and pain management. PTs evaluate your abilities and then use this information, along with the information you provide about your needs and priorities, to develop a treatment plan. The plan involves exercises to address your physical symptoms—fatigue, weakness, stiffness, impaired balance—as well as training in the use of the most appropriate mobility aids. In other words, they help you create the tool chest we talk about in Chapter 7—and, they're the world's best cheerleaders.

Occupational therapist

An *occupational therapist* (OT) helps you maintain the everyday skills that are essential to your activities at home and at work. OTs are among the most creative people on earth—they know a tool or workaround for any activity you can imagine. OTs know all the helpful gadgets, from easy-to-hold cooking utensils to pre-tied elastic shoelaces that save you from having to tie your shoes when your fingers are numb or tingly.

When an OT works with you, he or she will help in four main areas:

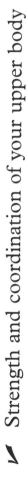

✔ Strength and coordination of your upper body

✔ The use of assistive technology to enhance your in-dependence and productivity at home and at work

✔ Fatigue management, with strategies to conserve your energy, simplify and expedite tasks, and manage your stress

✔ The use of compensatory strategies to deal with any problems you may have with thinking, sensation, or vision

OTs can evaluate your home space and work space, and then recommend ways to make those environments work comfortably for you.

Speech/language pathologist

Speech/language pathologists (S/LPs) evaluate and treat speech and swallowing problems that can be caused by im-paired muscle control in the lips, tongue, soft palate, vocal cords, and diaphragm. So, the goals of treatment are to help you communicate effectively, and to address any swallowing difficulties that may be affecting your health, comfort, and safety. S/LPs also evaluate and treat problems with memory, organization, and planning and problem-solving.

Vocational rehabilitation counselor

Vocational rehab counselors (also referred to as employment or career counselors) help people determine their work options. For example, by using information from other members of the rehabilitation team about your physical, cognitive, and emotional challenges, the counselor can make recommendations about disclosure, job accommodations, additional skills training, and retraining for alternative careers. While some rehab counselors work privately, others work in rehabilitation facilities and in state vocational rehabilitation offices.

The mental health specialists to help you keep your head on straight

When most people hear the words "mental health specialists" they usually think of only psychologists and psychiatrists. But, in fact, there are a variety of specialists in the mental health field. No matter what emotional challenges you're having, you're sure to find just the right professional to guide you.

In case you're thinking "I'm not crazy! I don't need any help from these kinds of doctors!" we'd just like to point out that these specialists come in handy even if you're healthy, happy, and sane. The mental health professionals who work in MS are used to working with healthy patients—those who were doing fine until the disease came along but then needed some education, coping strategies, emotional support, and problem-solving tools for dealing

126

with this new challenge in their lives. In fact, your friendly mental health professional can be a lot like your accountant or lawyer—someone you call when you have a problem to solve or an issue to discuss. The good thing about this type of setup is that in the event that you do begin to experience any of the emotional changes that MS can cause (see Chapter 9), your mental health professional can offer the treatment and referrals you need.

Fortunately, most insurance plans cover at least some outpatient mental services, but typically not at the same level that they cover medical services. Check with your insurance plan to see what types of mental health services it will cover and for how long.

Psychiatrist

Psychiatrists are physicians with a mental health focus. They diagnose and treat emotional changes (refer to Chapter 9 for details on handling MS-specific mood and emotional changes). In most states, psychiatrists are the only professionals in the mental health group that can prescribe medications. If a person who's being treated by a psychologist, social worker, counselor, or other psychotherapist needs medication to stabilize his or her mental health, the therapist will refer that person to a psychiatrist.

Clinical psychologist

Even though some *clinical psychologists* do neuropsychological testing and cognitive remediation, their primary work in the clinical setting involves individual, group, and family counseling to help people sort out challenging issues or relationships in their personal and professional lives.

Social workers

Social workers, depending on their licensure and area of interest, wear two hats: They offer individual, group, and family counseling in a variety of settings, and some also have special expertise in case management. When wearing their case management hat, social workers help people identify and coordinate the community resources they need.

Counselors and marriage and family therapists

Like psychologists and social workers, counselors and marriage and family therapists provide counseling in a variety of settings. These professionals can help family members deal with the impact that a chronic illness like MS can have on family life.

Even though their training and licensure vary considerably, all of these mental health professionals can provide invaluable support for your efforts to live comfortably with MS. Your local chapter of the National MS Society can refer you to therapists who are familiar with MS and the impact it can have on individuals and families who are living with its challenges. (Check out Chapter 15 for more information on making MS a part of your family).

Neuropsychologist

A *neuropsychologist* is a psychologist with special training and expertise in brain-behavior relationships. *Clinical neuropsychologists* assess, diagnose, and treat cognitive symptoms in people with MS. They evaluate a person's cognitive strengths and deficits and use this information, along with information provided by other healthcare providers, to plan and implement treatment strategies. Most insurance plans offer some coverage for cognitive evaluation, but coverage for the treatment of cognitive problems is spotty at best, so check it out carefully with your insurance plan.

The general medical doctors

Your family doctor, dentist, and—if you're female—the gynecologist are also key players in helping you take care of yourself. Chapter 11 is all about how to be healthy with MS. The main thing to remember is that having MS isn't a reason to neglect other aspects of your care.

Considering Comprehensive MS Treatment Centers

Beginning in the late '70s, experts in the MS field recognized the potential impact of MS on a person's physical, emotional, cognitive, social, and vocational well-being. They realized that a team approach was needed to provide the necessary care and support to individuals and families living with MS (think "it takes a village . . ."). Their idea was for each person with MS to be seen by a team of professionals who work collaboratively in a single place (think of it as one-stop shopping). Patients benefit from receiving coordinated, comprehensive care without having to find each of these specialists independently. Clinicians benefit because they can pool their expertise and support each other's efforts to provide optimal care.

Currently, you can find quite a few MS specialty centers around the country, each offering some variation on this ideal arrangement. You can find a list of National MS Society-affiliated clinics (by state) at www.nationalmssociety.org/clinics. In addition, the Consortium of MS Centers (CMSC), an organization for health professionals involved in MS care, lists its member centers at www.mscare.org/cmsc/index.php?option=com_people book&Itemid=500.

Even though many good MS centers exist, there certainly aren't enough. So, the reality is that you may need to create your own team. Your primary care physician may be willing to be your team manager, particularly if you have

129

other health issues besides your MS. If not, your neurologist may be willing to take the job. Otherwise, it's up to you. Putting your team together can be a challenge for even the savviest of consumers, so here are some strategies to keeping in mind:

- Get referrals (from your physician or the National MS Society) to professionals with experience and expertise in MS.

- Keep copies of all your medical records (you can request photocopies from your doctor's office, usually for a fee), and store your own MRI scans. No one will care about your MRI scans as much as you do, and they'll come in handy for your neurologist to make comparisons over time (or for you to take with you if you decide to change doctors or get a second opinion).

- Keep the members of your team in the loop by asking each clinician to copy the other key players on letters and reports.

- Make sure that each clinician is aware of your medical history—including your MS and any other conditions you're dealing with—and that he or she has a list of all the medications you're taking.

If, at any point, it all starts to feel unmanageable—if, for example, you're experiencing a lot of complications with your MS or have been unlucky enough to be diagnosed with more than one illness that requires complex care—you can contact the National MS Society for information about the care management services available in your area. *Care managers* are professionals who are trained to help coordinate your care and identify helpful community resources.

130

Part II
Taking Charge of Your MS

The 5th Wave   By Rich Tennant

"C'mon, Darrel! Someone with MS shouldn't be lying around all day. Whereas someone with no life, like myself, has a very good reason."

In this part . . .

Multiple sclerosis (MS) can't be cured yet, so the goal instead is to manage it comfortably. So, this part is all about working with your healthcare team to minimize the impact of the disease on your everyday life. We begin by mapping out all the strategies that go into treating a chronic illness, and then start you on the road to developing your own treatment plan. We also give you tons of tips on dealing with each of the specific symptoms that MS can cause.

Chapter 5

Developing Your Management Plan to Take Charge of Your MS

*A*s with many other situations in life, attitude is key when starting life with multiple sclerosis (MS). Feisty, determined, and stubborn are all good qualities to bring to the table. But, it's also important to make sure that you're fighting the right battles. Because MS can't be cured yet, winning the war against it isn't possible. So, setting out to "beat this thing" can be a setup for feelings of failure if the disease progresses in spite of your best efforts.

Here's what we recommend instead: Decide, beginning today, that you're going to take charge of your MS by meeting each of the smaller battles head on. We help you get started by outlining in this chapter the various treatment strategies recommended by MS specialists. Then we show you how to set realistic goals for your care and give you a

133

handy template for designing and implementing your treatment strategies.

It's important to work closely with your neurologist and the other clinicians on your healthcare team to design and implement the plan that best meets your needs. The information in this chapter will help you do just that.

Using Multiple Strategies to Manage MS

It wasn't very long ago that treatment options for people with MS were nonexistent. Patients diagnosed with MS were told to just go home and learn to live with it. Our mentor, Dr. Labe Scheinberg—acknowledged by many to be the father of comprehensive MS care—referred to that unfortunate time as the "diagnose and adios" era of MS treatment. Fortunately, the world of MS care has come a long way since then. Today, management strategies for MS fall into five main categories (sort of like an a la carte menu), which we discuss in the following sections. As you and your healthcare team work to manage your MS, you'll be using some or all of these strategies.

Modifying the disease course

Even though doctors still don't know how to cure MS, they now have several medications that have been shown to reduce disease activity (turn to Chapter 6 for more details). These medications help control the disease by:

➤ Reducing the number, frequency, and severity of acute *relapses* (which are also called attacks or exacerbations)

➤ Reducing the number of new brain lesions as shown

on magnetic resonance imaging (MRI)

✔ Possibly reducing or delaying future disability

The National MS Society's Disease Management Consensus Statement (www.nationalmssociety.org/consensus), which reflects the opinions of the nationally recognized experts on the Society's Medical Advisory Board, makes the following recommendations about early treatment with a disease-modifying therapy:

✔ Treatment with one of the disease-modifying therapies should be considered as soon as possible following a diagnosis of MS with active disease (for example, recent relapses or new lesions on MRI). Treatment may also be considered for some patients with a first attack who are at high risk of developing MS (this situation is known as *clinically isolated syndrome*, which is discussed in Chapter 2).

✔ Treatment should be continued unless the person is no longer benefiting from it, the side effects are intolerable, or a better treatment becomes available.

Managing acute relapses

Even though the disease-modifying therapies have been shown to reduce the number of relapses, they don't stop them completely. Because some relapses will still occur, managing them is an important aspect of MS care (see Chapter 6). When you have a relapse, you and your doctor can decide whether to treat it (usually with high-dose corticosteroids) or let it resolve itself.

Depending on the kinds of symptoms you experience during a relapse and the number of symptoms that remain after the relapse is over, you may also be referred for reha-

135

bilitation to help speed your recovery. Take a look at the section "Enhancing function through rehabilitation" later in this chapter for more information on the rehab team and the services it can provide.

Taking charge of your symptoms

Symptom management is a key element of MS care (check out Chapters 7, 8, and 9 for details). The process begins with your first visit to the MS doctor's office and continues for the rest of your life. Because MS doesn't significantly alter your life span, you and your doctor will be working together over the long haul to manage whatever symptoms you experience.

In order to manage your symptoms effectively, both you and your doctor have certain duties to fulfill: Your job is to keep the doctor informed of the symptoms and changes you experience, follow the treatment regimen he or she recommends, and report back on the outcome. Your doctor's job is to listen to the information you provide, suggest management strategies, and tweak those recommendations based on your feedback. Take a look at Chapter 4 for more information on how to work effectively with your physician.

Enhancing function through rehabilitation

Rehabilitation is a branch of medicine that focuses on a person's ability to function. The job of rehabilitation specialists, including physiatrists, physical therapists (PTs), occupational therapists (OTs), and speech/language pathologists (S/LPs), is to help you maintain the highest possible level of function, comfort, and safety, given whatever impairments MS may cause (see Chapter 4 for more info on the work of your rehab team). Beginning at the time of diagnosis, these specialists can help you manage your energy supply, identify strategies to help you function optimally at home and at work, and develop a personalized exercise regimen that's suited to your abilities and limitations.

Over the course of the disease, the rehab folks are the creative problem-solvers. They're the ones who help you identify the strategies and tools you need to keep doing the things that are important to you. Their ingenuity and know-how, combined with your determination and willingness to try new and different approaches to your daily activities, makes for a dynamic duo (take a look at the section "Tapping Your Creativity and Flexibility" later in the chapter for more on getting creative with your approaches).

Providing psychosocial support

Living with a chronic illness isn't anybody's idea of fun. And some days, your MS may ask more of you than you have to give. Fortunately, you don't have to go it alone. You have access to lots of support services—in your community, from the National MS Society (www.nationalms society.org) and other MS organizations, and from mental health professionals who specialize in helping individuals and families adapt to life with a chronic illness. (Check out Appendix B to discover some of these resources.)

 The biggest roadblock in getting these services will be your own attitudes toward them. If you consider reaching out for support a sign of weakness, you'll be depriving yourself of valuable partnerships. If, on the other hand, you see support services as one more tool you can use to manage MS, you'll feel more prepared to handle whatever comes your way.

The psychotherapists who specialize in chronic illness see themselves as consultants or coaches who can help you chart your course (see Chapter 4 to find out more about the members of your healthcare team). You may, for example, want to talk about your new diagnosis and plan your

137

next steps in an environment that's less nerve-racking than the doctor's office. Then, you may go back some time later to talk about changing symptoms, employment issues, or parenting challenges. And further down the road, you may go again to talk about retirement or long-term care options. Sometimes it just helps to have a place to deal with feelings and brainstorm some strategies.

If necessary, the mental health professionals are also available to help you with the mood and cognitive changes that are so common in MS (flip to Chapter 9). Psychotherapists work with you to identify and manage any mood changes you're experiencing, and they can refer you to a psychiatrist if further evaluation or medication is needed. Neuropsychologists evaluate and treat cognitive changes.

Taking care of your health

All of the MS treatment strategies in the world won't do you a bit of good if you neglect your overall health. We think this is so important that we devote Part III of this book to guidance on how to be healthy and feel well.

A word to the wise: MS can take up so much of your attention and your doctor's that other important aspects of your health are neglected. The tendency will be for you and others to attribute everything to your MS even though other things can happen as well. MS doesn't provide any protection from cancer, heart disease, or stroke (which are the primary causes of death for people with and without MS). Your best bet is to rely on your MS healthcare team for your MS care, but also to maintain an ongoing relationship with your family doctor, your optometrist, and your dentist (and gynecologist if you're a woman) for full tune-ups on a regular basis.

And remember that inactivity caused by MS fatigue and mobility problems can lead to weight gain. Those extra

138

pounds aren't good for anyone's overall health, and they tend to increase the fatigue and make it even more difficult for you to get around. To avoid that vicious cycle, talk to your doctor or a nutritionist about a healthy diet that's right for you.

It's a good idea to sort out early on who's going to oversee your healthcare. In the good old days, the family doctor took on that role—checking you over from head to toe, making referrals to specialists when needed, and generally ensuring that the right hand knew what the left was doing. In today's system, however, healthcare is much more specialized and fragmented. So, you need to find out who's handling the job for you—your neurologist, your family doctor, or even you. If you find the responsibility seems to be all yours, the National MS Society can point you to community resources that may be able to help with the process. Contact the Society by calling (800) FIGHT-MS (800-344-4867).

Tapping Your Creativity and Flexibility

Even with optimal use of the available treatment strategies, there's still no magic bullet. MS is a chronic disease that's likely to progress over time, and most people can expect to experience at least some change in their physical or cognitive abilities (or both). So you may be called upon to learn how to do things differently than you did in the past. Not too surprisingly, this task of relearning is a huge hurdle for some folks—particularly for those who feel that things that have to be done differently just aren't worth doing any more.

Grieving, which is a normal (and healthy) process that people go through when they need to let go of someone or something, is an essential part of living well with MS. When you grieve, you're letting go of "the way things were" in order to think about "the ways things can be." (See Chapter 3 for more on the role of grieving in MS.)

The possibilities are limitless after you're able to wrap your head around the idea of doing things differently. The world of *assistive technology* (AT) offers tools and gadgets to help you manage virtually every aspect of daily life. Pay a visit to www.abledata.com, which provides information about AT, or go to an abilities fair in your area to get an idea of the range of stuff that's available. Your rehab specialists will be your "lifeguards," making sure that you find the right tools and learn how to use them safely and effectively. (Refer to Chapters 7 and 9 for more on how AT can help you keep doing the things that are important to you.)

Creating Your Own Treatment Template

Given all the treatment strategies you're likely to need over the course of your MS, you're probably wondering how to figure out what to do and when you should do it. Of course, your neurologist will likely be guiding you—but we thought a treatment template would be useful to help you:

➤ Think about the types of treatment you need

➤ Identify the professionals who are most qualified to provide your treatment (Check out Chapter 4 for a description of the professionals involved in MS care.)

➤ Facilitate conversations with your doctor and other healthcare providers

The following steps will help you use the template most effectively:

1. **Identify the problem you're trying to solve.**

For example, deciding to start a disease-modifying therapy, learning to self-inject, identifying helpful job accommodations, choosing a mobility aid to help with balance problems, figuring out how to manage your fatigue, or finding out how to talk to your kids about MS.

2. **Determine which kind of intervention(s) you think you need.**

   For example, disease management, relapse management, symptom management, rehabilitation, or psychosocial support.

3. **Identify the appropriate health professional.**

   For example, a neurologist, an MS nurse, a rehabilitation specialist, a mental health professional, a family doctor, or another specialist.

The treatment template can provide a kind of roadmap as you look for solutions to the challenges you encounter. Your access to the treatment interventions described in this chapter depends on the availability of MS specialists in your area and the kind of health insurance coverage you have. It's a good idea to check over your insurance policy carefully to see exactly what kinds of treatments and services are and aren't covered. The National MS Society (800-FIGHT-MS) can refer you to local MS specialists.

Figure 5-1 provides a sample template, showing how you might fill in the blanks. Figure 5-2 is a blank template for you to photocopy and fill in with your own information. We suggest making multiple copies of the blank template so that you can start with a fresh template every year.

	Neurologist	MS Nurse	Rehab. Specialist (PT, OT, SLP)	Mental Health Specialist	Family Doctor
Disease Management	Disease modifying therapy?	Giving myself injections; site reactions	Regaining function after an attack	Scared of needles	
Relapse Management	Is this a relapse?	Handling the corticosteroids	Getting back on my feet!	Scared of relapses	
Symptom Management	Evaluation of new symptoms; treatment strategies	Managing medications; coordinating specialists	Stretching exercises; mobility aids; gait training	Mood swings; depression	
Rehabilitation	Referral to PT	Coordinating my care	Exercise; fatigue management	Cognitive remediation	
Psychosocial Support	Education about MS	Education about MS	Education about MS	Grief; coping skills	
General Health	Sorting out what's MS and what's not	Education about health/ wellness	Exercise recommen-dations	Stress management skills	Schedule a physical; maintain weight/ healthy diet

Figure 5-1: Sample treatment template.

142

	Neurologist	MS Nurse	Rehab. Specialist (PT, OT, SL/P)	Mental Health Specialist	Family Doctor
Disease Management					
Relapse Management					
Symptom Management					
Rehabilitation					
Psychosocial Support					
General Health					

Figure 5-2: *Personal treatment template.*

143

Chapter 6

Managing the Disease Course and Treating Relapses

*J*ust because there's no cure for multiple sclerosis (MS) doesn't mean that there's no treatment for it. In fact, a variety of treatment strategies have been shown to make MS much easier to deal with. In Chapter 5, we outline a comprehensive plan for managing your MS—including the five basic treatment strategies that you and your healthcare team can use to manage your MS and help you feel your best. In this chapter, we take a closer look at two of those strategies—managing the disease course and treating relapses—both of which are important right from the get-go.

First, we describe the six FDA-approved medications that have been shown to have a positive impact on the course of MS, and explain how you and your doctor can decide if you're a good candidate for one of them. We also talk about what you can expect from these medications in terms of treatment benefits, side effects, and possible risks, and we emphasize the importance of starting treatment early in the disease course.

Then we give you a heads up about MS relapses (also called attacks, exacerbations, flare-ups, or episodes)—including what they are, how they're diagnosed, and how the decision is made to treat a relapse or not. Because corticosteroids are the first-line treatment for significant relapses, we make sure you know what to expect in terms of their benefits and side effects.

Even though having more treatment options to choose from is a good thing, it also tends to make people a little anxious about picking the right one. So our goal in this chapter is to give you the information you need to talk comfortably with your healthcare team about the treatment options that are best for you.

Managing the Disease Course

Managing MS is a little like managing an unruly toddler—sometimes it's difficult to tell who's winning but it's up to you to do everything you can to maintain control. To help you maintain control of your MS, in this section, we give you the lowdown on early treatment, and then introduce you to the medications that have been shown to slow or modify the disease course (which is why they've been given the catchy name "disease-modifying therapies" or DMTs for short). We start with the immunomodulating medications because they're the ones your doctor is most likely to recommend early on, and we finish with a discussion of the immunosuppressant medications that are available for folks with a more progressive disease course. While *immunomodulators* alter selected actions of the immune system, the *immunosuppressants* temporarily shut down the body's nor-

145

mal immune functions (flip to Chapter 1 to read about what's up in your immune system).

Keep in mind as you read about these medications that none of them is considered safe for use during pregnancy or breastfeeding. Be sure to let your doctor know if you're thinking about getting pregnant so that your treatment planning can take into account your best interests as well as your baby's (check out Chapter 16 for more info about pregnancy and MS).

Understanding the whys and wherefores of early treatment

Here's one of the trickiest things about MS: Even before you know you have this disease or before it has caused you any significant symptoms or problems, it's having a field day in your *central nervous system* (CNS). Studies with magnetic resonance imaging (MRI) have shown that a significant amount of damage to the myelin coating around the nerve fibers in your CNS, as well as to the nerve fibers (axons) themselves, begins early on. In fact, five to ten times more disease activity is detectable by MRI than is clinically detected by you or your doctor. And this sneaky disease activity may eventually translate into clinical symptoms and disability. Although the myelin in the CNS has some ability to repair itself (see Chapter 1), the damage to the nerve fibers—referred to as *axonal loss*—appears to be more permanent. This nerve fiber damage is most likely the cause of the progressive disability that occurs in MS.

What all this means for you is that even though there are no guarantees with this unpredictable disease, the earlier you begin treatment with one of the disease-modifying therapies, the better shot you have at slowing disease activity and reducing future disability. Another good reason to start treatment early is that all of the DMTs we describe in this part of the chapter primarily target inflammation in the CNS, and you guessed it: Inflammation is most common during the early stages of the disease. Therefore, the earlier you get started with treatment, the more effective these medications are likely to be.

Getting familiar with the immunomodulators

Five immunomodulating medications, which alter certain functions of the immune system, have been approved by the FDA for the treatment of MS. Of those medications, four are considered *first-line options*—the ones that your doctor may discuss with you right off the bat. The fifth is more likely to be recommended only if none of the first-line medications seem to be effective for you.

All of these drugs—which are taken on an ongoing basis—are expensive. And although much of the cost may be covered by your health insurance, not every insurance plan includes all five drugs in their formulary. You may find, for example, that your plan covers two or three of the immunomodulating medications but not the others. You and your doctor can take that into consideration when making the decision about which of the medications is best for you. You may also find that your monthly co-payment is significantly different—higher or lower—than someone else's for the same drug. This difference in co-payments occurs because the manufacturers of the drugs negotiate different deals with different insurance companies (flip to Chapter 19 for more information about health insurance). Your best strategy for finding out your cost for any of these medications is to consult your insurance plan. But, keep in mind that medication prices can change frequently because the manufacturers are free to raise or lower them whenever they choose.

147

Each of the drug companies runs a program designed to help people apply for and use all the state and federal programs for which they're eligible. These companies also help people who are uninsured or underinsured (and who meet certain income-and-assets criteria) through patient assistance programs. Because these criteria take into account many factors, including high healthcare costs, many middle-income people are eligible for assistance. The companies invite you to call the toll-free numbers listed in the following section for information about financial assistance.

Injectable immunomodulating medications: First-line treatments

Avonex, Betaseron, Copaxone, and Rebif are the four injectable immunomodulating medications available for the treatment of MS. These medications, which primarily target inflammation in the CNS, are generally recommended for any person who experiences relapses—whether he or she has *relapsing-remitting MS* (RRMS), *secondary-progressive MS* (SPMS), or *progressive-relapsing MS* (PRMS). They aren't recommended, however, for people diagnosed with *primary-progressive MS* (PPMS) because PPMS—which has no relapses or remissions—has not been shown to respond to any of these medications. (Check out Chapter 1 for a description of the four disease courses in MS.)

None of the four injectable immunomodulating medications is head and shoulders above the others, so you don't have to worry about making the "best" choice. None of them stops the disease in its tracks either. But, each has been shown to reduce the frequency and severity of MS relapses and the number of *new lesions* (also called plaques or scars,) seen on MRI scans. Studies indicate that some or all of these meds may also slow disease progression and the accumulation of disability.

The debate about neutralizing antibodies

Antibodies are immune system proteins that develop in response to foreign substances, such as viruses and bacteria. Some — but not all — people who take an interferon beta medication (Avonex, Betaseron, Rebif) develop a form of antibody known as a *neutralizing antibody* (NAb), so called because it interferes with the biological activities of the interferon. When they occur, NAbs typically develop 12 to 18 months after the start of treatment. Even though NAbs seem to have an impact on relapse rates, the development of new lesions in the CNS, and perhaps on disease progression, neurologists are still learning how best to use this information in treating their patients. Here are the factors that doctors must take into consideration:

➤ The higher-dose, more frequently administered interferons (Betaseron and Rebif), which have been shown to produce more NAbs than the lower-dose interferon (Avonex), may also provide greater short-term benefit than the lower-dose interferon.

➤ Some people seem to do well on their interferon medication in spite of developing NAbs, while others do poorly on an interferon medication even without developing NAbs.

For these reasons, most MS specialist neurologists believe that treatment decisions are best made by evaluating how a person is feeling and functioning rather than by measuring NAbs. If a person's MS remains very active in spite of being on an interferon medication *and* he or she tests positive for NAbs on more than one occasion, the doctor may recommend that the person switch to a non-interferon medication.

149

The following list describes how each medication works.

▶ **Interferon beta medications:** Although no one is exactly sure how the interferon beta medications work in MS, they seem to impact the immune system in several ways—including slowing the trafficking of immune cells across the *blood-brain barrier* into the CNS and decreasing production of the messenger proteins that cause inflammation.

The interferons should be used with caution by anyone who's depressed or has a history of depression because some evidence indicates that these meds may increase depressive symptoms. So, if you're feeling depressed or have a history of depression, be sure to let your physician know about it. This conversation will help you and your doctor make the best possible treatment decisions for you while also keeping an eye on your mood (see Chapter 9 for more on MS and depression).

The interferon beta medications include the following:

• **Avonex** (interferon beta-1a): Avonex has been shown in clinical trials to reduce the frequency of relapses and the number of new or active lesions on MRI scans, and to slow disease progression. It's approved to treat relapsing forms of multiple sclerosis (which includes secondary-progressive MS in those people who continue to have relapses). Avonex has also been shown to delay the onset of MS in people who have experienced one clinical episode of *demyelination* (damage to the myelin in the CNS) that puts them at risk for developing MS (look at Chapter 2 for more information about *clinically isolated syndrome*, or

150

CIS). The FDA has approved Avonex for this purpose.

For more information, contact Avonex Alliance at (800) 456-2255, or online at www.avonex.com, www.msactivesource.com, or www.healthtalk.com.

- **Betaseron** (interferon beta-1b): Betaseron has been shown in clinical trials to reduce the frequency and severity of relapses and reduce the number of new or active lesions on MRI scans. It's approved in the U.S. to treat relapsing forms of MS (which includes secondary-progressive MS in those people who continue to have relapses). Like Avonex, Betaseron has also been shown to delay the onset of MS in people with CIS and has been approved by the FDA for this use.

For more information, contact Pathways at (800) 788-1467 or (800) 948-5777 (for financial issues). Or, you can research Betaseron online at www.betaseron.com, www.mspathways.com, or www.championsofcourage.org.

- **Rebif** (interferon beta-1a): Rebif has been shown to reduce the frequency of relapses and the number of new or active lesions on MRI scans, and slow the progression of disability. It's approved in the U.S. to treat relapsing forms of MS (which includes secondary-progressive MS in people who continue to have relapses). Like Betaseron and Avonex, Rebif has demonstrated its ability to delay the onset of MS in people with CIS, but it isn't FDA approved for this use.

For more information, check out www.rebif.com or contact MSLifeLines at (877) 447-3243 or online at www.mslifelines.com.

▸ **Copaxone (glatiramer acetate):** Copaxone has been shown to reduce the frequency of relapses and the number of new or active lesions on MRI scans. It's approved in the U.S. to treat relapsing-remitting MS. As with the interferons, no one is sure exactly how Copaxone works, but it's believed that it works by changing "bad guy" lymphocytes into "good guy" lymphocytes. These good guys cross the blood-brain barrier into the CNS to suppress inflammatory activity.

For more information, contact Shared Solutions at (800) 887-8100 or online at www.sharedsolutions .com or www.mswatch.com.

For a simple way to think about the possible actions of the interferons and Copaxone, picture a barroom: The interferons guard the door (which in MS terms is the blood-brain barrier) so that the bad guys can't get in. Copaxone makes up the good guys (bouncers) who work inside the bar to break up fights.

Although the medications have all been shown to reduce disease activity in people with relapsing forms of MS, they differ in the following ways:

▸ In the dosing, frequency, and route of delivery:

- **Avonex:** 30 micrograms once a week by *intramuscular* (into the muscle) injection
- **Betaseron:** 250 micrograms every other day by *subcutaneous* (under the skin) injection
- **Copaxone:** 20 milligrams (or 20,000 micrograms) every day by subcutaneous injection
- **Rebif:** 44 micrograms three times a week by subcutaneous injection

152

✔ In the side effects they cause:

- **Avonex:** Flu-like symptoms following injection (which lessen over time for many people). Rarer: depression, mild anemia, elevated liver enzymes, and liver toxicity.

- **Betaseron:** Flu-like symptoms following injection (which lessen over time for many people); injection-site reactions. Rarer: depression, elevated liver enzymes, and low white blood cell counts.

- **Copaxone:** Injection-site reactions. Rarer: a reaction immediately after injection, which includes anxiety, chest tightness, shortness of breath, and flushing. This reaction lasts 5 to 10 minutes and has no known long-term effects.

- **Rebif:** Flu-like symptoms following injection (which lessen over time for many people); injection site reactions. Rarer: Elevated liver enzymes, liver toxicity, and low white blood cell counts.

You may find it difficult to get excited about these injectable medications, but the fact is that they're all quite manageable (and the good news is that some oral medications are currently being evaluated in clinical trials). You can learn to do the shots yourself, on a schedule that's convenient for you. And you can do them in the comfort of your home or office. Even though each has advantages and disadvantages to consider in terms of frequency and route of injection and side effects, they all offer significant benefits.

Your job is to work with your doctor to figure out which medication will be most effective and easiest to manage given your particular needs, preferences, and lifestyle. The best medication for you is the one that you can take on a

153

consistent basis until something more effective comes along.

Tysabri: A first-line alternative

Tysabri (natalizumab), the newest of the immunomodulating options, was initially approved by the FDA in 2004, but then it was withdrawn from the market by the manufacturer (Elan) because of safety concerns. It was approved by the FDA for return to the market in June 2006 for use by people who have relapses—which means that folks who have primary-progressive MS or secondary-progressive MS without relapses aren't candidates for this medication.

Tysabri is delivered every four weeks by *intravenous infusion*, (a slow drip through a needle inserted into a vein). The most common side effects include headache, fatigue, urinary tract infections, lower respiratory tract infections, joint pain, and chest discomfort. This medication is designed to hamper the movement of potentially damaging immune cells from the bloodstream, across the blood-brain barrier, and into the brain and spinal cord. Tysabri has been shown to reduce the risk of progression of disability, the number of relapses, and the development of new or enlarging lesions on MRI scans.

Even though Tysabri has never been compared directly with the injectable medications, the clinical trial data suggest that it's more effective in reducing relapses, lesions on MRI, and the risk of disability progression. However, these benefits come with significantly greater risks. Three people who had been in clinical trials involving Tysabri (two in a trial for MS and one in a trial for Crohn's disease) developed a rare, but rapidly progressive brain disorder called *progressive multifocal leukoencephalopathy*, or PML. Two of the people died, including one person who had been diagnosed with MS (but the diagnosis in now in question). PML is thought to be caused by the *JC virus* (JCV). Most

154

people are exposed to this virus in childhood and carry it in a dormant state but never become ill. PML occurs almost exclusively in individuals with suppressed immune systems (such as people with AIDS or those who take immunosuppressant medications to treat cancer or receive an organ transplant). The immune suppression allows the virus to cause disease. The symptoms of PML include mental deterioration, vision loss, speech disturbances, loss of coordination, paralysis, and ultimately coma and usually death.

The people in the MS clinical trial who developed PML were taking Tysabri in combination with Avonex. Right now, no one knows the precise risk of developing PML while on Tysabri alone or in combination with another DMT, but the risk within the clinical trials group equaled about one in one thousand. The FDA has assumed that same level of risk in their approval for Tysabri's return to the market.

Because of the significant risks involved, Tysabri isn't typically used as a first-line treatment. The FDA recommends that it only be offered to people who haven't received adequate benefit from the first-line MS medications or have been unable to tolerate the injections or the side effects associated with those medications.

In accordance with the FDA's requirements, the drug's manufacturers (Biogen Idec and Elan) have developed procedures for the careful tracking of *adverse events*, which generally translates to mean "when bad things happen to good people while undergoing a particular treatment." They also have established a large observational study to help evaluate the long-term safety of Tysabri. In addition, the FDA included the following requirements in their approval of Tysabri's return to the market:

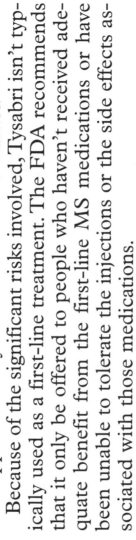

✔ Tysabri is not to be given to people who have weakened immune systems (for example, from leukemia or lymphoma) or who are taking any other im-

155

munomodulatory or immunosuppressive medication, including the DMTs described in this chapter.

➤ Tysabri is available only to patients who have enrolled (along with their physicians) in a mandatory registry program called "TOUCH."

➤ Tysabri will be given only at registered infusion centers where the medical personnel have been trained in its proper use and in the risks of PML.

➤ Prior to each infusion, the patient and infusion nurse must complete a checklist to identify any new signs or symptoms that require evaluation by a physician.

➤ The prescribing physician should evaluate patients at 3 and 6 months after the first infusion of Tysabri and every 6 months thereafter.

As you read the information about Tysabri, some of you undoubtedly said "One in thousand—I'd take that risk in a minute if it was offered to me!" However, others of you said "I wouldn't touch that drug with a 10-foot pole!" This is one of those situations where the right and wrong answers aren't clearly marked. Should the situation arise, you'll be weighing the risks and benefits with your healthcare team and family members in order to make the choice that's right for you.

Turning to immunosuppressants

Immunosuppressant medications, which shut down the body's immune system, are primarily used to treat certain types of cancer. Some are also used to treat MS when the first-line medications described in the previous section have been ineffective. For this reason, they're sometimes referred to as *rescue therapies*.

Novantrone

Novantrone (mitoxantrone) was approved by the FDA to treat people with relapsing-remitting MS that's rapidly getting worse, as well as people with progressive-relapsing or secondary-progressive MS (check out the disease courses in Chapter 1). This medication appears to work by suppressing the activity of the cells that lead the attack on myelin in the CNS. In the clinical trial leading to its approval, Novantrone was found to delay the onset of the first relapse requiring treatment with corticosteroids (see the section "Treating an acute relapse" later in the chapter), and to delay the time to increased disability. It also was shown to reduce the number of relapses requiring treatment and the number of new lesions seen on MRI scans. This medication is given by intravenous infusion every three months.

Novantrone can cause damage to the heart, so it's only recommended for those people whose heart function is completely normal. But don't worry—your doctor will carefully evaluate the health of your heart with an echocardiogram or a multiple-gated acquisition (MUGA) scan before prescribing this medication to you. Here's the lowdown on these tests:

✔ An *echocardiogram* is a non-invasive test that uses sound waves to evaluate heart function.

✔ The *MUGA scan* is a different kind of non-invasive test that evaluates the health of the heart wall and the *ventricles* (the heart's pumping stations).

As an added measure, the use of Novantrone is limited to 8 to 12 doses over 2 to 3 years, and repeat cardiac testing is recommended prior to each dose. In addition, Novantrone carries with it an increased risk for *secondary* acute myelogenous leukemia. However, this condition is thought to occur more commonly in patients who have been treated previously with another immunosuppressant or who have been using Novantrone in combination with other chemotherapy or radiotherapy.

Other immune-suppressing drugs

In addition to Novantrone, several other immunosuppressants are used to treat a case of MS that doesn't seem to be responding to the first-line treatments. Even though their specific use in MS hasn't been approved by the FDA, the following immunosuppressants are used:

- ✔ **Cytoxan (cyclophosphamide):** Cytoxan is a potent immunosuppressive drug that's usually given to treat cancer. It has been used for treating MS for many years, but mostly in uncontrolled studies where it was often (but not always) reported to improve the condition of people with primary- or secondary-progressive MS.

- ✔ **Imuran (azathioprine):** Imuran suppresses the immune system and is commonly used to treat autoimmune diseases such as rheumatoid arthritis. It's also part of the chemotherapy regimen for some cancers.

- ✔ **Leustatin (cladribine):** Leustatin is a medication that has been used to treat hairy cell leukemia. Pilot studies suggested a benefit in both relapsing-remitting MS and progressive MS.

- ✔ **Methotrexate:** Methotrexate is a synthetic immunosuppressive drug that's highly effective in the short-term against rheumatoid arthritis. At least one study found it useful in treating secondary-progressive MS.

158

If you're a woman or man of baby-making age, you need to consider the possible impact of any of these immunosuppressant medications on fertility. (See Chapter 16 for more information about how to guarantee a good supply of those eggs and sperm). Because immunosuppressants can temporarily or permanently interfere with the menstrual cycle or damage eggs and sperm, you may want to consider storing some of your eggs or sperm for future use. And, remember, none of these medications are safe for use during pregnancy because they can harm the developing fetus.

Setting realistic expectations for the DMTs

One of the keys to success with the DMTs is knowing what you can reasonably expect from them, and what you can't. So here it goes:

✔ These medications aren't cures for MS, and they aren't designed to make you feel better.

✔ When effective, these medications can help reduce the number and severity of relapses and decrease the numbers of new lesions that appear on your MRI scan.

✔ With these medications, you're still likely to experience a relapse every now and then, and you'll probably find new lesions on the MRI (although not as many new ones as before). You may also still have a lot of the same old symptoms.

The fact is that on a day-to-day basis you aren't going to know whether the medication you're taking is actually "working" for you. Because the goal of the disease-modifying medications is to slow disease activity, you and your doctor will determine the effectiveness of your treat-

Using your resources to dig up additional info about the DMTs

Getting a handle on the available disease-modifying therapies is no easy task, but several resources are available to help you. You can contact the National MS Society at 800-FIGHT-MS (800-344-4867) to ask questions about any of the medications. In addition, the Society offers the following publications to assist you in finding out about the medications and discussing them with your healthcare team:

➤ *The Disease Modifying Drugs:* This handy pocket-size brochure gives you an overview of the disease-modifying therapies in MS. You can find this brochure at www .nationalmssociety.org/dmd.

➤ *Putting the Brakes on MS:* This brochure provides an extensive discussion of the medications, including some vignettes describing a few people's experiences. To take a look at this brochure, go to www.nationalmssociety.org/dmddecide.

You can also contact the manufacturers of the medications for such information as administration procedures, side effects, and the availability of financial assistance. The telephone numbers and Web sites for each of the companies can be found in the section "Injectable immunomodulating medications: First-line treatments" earlier in this chapter. Keep in mind, however, that the companies are marketing their products to you at the same time that they're providing information and support. Be sure to discuss any questions you have with your healthcare team.

160

ment by tracking your relapses, keeping an eye on your symptoms, and perhaps repeating your MRI scans on a yearly basis.

You're taking a DMT based on the assumption that the medication will do for you what it did for the people in the clinical trial that evaluated it—which is to slow disease activity. By keeping your expectations realistic, you'll be able to stick with the program no matter what medication you're on. In the event that your physician determines that the treatment isn't helping sufficiently to slow your disease, he or she will suggest trying another one of the medications to see if it does the trick. Clinical trials are currently in progress to determine whether any of these medications can be used safely and effectively in combination.

A word about primary-progressive MS

If you've been diagnosed with primary-progressive MS, we know that you're impatiently waiting to hear what's out there to treat your condition (flip to Chapter 1 for information on the many disease courses). We don't blame you either. The entire MS community—including healthcare professionals, scientists, and people with MS—is waiting along with you. The treatments we discuss earlier in this chapter primarily target inflammation in the CNS. And because little or no inflammation is involved in primary-progressive MS, these medications aren't effective for you. Of course, there's still a lot you can do to take care of yourself. For example, the symptom management strategies we describe in Chapters 7, 8, and 9 and the rehab strategies in Chapter 13 can help you feel and function at your best. Scientists and clinicians are working to understand the underlying mechanisms of primary-progressive MS in order to develop effective treatments.

Managing Relapses

The majority of people with MS (except those with primary-progressive MS) experience relapses (also called attacks, exacerbations, or flare-ups) during the early phases of the disease. Folks often call them "exasperations," either by accident or on purpose, and for good reason: They never come at a good time, they generally produce one kind of discomfort or another, and more often than not they interfere with everyday life at least to some degree. So that you can get on with your life as quickly as possible, we filled the following sections with information about what relapses are (and aren't) and how they're treated.

Defining a relapse

A *relapse*, which is defined as the appearance of new symptoms or the aggravation of old ones, lasts at least 24 hours (more often a few days or weeks) and is associated with inflammation and demyelination in the brain or spinal cord. (Check out Chapter 1 for more information about demyelination in the CNS.)

The first key point in the relapse definition is that the symptoms you experience during a relapse are caused by disease activity in the CNS—in other words, they're the outward sign of changes in your brain or spinal cord. The second key point is that the episode needs to last for at least a day to be considered the real thing. These key points are important to keep in mind because, as you've probably noticed, MS symptoms frequently act up for short periods of time—minutes, hours, or maybe even a day or two. But, most of these wannabe relapses aren't true relapses. When symptoms act up for reasons other the disease itself, they're called *pseudoexacerbations*.

162

Recognizing the relapse wannabe

Symptoms can act up for a variety of reasons—most of which are in response to a temporary increase in your body temperature instead of any underlying disease activity.

Even a half-degree elevation in your core body temperature can cause a pseudoexacerbation. For example, you may notice some discomfort in the following situations:

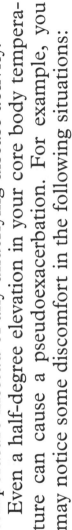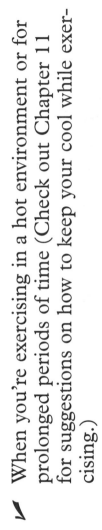

✔ When you're exercising in a hot environment or for prolonged periods of time (Check out Chapter 11 for suggestions on how to keep your cool while exercising.)

✔ When you're running a fever caused by a virus or some kind of infection—most commonly a urinary tract infection (UTI)

✔ When the weather is hot or humid or both

If you experience a heat-related pseudoexacerbation, don't panic—your MS isn't progressing. The symptoms will gradually subside as your body temperature returns to normal. Keep in mind, though, that if your flu or urinary tract infection lasts several days, the pseudoexacerbation isn't likely to simmer down until the infection is gone.

You may also find that your symptoms act up when you're particularly tired or stressed out. This reaction isn't too surprising considering that most people (with MS or without) tend to feel crummy when they're exhausted or under pressure. So, again, don't panic—this blip in your symptoms doesn't mean that your MS is getting worse. Chances are that you'll begin feeling better after a good night's rest or after a little fun and relaxation. You can read about strategies for managing your fatigue in Chapter 7 and your stress in Chapter 12.

163

Knowing when to call the doctor

If your symptoms suddenly take a turn for the worse, or you experience a symptom that you've never had before, take a minute to think about what might be causing it. If you're overheated, tired, or particularly stressed out, take a little time to chill out. If the situation doesn't improve by the next day or so, it's time to check in with your neurologist. Just remember: Virtually nothing that happens in MS is a dire emergency, so don't feel that you have to rush to the ER or call the doctor at 2 a.m.

Because any kind of infection can cause MS symptoms to flare up, your doctor will probably first check to see if you have a UTI that may be causing the problem. UTIs are very common in MS (check out Chapter 8 for more information about urinary symptoms and UTIs), and they can aggravate other symptoms even before you're aware of the bladder problem. After the UTI is treated, your other symptoms will quiet down.

While you're visiting his or her office, the doctor will also do a neurologic exam (see Chapter 2 for a description of the exam) to look for anything that has changed significantly since your last exam. These findings, in combination with the information you provide about the changes in your symptoms, enable the doctor to determine whether you're experiencing a true relapse.

Treating an acute relapse

The fact is that most MS relapses gradually resolve on their own over a period of days, weeks, or months. In other words, the inflammation underlying the relapse eventually dies down, taking with it all or some of the symptoms it caused. So, following a relapse, you may feel and function just like your old self, or you may find that some of your symptoms stick around for a long time or even forever.

Given that most relapses gradually get better on their own, you're probably wondering how your doctor decides whether to treat a relapse or not. Here's the bottom line answer: In general, neurologists will treat the relapse with corticosteroids if it's interfering significantly with your daily life.

For example, if your vision or ability to walk are impaired—and you can't drive your car, function at work, or take care of your kids—your doctor is likely to recommend treatment. If, however, your symptoms are less invasive—maybe you're experiencing increased fatigue, some numbness or tingling on your left side, or *spasticity* (increased stiffness)—the recommendation may be to treat whatever symptoms you're having and let the relapse resolve on its own. The main reason that doctors don't treat every relapse that comes along is that the corticosteroids that are used are more of a quick fix than a long-term solution—and they can pose problems of their own (see the upcoming section "Managing the side effects of corticosteroids" for details).

Understanding corticosteroid treatments

Corticosteroids are hormones that are produced in the human body by the adrenal glands (these are very different from the anabolic steroids used by athletes, so don't get your hopes up for next year's World Series). When prescribed as a medication, these hormones have a number of physiologic effects on different organ systems, but they're most widely used for their anti-inflammatory actions. For example, in MS, corticosteroid medications help reduce the inflammation that occurs during a relapse so that the relapse comes to an end more quickly. A study is currently underway to determine if these meds also have some long-term benefit on the progression of the disease.

Some corticosteroid medications, such as prednisone, are

165

generally given orally. Others, such as Solu-Medrol (methylprednisolone) and Decadron (dexamethasone) are given by intravenous infusion. Most MS specialists recommend a three- to five-day course of high-dose intravenous (IV) steroids as the treatment of choice for severe MS attacks because this regimen seems to provide maximum benefit with the fewest side effects. This treatment may require hospitalization, but it's also common to have the intravenous treatment on an outpatient basis. Your doctor may also prescribe what's called a steroid taper—a gradually decreasing dose of oral steroids over a one- to two-week period—to prolong the benefit of the medication while easing you off it more slowly.

As an alternative to IV steroids—particularly for attacks that aren't quite as severe—a short course of high-dose oral steroids may also be appropriate. Your neurologist will work with you to figure out the best option for your particular circumstances.

What to expect from corticosteroids

The physician's goal in prescribing corticosteroids is to help you get back on track more quickly—especially if your relapse is interfering with your daily activities. In other words, the corticosteroids jump-start your recovery from the attack. But, they don't have any impact on your ultimate level of recovery from the attack.

While most people do well with these medications, it's difficult to predict exactly what your response will be. You may, for example, feel dramatically better within a couple of days—so good and energized, in fact, that you wish you could stay on corticosteroids forever (one woman commented that her closets are always at their cleanest when she's on corticosteroids). Or, you may experience little relief from your symptoms, in which case you and your doctor will focus on managing your symptoms and wait for the

166

relapse to resolve itself. Or, if the relapse is particularly severe, your neurologist may recommend another treatment strategy (see the section "Alternatives to corticosteroids" later in the chapter).

You may find corticosteroids easy to tolerate and you may enjoy the energy boost, or you may find yourself struggling with some pretty intense irritability or mood swings ranging from "high" and energized during the treatment to down and depressed as you come off the medication.

It's important to be aware of the range of possible corticosteroid reactions because they can all happen to anyone at one time or another. In other words, responding positively to corticosteroids during one relapse doesn't necessarily mean that you'll respond positively the next time, and having one negative experience doesn't mean they'll all be negative.

Managing the side effects of corticosteroids

Although most people tolerate treatment well, corticosteroids can produce a variety of side effects—both immediate and long-term—and it's because of these side effects that doctors recommend the short three- to five-day course. The immediate side effects can include stomach irritation, elevation of blood sugar, water retention/weight gain, restlessness, difficulty sleeping (which is why the closets get cleaned), and mood swings. Chances are that you won't run into any problems, but your doctor can prescribe medication to help you sleep or to minimize stomach irritation if necessary.

Corticosteroids should never be used on an ongoing basis because they can cause acne and unwanted hair growth, along with much more serious and debilitating problems such as stomach ulcers, cataracts, and *osteoporosis* (thinning of the bones).

167

Alternatives to corticosteroids

For anyone who can't obtain corticosteroids (shortages have occurred in the past) or who is unable to tolerate the side effects, the FDA has approved the use of a medication called H.P. Acthar Gel, which is made from *adrenocorticotropic hormone*, or ACTH for short. Like corticosteroids, ACTH treats the relapse but doesn't affect the ultimate outcome or natural history of the MS. It's administered by daily intramuscular injection over a two- to three-week period. The possible side effects include vomiting, changes in appetite, diarrhea, constipation, restlessness, difficulty sleeping, and sweating. And like corticosteroids, ACTH shouldn't be used on an ongoing basis.

Intravenous immunoglobulin (IVIg), which is a medication that's generally delivered by monthly intravenous infusion, is another option for people who can't tolerate, can't obtain, or don't respond well to corticosteroids. However, MS specialists vary considerably in their opinions about the effectiveness of IVIg. And *plasmapheresis* (plasma exchange) is available for someone who's experiencing a particularly severe relapse that won't respond to treatment with high-dose corticosteroids.

Bringing in the rehab team

In spite of whatever treatment your doctor prescribes for a relapse, some symptoms may remain. This is an ideal time to call on the expertise of the rehabilitation professionals (see Chapter 4). If, for example, you're left with weakness in one or both legs, problems with balance, or more fatigue than you've been used to dealing with, a physical therapist can help. He or she can work with you to improve your walking and to identify the mobility aid that could best help you maintain your balance and conserve your energy (flip to Chapter 7 for more on managing physical symptoms).

The occupational therapist can recommend modifications to your home or work space to make it easier for you to get around and get stuff done. If your relapse left you with some memory or attention problems, your best ally is a neuropsychologist who can scope out the problem and recommend some ways to compensate (check out Chapter 9 for strategies dealing with memory problems and other cognitive changes). As you can see, after a relapse is over, there's a lot you can do to help yourself get back in the groove.

Getting Comfortable with Your Treatment Decisions

Any good MS doctor will tell you that treating MS is as much an art as it is a science—in other words, it's more creative problem-solving than hard-and-fast rules. Even though tremendous progress has been made toward understanding the disease and developing medications to treat it, there's no cure at this time and no single treatment plan that works for everyone.

The artistry involves you and your healthcare team working together to develop a treatment plan that meets your needs (take a look at Chapter 5 for suggestions on creating your personal disease management plan). And although your treatment plan will probably include some of the medications described in this chapter, keep in mind that none of them are cure-alls or magic potions—they slow things down, but they don't stop 'em. You'll probably experience relapses even while taking a DMT, and your symptoms are going to continue to do their thing. But this doesn't mean that you've failed in any way or chosen the wrong treatment. When docs use that terrible term "treatment failure," they don't mean you! You didn't fail the treatment—the

169

treatment failed you by not doing all that you hoped and expected. Rest assured, when treatments fail, your physician will work with you to figure out what other treatments to try.

In the meantime, keep your eye on the big picture: Work with your healthcare team to manage your symptoms (check out Chapters 7, 8, and 9), and remember that feeling healthy is about more than just your MS. See Chapter 11 for tips on how to make exercise and healthy eating a part of your wellness strategy and Chapter 12 for suggestions on how to manage the stresses of everyday life.

Chapter 7

Managing Fatigue, Walking Problems, Visual Changes, and Tremor

In This Chapter

▲ Understanding and addressing the causes of MS fatigue
▲ Dealing with visual changes
▲ Enhancing mobility and independence
▲ Minimizing the impact of tremor

*M*ultiple sclerosis (MS) can cause a whole slew of symptoms. While most people experience only a few of them over the course of the disease, others have to deal with many more. Unfortunately, there's no way to predict which symptoms you may experience or to what degree, but our goal is to help you feel more prepared to manage whatever symptoms do occur.

In this chapter, we focus on four MS symptoms—fatigue, visual changes, walking problems, and tremor. Even though these symptoms may not seem to have anything in common—other than being annoying—the management of each of them relies, at least in part, on the marvels of *assistive technology* (AT). AT refers to all of the tools, products, and devices—from the simplest to the most complex—that can make functioning (and therefore daily life) easier for you.

Don't let this chapter overwhelm you. The strong message here is that there are many strategies to manage problems with fatigue, walking, vision, and tremor. And you don't have to handle any of it alone. Your rehab team members are sure to be your closest allies—they'll help you be in the best shape you can and they'll show you how to use AT to the max. Think of it this way: You wouldn't try to build a house without a tool chest full of good stuff, so there's no need to manage MS without a full set of tools either.

Foiling Your Fatigue

Fatigue is the most common (and often the most disabling) symptom reported by people with MS. In fact, somewhere between 75 and 90 percent of people with MS complain about fatigue, with a good 50 percent identifying it as the symptom having the greatest impact on their daily lives. Fatigue is one of those frustrating symptoms that you can feel but others can't see. So, you need to be ready to educate the important people in your life—your family members and friends, your boss, and even your doctor—about how your fatigue feels and how it affects your day-to-day activities. Check out Chapter 14 for suggestions on how to talk to others about what's up with your MS.

Along with cognitive impairment, fatigue is a primary cause of early departure from the workforce, so effective fatigue management needs to be high on everyone's priority list from the get-go. The good news is that there are strategies to help you deal with whatever level of fatigue you're experiencing.

The critical point about fatigue management is that it's an ongoing process. In other words, you'll have to tweak it as the fatigue, your activities, or your priorities change.

Identifying and dealing with the causes of fatigue

People with MS can feel tired for a lot of reasons. The trick is to identify all the factors that are contributing to your fatigue and then take steps to address each one of them. The following sections explain some of the most common causes of fatigue.

The extra effort required by everyday activities

When symptoms of MS, such as weakness, balance problems, stiffness, or vision problems, make carrying out daily activities more difficult, you may find yourself having to work harder to do the same things that you did before—which will probably leave you feeling a lot more tired. If, for example, it takes more time and effort to get dressed, make breakfast, climb in and out of your car, and walk from your car to your office, you may have used up all your energy before the day even starts. Your energy supply is similar to a bank account: The larger and more frequent your withdrawals, the sooner you run out of resources (for some great "banking" tips, take a look at the "Managing your energy bank to help put your sleepiness to bed" section later in this chapter).

The best approach to managing your fatigue is to begin thinking creatively about how you carry out your daily activities. The following list suggests ways to help you streamline those activities and make the best use of your energy supply. As you think about how to apply these ideas at home and at work, remember that the rehabilitation specialists on your healthcare team are great resources. They're

173

Other valuable resources for symptom management

Take a look at the National MS Society's list of publications (www.nationalmssociety.org/PubCatalog) to find brochures about each of the symptoms in this chapter. You can download the publications from the Web site or request them by calling (800) FIGHT-MS (800-344-4867).

Other valuable resources include:

↘ *Multiple Sclerosis: A Self-Care Guide to Wellness*, 2nd edition, by Nancy Holland and June Halper (Demos Medical Publishing, 2005).

↘ *Multiple Sclerosis: The Questions You Have; The Answers You Need*, 3rd edition, by Rosalind Kalb (Demos Medical Publishing, 2004).

↘ *Managing the Symptoms of Multiple Sclerosis*, 4th edition, by Randall T. Schapiro (Demos Medical Publishing, 2003).

the experts when it comes to energy management and labor-saving strategies (you can read more about the role of physical and occupational therapists in Chapter 4). Here's the list of tips:

↘ **Open up the tool chest.** The perfect time to put AT to use is when your fatigue is negatively affecting your daily life. Why stand in the shower when you can sit on a shower chair? Why use a manual can opener when an electric one can do the job faster and with less effort? Take a careful look at all the gadgets that have been designed to make life easier for you. Visit Abledata (www.abledata.com) to discover what AT has to offer, and check out service.maddak.com/catalog.asp and www.independentliving.com for a quick look at some creative gadgets and tools for everyday use.

Using a mobility aid, such as a cane or motorized scooter, can help you conserve energy for the important things. What's the point of using all your energy to get from point A to point B if you're so tired once you get there that you can't enjoy yourself or be productive? We talk more about mobility aids in the section "Getting Around Walking Problems" later in the chapter.

↙ **Substitute organization for effort.** Make sure that your work spaces at home and at the office are well-organized and readily accessible. For example, why put the items you use most in out-of-the-way places? And why put the tools you need for a particular task in six different places when you can store them together?

↙ **Ask for reasonable accommodations in the workplace.** Think how much energy and effort you would save if you had a parking spot closer to the building, an office closer to the bathroom, and a flex-time schedule that allowed you to work during your high-energy hours. (Flip to Chapter 18 for more information about asking for reasonable accommodations in the workplace.)

↙ **Make things easier for yourself—not more difficult.** For example, plan meals that require a minimum of preparation, and gather all your ingredients in one place before starting to cook. Make your bed one side at a time to avoid trips back and forth.

Throw the laundry bag down the basement stairs rather than trying to carry it. The possibilities are endless. Check out the book by Shelley Peterman Schwarz called *300 Tips for Making Life with Multiple Sclerosis Easier*, 2nd edition (Demos Medical Publishing, 2006).

- **Give yourself permission to do things differently and ask for assistance when you need it.** One of the biggest hurdles to dealing with MS fatigue is getting used to the idea that you may not be able to do everything the way you did it before. After you've decided that it's okay to adapt to the changes, you'll be able to come up with creative strategies and workarounds to save energy and time.

The side effects of medications

People with MS often take a variety of medications, many of which have sleepiness as a side effect. So, the more medications you're taking, the more likely it is that they're contributing to your feelings of fatigue. Here are some examples of medications that can cause feelings of fatigue or drowsiness:

- The three disease modifying therapies made from interferon beta—Avonex, Betaseron, and Rebif. Fatigue is most common right after the injection.

- Medications used to treat *spasticity* (stiffness), including baclofen, Zanaflex (tizanidine), and Valium (diazepam).

- Medications used to treat pain, including Neurontin (gabapentin), Tegretol (carbamazepine), Klonopin (clonazepam), and Cymbalta (duloxetine).

- Some of the medications used to treat depression,

including Zoloft (sertraline), Paxil (paroxetine), and Effexor (venalfaxine).

If fatigue is a problem, talk with your physician about your medications and medication schedule. It may be possible to reduce the side effects by adjusting the dose or dosing schedule of some of the medications. Your doctor may even be able to substitute a different medication that causes less fatigue or drowsiness.

Sleep disturbances

Disrupted sleep isn't restful or refreshing—so you probably want to do something about it as soon as possible. The first step in dealing with sleep problems is to talk about them with your doctor. Sleep problems are one of those subjects that can easily be forgotten during a busy office visit, so add it to your list of questions if it's an issue for you. The next step is to work with your doctor to address all the factors that disrupt your sleep. For example, any of the following can interfere with a good night's rest:

- ✔ **Corticosteroids:** The corticosteroids used to treat some MS relapses are notorious for interfering with sleep. The energy boost they provide may help you get your closets cleaned, but they won't let you sleep very much (check out Chapter 6 for more information about relapse management).

  If corticosteroids prevent you from sleeping, your doctor can prescribe a sleep medication for the time period that you're taking them.

- ✔ **Frequent nighttime urination:** This condition, which is called *nocturia*, can really interfere with a good night's sleep (take a look at Chapter 8 for information about bladder management).

So, if your bladder is giving you too many wake-up calls, a referral to a urologist is definitely a good idea.

✔ **Spasms:** Painful nighttime spasms caused by spasticity in your legs can jolt you right out of a good night's sleep (we talk more about pain management in Chapter 8).

For painful spasms in your legs, your doctor can prescribe an anti-spasticity or muscle relaxant medication.

✔ **Periodic limb movements (PLMs):** PLMs, which include jerkiness or spasms that occur only during sleep, are more common in people with MS than in the general population. These movements can disrupt your sleep even if you aren't aware of them (your sleep partner will be sure to tell you about them though!). Although these movements can sometimes be very slight—such as a flexion of your big toe—they may be intense enough to interrupt your regular sleep cycle.

Your doctor can prescribe a medication such as Lioresal (baclofen), Klonopin (clonazepam), or Neurontin (gabapentin) to reduce the number of PLMs and help you sleep soundly through the ones that do occur.

✔ **Depression and anxiety:** Although some depressed people feel like sleeping all the time, many find it difficult to fall asleep or stay asleep. (Go to Chapter 9 for information on treating depression.)

If you or your physician think that depression or anxiety may be responsible for your sleep problems, a referral to a mental health professional for an evaluation is the best next step.

The effects of deconditioning

People who don't get enough exercise gradually get out of shape, which means that their muscles are weaker and less toned and their cardiovascular system doesn't function as efficiently as it did before. This kind of deconditioning is pretty common in anyone with MS whose mobility has been impaired. If you're unable to get around as easily as you used to, you may find that physical activity wears you out much more quickly.

In the old days, people with MS were told that they shouldn't exercise. However, it's now known that a regular exercise program, geared to your abilities and limitations, can reduce fatigue, increase your cardiovascular fitness, and enhance your mood (take a look at Chapter 11 for more information about exercise). A physical therapist or personal trainer who's familiar with MS can design a program to help you get back in shape.

Primary MS fatigue

In addition to all the other things that can make you feel tired or sleepy, you can add to the list another type of fatigue, commonly referred to as *lassitude*, that's unique to people with MS. Lassitude is thought to result from poor nerve conduction caused by damage to the myelin around the nerve fibers in the central nervous system, or CNS (check out Chapter 1 for an overview of what happens to myelin in the CNS). Because of the demyelination, your body has to work harder just to transmit messages between your brain and other parts of your body. Unlike normal fatigue, MS lassitude

✔ Tends to come on suddenly

✔ Generally occurs on a daily basis

179

- Can occur at any time of day, even in the morning after a restful night's sleep

- Generally increases as the day progresses

- Can worsen temporarily with heat and humidity

- Is much more likely to interfere with everyday activities

Lassitude may respond well to medication, so talk to your doctor about whether a prescription would work for you. Even though no medications have been approved specifically for the treatment of MS fatigue, several are known to provide relief for some people. For example, talk to your doctor about the following medications:

- **Amantadine:** This antiviral medication has been found to relieve fatigue in some people with MS.

- **Provigil (modafinil):** This medication is FDA-approved for the treatment of narcolepsy. The trials in MS have had mixed results, but many people find that it reduces feelings of sleepiness and tiredness.

- **Prozac (fluoxetine):** This antidepressant may reduce feelings of fatigue, particularly if you're also experiencing depression.

- **Ritalin (methylphenidate):** Some people find this stimulant very beneficial for managing their fatigue.

While one or another of these medications may be helpful, it's usually a process of trial and error to find the one that's best for you. No medication, however, can

180

take the place of adequate rest and exercise, the creative use of assistive technology, and other energy-saving strategies.

Managing your energy bank to help put your sleepiness to bed

As a person with MS, energy will always be one of your most precious resources—so don't waste it. Your best overall strategy for managing MS fatigue is to monitor your energy use as carefully as you monitor the use of your money. Think of yourself as having an energy bank account, complete with deposit and withdrawal slips. Your goal is to keep a good supply of energy in your account at all times, which means that if you make a pretty good-sized withdrawal, you need to be ready to make a deposit or two to make up for it. For example, if you know you're looking forward to a night on the town, you probably want to schedule in a rest time that afternoon and an extra hour to sleep the next morning. Here are some tips for managing the bank:

✔ **Keep an energy log for a week or two, making note of your peak energy and fatigue periods over the course of each day.** This log will help you plan your calendar more wisely, with high-energy activities scheduled during your best hours, and easier, more restful activities scheduled during your low points.

✔ **Set priorities so that you save your energy for the stuff that's most important.** Learning to let go of the less important things (or delegating them to someone else) is a great way to conserve your energy.

- **Pay attention to the signals your body sends you.** If you start to feel tired, take a breather. You'll be surprised how much better you feel after a few minutes in a quiet place with your feet up.

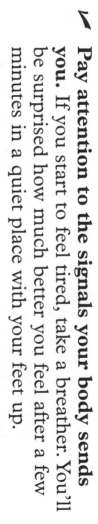

- **Don't over-do it.** If you push yourself to the max on a good day, you may hit a wall and end up paying for it over the next week. It's a much better strategy to spread your energy usage more evenly over the week—keeping your withdrawals and deposits as even as you can.

  If you do push too hard and suddenly feel your symptoms begin to flare up (feeling tingly or numb or noticing a change in your color vision, for example), don't panic—the symptoms will subside as you rest and your body cools down. This is called a *pseudoexacerbation* (see Chapter 6) because it mimics the changes you might experience with a real relapse or exacerbation. However, these wannabe relapses are caused by a temporary elevation in your core body temperature rather than by disease progression.

- **Make full use of the tools and devices that are available.** Doing so isn't giving in to MS, it's taking charge of it. Check out the section "Using aids to take charge of your mobility" later in the chapter for more details on these helpful tools.

- **Eat a balanced diet to ensure that your body is getting the appropriate nutrients.** A high-fiber, low fat diet not only supplies the fuel for your energy bank, but it also helps you maintain a healthy weight. Nothing causes more fatigue than dragging around extra pounds. Go to Chapter 11 for recommendations about diet.

182

Envisioning Solutions to Vision Problems

Visual symptoms are common in MS. In fact, eighty percent of people with the disease experience some type of visual problem at one time or another, and it's the first symptom for many. These symptoms can come and go over the course of the disease as a result of inflammation in the optic nerve or parts of the brainstem. They also may worsen temporarily when your body temperature is elevated by exercise or a fever. Knowing about the kinds of changes that can occur is important for a couple of reasons: First, the changes can be abrupt and frightening, and second, vision problems can interfere with everyday activities in a significant way. Being knowledgeable about the available treatments and resources helps you feel a bit more prepared and helps you get back on track more quickly if these symptoms do happen to you.

In the following sections we describe the vision problems that are common in MS and clue you in on the strategies for handling them.

Managing visual symptoms

The visual symptoms that occur with MS can be divided into two types—those that affect vision directly and those that affect eye movement. Neither type can be addressed with standard eyeglasses because the underlying causes are related to damage in the CNS. MS vision problems are treated by your neurologist or a *neuro-ophthalmologist* (a physician who specializes in eye problems that are neurologic in origin) rather than your regular eye doctor.

Whether you have MS-related eye problems or not, you need to continue receiving standard eye and vision care from your optometrist or ophthalmologist.

Vision problems

Optic neuritis, or inflammation of the optic nerve, is the most common visual disorder associated with MS, and it's often the first symptom that people experience. With optic neuritis, you can have any or all of the following problems:

- ✔ Vision loss in one eye (Even though loss in both eyes simultaneously is rare, it isn't uncommon for visual changes in the other eye to occur during subsequent episodes of optic neuritis.)

- ✔ Blind spots in the center of the visual field

- ✔ Faded or washed-out color vision

- ✔ Reduced contrast sensitivity, which makes it difficult to see things that don't contrast sharply with their background (for example, gray print on blue paper)

- ✔ Pain behind the affected eye

- ✔ Visual phenomena, such as flashes of light

- ✔ Slowed response of the pupils to changes in light

Your symptoms are likely to worsen over the course of a few days or weeks and then gradually improve. Some people recover within a month while others need up to a year or more. Most people regain normal or near-normal vision, but you may find that the quality of your vision, including contrast sensitivity and color vision remains somewhat off. Keep in mind that any of the changes can affect your daytime and nighttime driving.

Optic neuritis may resolve on its own, meaning that patience is all you need. However, a regimen of high-dose, intravenous corticosteroids—for example, a three- to five-day course of Solu-Medrol (methylprednisolone), which is sometimes followed by several days of a tapering dose of oral steroids—can speed your recovery.

So, the question becomes whether or not to treat. Because corticosteroids don't have any long-term benefit, and because they can have unpleasant side effects for some people, waiting it out is a reasonable option (flip to Chapter 6 for more information about relapse management). If, however, your ability to function at home or work is being compromised by the changes in your vision, most MS specialists recommend treatment. Most specialists also recommend treatment if the optic neuritis is your first MS symptom because IV corticosteroids given at that time can delay a second demyelinating event in some people—and therefore the diagnosis of MS (take a look at Chapter 2 for an overview of the diagnostic criteria). In the short-term, we suggest marking doorways, stairs, and steps with high-contrast tape, turning up the lights as high as you can, and eliminating glare by moving mirrors and other shiny objects and by wearing glasses with polarizing lenses.

Inflammation of the optic nerve can also occur without causing any symptoms. In other words, the damage occurs to the optic nerve without you noticing any changes in your vision. That's why the *visual evoked potential test* (see Chapter 2) can be so useful in making the MS diagnosis. This test can detect evidence of demyelination even though you're unaware of the problem.

The symptoms of optic neuritis can flare up when your body is overheated, whether it's from exercise, hot, humid weather, or a fever. This phenomenon is so common that it has a name—Uhthoff's phenomenon. Even if you were unaware of ever having had optic neuritis, you could experience a temporary flare-up of the symptoms, which resolves fairly quickly after your body temperature returns to normal. Uhthoff's phenomenon is an example of a pseudoexacerbation that can occur when your body is overheated (see Chapter 6 for more on pseudoexacerbations).

Because it only takes a small elevation in core body temperature to cause this phenomenon in some people, it's a good idea to keep yourself cool with air conditioning and cold drinks, particularly when exercising or during periods of hot weather.

Eye movement problems

Several different muscles control your eye movements. So, in order for your eyes to move in a coordinated fashion, these muscles must be perfectly in synch with one another. The most common problems caused by incoordination in these muscles include the following:

➤ **Nystagmus:** This tiny repetitive movement of the eye (generally up and down or side to side) occurs in 40 to 60 percent of people with MS. These movements can be so small that you're unaware of them, or significant enough to cause impaired vision (with objects appearing to jump around), nausea, loss of balance, and disorientation. In other words, the world can feel pretty wiggly.

The problem may resolve on its own (though it's unlikely) or it might respond to a regimen of high-dose IV or oral corticosteroids. Unfortunately, nystagmus can be pretty persistent. Some medications have been helpful for some people, including baclofen, Klonopin (clonazepam), Neurontin (gabapentin), and Transderm Scop (scopolamine), but the results aren't earth-shattering. Work is being done on optical devices to stabilize the jiggling visual environment of people with nystagmus, but these de-

Low vision resources

The good news is that if you're dealing with vision problems, you don't need to do it alone. Check out these helpful sources of information, support, and assistance:

✓ The National MS Society (phone: 800-FIGHT-MS or 800-344-4867; Web: www.nationalmssociety.org)

   More specifically, check out the National MS Society's brochure *Vision Problems: The Basic Facts* at www .nationalmssociety.org/specificissues (or you can call using the telephone number given above).

✓ American Foundation for the Blind (phone: 800-AFB-LINE or 800-232-5463; Web: www.afb.org)

✓ American Nystagmus Network (Web: www.nystagmus.org)

✓ American Printing House for the Blind (phone: 800-223-1839); Web: www.aph.org)

✓ The Lighthouse (phone: 800-829-0500; Web: www.light house.org)

✓ The Low Vision Gateway (Web: www.lowvision.org)

✓ Low Vision Information Center (phone: 301-951-4444; Web: www.lowvisioninfo.org)

✓ The National Association for the Visually Handicapped (phone: 800-677-9965; Web: www.navh.org)

✓ The National Federation of the Blind (phone: 410-659-9314; Web: www.nfb.org)

✓ The National Eye Institute (phone: 301-496-5248; Web: www.nei.nih.gov)

✓ Public Broadcasting Service's Descriptive Video Service (phone: 617-300-3600; Web: www.wgbh.org/dvs)

vices aren't available yet. In the meantime, a magnifying glass, large-print materials, and other low-vision aids may be useful (take a look at the upcoming section "Exploring longer-term management strategies").

✔ **Diplopia (double vision) and blurry vision:** These problems are caused by eyes that don't dance well together. In other words, each eye is doing its own thing. The doctor may prescribe a course of steroids to try and resolve the problem quickly. Like nystagmus, however, these problems don't tend to respond to corticosteroids as well as optic neuritis does.

You can patch one eye or frost one lens of your eyeglasses to eliminate the second image. It doesn't matter which eye you cover, the second image will disappear—and there's no reason to alternate the eye you patch. The opinions about how often or how long you should use an eye patch aren't unanimous. Some physicians encourage patching only while driving or reading, in hopes that the brain will gradually adapt to the two images and merge them into one. Other doctors feel that patching is fine, no matter how often or how long you do it.

Mechanical or surgical interventions may also be helpful with the double vision. For example, a prism can be added to the surface of your eyeglasses or to the prescription itself to help align the images from your two eyes, or surgery on the muscles of the eye may help to realign your vision. However, these interventions shouldn't be tried if your symptoms are fluctuating a lot; waiting until your vision has stabilized will avoid multiple prescription changes or the need to repeat surgery.

Exploring longer-term management strategies

Unfortunately, there are no quick fixes for some of the vision problems that can occur with MS. So, if your vision remains impaired in spite of all of the interventions mentioned earlier in this chapter, contact a low-vision specialist. Unlike the neurologist or neuro-ophthalmologist who focuses primarily on diagnosing your symptoms and trying to manage them medically, low-vision specialists zero in on how your vision problems affect your everyday life.

Low-vision specialists are licensed optometrists or ophthalmologists with a special expertise in analyzing and addressing the impact of vision loss on daily activities. They pay special attention to your activities at home and work, as well as your hobbies and interests, and recommend aids and strategies to help you make the most of the vision you have. The specialist may be able to prescribe or recommend optical devices that meet your specific needs.

One particularly useful visual aid is the closed circuit television (CCTV), which magnifies right onto a TV screen hard-to-see things, such as photos, letters, book pages, and labels on your prescription medications. Your computer can also be modified to magnify text or translate text into voice and vice versa. The Low Vision Gateway, a Web site sponsored by the Internet Low Vision Society, provides a list of computer programs for people with low vision (see the upcoming sidebar "Low vision resources" for contact info).

Getting Around Walking Problems

"Am I going to end up in a wheelchair?" is one of the questions that MS doctors hear most. The simple answer is that most people don't become severely disabled by

189

their MS or need to use a wheelchair on a full-time basis. However, two-thirds of people eventually need some kind of mobility device—such as a cane, walker, or scooter—to help them be as active as they want to be. In other words, walking may be somewhat impaired, but *mobility* doesn't have to be.

In the following sections we describe the many ways in which a person's walking can be affected by MS, and describe the management strategies and tools that can be used to help you stay comfortably mobile.

Addressing the sources of the problem

When you have MS, many different factors can affect your ability to walk easily and safely, so the first step is to identify the sources of the problem. Read on for an overview of the things that can trip you up.

Fatigue

As we talk about in the section "Foiling Your Fatigue" at the beginning of the chapter, lassitude and fatigue resulting from overexertion or deconditioning can make it difficult for you to do the things you want to do—including walking. Activities like climbing the stairs or walking around the block, which used to feel easy, may begin feeling like marathons. So, it's important to remember that managing your fatigue will also help your walking.

Spasticity

Spasticity or stiffness in your limbs, which is the result of increased muscle tone caused by demyelination, can interfere with walking. Limbs that are stiffened by spasticity are more difficult—and therefore more tiring—to move. The most common sites for spasticity are the muscles of the calf, thigh, buttock, groin, and sometimes the back. The

190

stiffness can range from mild and barely noticeable to severe and painful.

Here's the tricky thing about spasticity: If you're experiencing any weakness in your legs, a little bit of stiffness can actually help you stand and walk. Too much stiffness, on the other hand, is uncomfortable and tiring. So, the goal is to manage your spasticity in such a way that you have just the right amount. Here are some tips for managing your spasticity:

✔ **Treat the problems that are known to increase spasticity.** These problems include a distended bladder or bowel, urinary tract or other types of infections, pain of any kind, and pressure sores (take a look at Chapter 13 to find out more about complications of MS).

✔ **Ask your physical therapist to recommend a stretching plan.** The plan should include both active stretching (that you do on your own) and passive stretching (that you do with a helper who stretches some muscles for you).

Take a look at the National MS Society's stretching booklets online at www.nationalmssociety.org/stretching and www.nationalmssociety.org/stretching help or by calling (800) FIGHT-MS (800-344-4867).

✔ **Ask your doctor about medications to treat your spasticity.** The most commonly used medications are Lioresal (baclofen) and Zanaflex (tizanidine). Just remember that dosing is important because too little medication won't provide relief and too much will make you tired and weak. The best plan is to start low and work up gradually until the optimal degree of spasticity (not too much and not too little) is reached. Be patient—it may take some time to reach this optimal point.

Severe spasticity that doesn't respond to tolerable doses of these oral medications is best managed with a surgically-implanted pump that delivers baclofen directly to the spinal cord. Because the medication goes straight to the spinal cord, this recent miracle of modern medicine relieves spasticity with a much lower dose of medication—thereby avoiding the unpleasant side effects of fatigue and weakness.

Dizziness and vertigo

Although *dizziness* (a sensation of light-headedness or inability to maintain balance) and *vertigo* (a sensation that you're spinning or the world is spinning around you) don't directly affect walking ability, they sure can make it unpleasant to move around. They generally occur in MS for one of two reasons: demyelination in areas of the brain stem that control balance, or demyelination that interferes with messages from the inner ear to the brain. Because both of these problems can occur for other reasons, it's important to rule out other causes before assuming that MS is the culprit.

Here are some tips that may help get you back on your feet:

- ✔ If the sensations are worse when you change position, a physical therapist can give you exercises that help build your tolerance to motion.

- ✔ Niacin, a component of the vitamin B complex that dilates blood vessels, sometimes provides relief.

- ✔ Antihistamines, such as Benadryl (diphenhydramine), Antivert (meclizine), or Dramamine (dimenhydrinate) may relieve mild dizziness or vertigo.

192

↙ Medications in the benzodiazepine family such as Valium (diazepam), Klonopin (clonazepam), Ativan (lorazepam), and Xanax (alprazolam) may suppress the workings of the inner ear that can cause dizziness.

The dilemma you face in trying to manage dizziness and vertigo is that the medications that provide the best relief—the antihistamines and benzodiazepines—are also known to cause drowsiness. So work with your doctor to find the lowest possible dose that relieves your discomfort without zonking you out.

Weakness

Weakness is a tricky symptom. Like fatigue, you have to figure out what's causing it in order to manage it effectively. Weakness can be caused by the following:

↙ **Deconditioning:** This type of weakness, which results from impaired mobility or couch potato-itis, can be improved with exercise (take a look at the section "Foiling Your Fatigue" earlier in the chapter). Progressive resistive exercise with weights will gradually strengthen a muscle that's weak from lack of use.

↙ **Demyelination of the nerve fibers that stimulate the muscles:** This is a different kettle of fish because with this kind of weakness, the muscles are fine but the nerves that transmit signals to them are damaged. Without those signals, the muscles can't do their thing. Even though it's important to keep these muscles toned with appropriate exercise, lifting weights won't improve their strength because the nerves providing signals to those muscles aren't working. The good news is that exercise can

193

strengthen the surrounding muscles that are being used to compensate for the weakened ones.

Managing weakness involves a balancing act: In order to minimize weakness, you first have to make sure that your fatigue and spasticity are under control. Then you have to figure out which exercises will be beneficial and which may make things worse. A physical therapist can work with you to develop an exercise program to meet your needs. For example:

✔ An aerobic program tailored to your level of ability can improve your overall strength and conditioning.

✔ Weight-resistance training can strengthen muscle groups that are weak from a lack of use.

✔ Passive range-of-motion exercises performed by the physical therapist can help keep all of your muscles flexible and toned even if they aren't receiving adequate messages from impaired nerves.

To manage your weakness most effectively, you also need to take advantage of the tools and mobility aids available to enhance your safety and conserve your energy. For example, if weakness in your foot and ankle is causing your toes to drag, not only will you trip a lot, but you'll also use a lot of valuable energy trying to lift those toes up all the time. An *ankle-foot orthosis* (AFO) is a lightweight plastic brace worn inside your shoe that keeps your foot and toes at the appropriate angle so that you don't have to work so hard. An AFO is made-to-order for you by an *orthotist* (a person who designs, fabricates, and fits braces and other orthopedic devices prescribed by your physician). Even though an AFO may not seem all that appealing at first (women like to cover them up with slacks), you'll pretty quickly find that

194

its pros outweigh its cons.

Mobility aids such as canes, crutches, walkers, and motorized scooters also help compensate for weakness. No one likes to think about needing these kinds of aids, but they're valuable tools for anyone who's experiencing a lot of weakness These aids can make it possible for you to conserve your energy for the big stuff. And, besides, walking isn't always the smartest or safest way to get where you want to go. (Take a look at the section "Using Aids to take charge of your mobility" later in the chapter.)

Sensory changes

Sensory changes such as numbness and pins-and-needles sensations in your legs and feet can also interfere with walking. For example, it's difficult to walk comfortably and safely when you can't feel the ground. Unfortunately, no medications specifically deal with numbness. However, pins and needles may respond to a medication like Neurontin (gabapentin) or Lyrica (pregabalin).

The best strategy is to wear whatever shoes provide you with the most comfort and the best "feel" for the ground. You also need to closely watch where you're going in order to avoid stubbing or stepping on surfaces that are too hot or too sharp. If the sensory changes in your feet cause you to feel less secure, a cane will provide greater stability.

Balance problems

Most problems with balance are caused by lesions in the cerebellum. Like numbness, there are no medications to improve your balance. However, if you find yourself stumbling, contact a physical therapist. He or she can recommend exercises to help improve balance.

For severe balance problems, mobility aids are the tools of choice. The specific tool depends on how much support you need to be safe on your feet. A cane, which provides support on one side of your body, may be sufficient. But, if one-sided support isn't enough for you, you can increase the support by using two canes, crutches, or a walker. Each has its particular charm—check out the "Using aids to take charge of your mobility" section to see what tweaks your fancy. A physical therapist can help you identify the best tool for you and teach you how to use it effectively.

Vision problems

If you can't see where you're going, you surely can't walk around safely and comfortably. Look at the section "Envisioning Solutions to Vision Problems" earlier in the chapter for details on managing any visual symptoms that may be interfering with your mobility.

Using aids to take charge of your mobility

Walking around is much more complicated than most people realize. If you want walking to be safe and comfortable, a lot of stuff needs to be in good working order. The thing is—and we mean this in all sincerity—walking can be overrated. People walk to get where they want to go and do something important after they get there. But, in all likelihood, you can still do those things even if you use a different way to arrive at your destination.

Your best strategy is to think in terms of maximizing your mobility, even if your walking isn't as reliable as it used to be. Mobility aids come in all shapes and sizes. They're tools, just like lawn mowers, dishwashers, computers, and vacuum cleaners. They (like lawn mowers, dishwashers, and any other tool you can think of) exist to conserve energy and time and to help you do something more easily and efficiently. Your physical therapist can help you pick the tools that will get you where you want to go.

196

MS is highly variable and unpredictable. You may need a mobility aid today but not tomorrow, or this month but not next. Yes, MS is generally a progressive disease, but it often travels in a roundabout path. For example, you may need to use a walker or wheelchair during a severe exacerbation, but you may be fine without one after the exacerbation has subsided. Luckily, rehabilitation specialists help you figure out what tools you need to remain mobile during the attack, while also giving you an exercise regimen to get you back on your feet ASAP.

Canes

A cane is used to support your weaker side, so the best strategy is to hold it in your opposite hand. However, any old cane won't do. While the style is pretty much up to you, the cane definitely needs to be the right height to provide the support you need. Your physical therapist can help you figure out what size cane you need.

People generally want a cane that looks as little like a cane as possible. So, they look for decorative walking sticks (or do the decorations themselves) or collapsible canes that can remain out of sight until needed. Keep in mind, however, that a cane won't be useful unless it does what you need it to do. So, decorate it all you want, but make sure that the cane is sturdy enough to support you, that the handle is comfortable to hold and gives you enough surface to grip firmly, and that the tip doesn't slip easily. If you need more support than a regular cane can provide, you have the option of using a *quad cane*, which has four small feet attached to a platform in place of the tip. Or you can use two canes instead of just one.

A cane stored in your briefcase, the trunk of your car, or the back of your closet doesn't provide a whole lot of support. If you need it, bring it out of storage and use it.

197

Forearm crutches

Forearm crutches (also called Lofstrand or Canadian crutches) are good if you need more support than a cane can offer. They differ from standard crutches in that they have a cuff that goes around your lower arm and a handle perpendicular to the crutch that helps support your weight. Forearm crutches don't require as much upper arm strength as regular crutches or canes so they help conserve valuable energy.

Walkers

A walker, which moves in front of you instead of to the side of you, provides much more stability and requires much less energy than crutches or canes. But, no one likes the idea of walker because the first image that comes to mind is always an elderly person shuffling along with an aluminum walker that makes quite a bit of noise. Fortunately, the walker options have increased. Depending on your needs, you have the option of many brightly-colored styles, complete with four wheels, handbrakes, a convenient seat for resting when you get tired, and a basket to hold stuff.

Motorized scooters

Believe it or not, motorized scooters are actually designed primarily for people who can walk! Scooter-lovers simply want a way to conserve energy over long distances—sightseeing trips, visits to zoos and museums, long "walks" in the country, and exhausting trips to the grocery store or mall. In fact, many department stores and malls provide scooters on a first-come, first-served basis for their customers. After you get where you want to go, you can park your scooter and walk, with or without a cane for support. In other words, a scooter is like a golf cart for everyday use. Motorized scooters come in three-wheeled and four-wheeled styles, with a wide variety of options in terms of size, weight, battery life, type of tire, and color. Each style has its pluses and minuses, so it's important to think carefully about how you're going to use it. For example, a lightweight scooter that goes easily in and out of the trunk of your car will have less battery power than a heavier machine with bigger batteries. A scooter with heavy-duty tires is ideal for outside use but unnecessary for inside your home or office. And finally, a three-wheeled scooter may look more attractive to you, but they generally offer less stability on turns and bumps than those with four wheels.

Here's something else to keep in mind about a scooter: Even though you may worry that using one will make you look "disabled," people generally find that driving a scooter helps them feel and look stronger, more stable, and more in control. When you're confidently driving around in your spunky-colored scooter, your loved ones don't have to worry about you tripping or falling or being able to keep up. In fact, they'll generally have to run to keep up with you.

Wheelchairs

Before you panic at the mere thought of using a wheelchair, just remember that sitting in one doesn't mean that your butt gets glued there. You can use a wheelchair when and if you need it, without worrying that sitting down from time to time will cause your legs to get weaker or your walking to get worse. And, you can use a wheelchair for short distances or long. Lots of people opt to keep a folding chair in the trunk of the car in case they "run out of gas" or know they're going to be doing something strenuous.

Wheelchairs come in a variety of motorized and non-motorized styles, depending on your needs and preferences. Motorized wheelchairs offer more support and positioning options (sort of like the seat of your car) than manual wheelchairs or scooters but are generally heavier and less portable than the other options. Although most people never need to use a wheelchair on a full-time basis, it's good to know that there are safe, comfortable chairs that allow people to work full-time, take care of their kids, travel around the world, play sports, and even dance if they want to.

Even though most insurance policies do cover the cost of a wheelchair or scooter, they generally don't cover both. So, you need to think about which type of mobility aid best meets your needs. If you decide that you need more than one type, you'll have to pay for the additional ones on your own.

Taming Tremor

Tremor is tough—of all the symptoms of MS, it's probably the one with the least satisfactory treatment options. It's a close relative of the balance problems caused by demyelination in the cerebellum. The most common tremor in MS is called an *intention tremor*. This type of tremor is a relatively slow back-and-forth movement of the hands, arms, or legs that occurs when you make a purposeful (intentional) movement, such as reaching out to pick something up. When your doctor has you do the finger-to-nose test (touching your index finger to the tip of your nose several times rapidly), he or she is looking for tremor.

Folks with tremor can have a difficult time with daily activities, so it's important that you find healthcare professionals (generally a neurologist and an occupational therapist) who'll work with you to find a solution. The following strategies are used for managing tremor:

✔ **Medication:** The challenge here is that many of the medications that have been used to manage tremor

200

are also pretty sedating, so you may be trading tremor for sleepiness. The trick is to start with a low dose and work up gradually until you get some relief. You may need to try several different types of medication before you find something that works for you. Here are some of the most commonly used medications:

- **Atarax (hydroxyzine):** Antihistamines such as this one may be useful if your tremor is worsened by stress.

- **Klonopin (clonazepam):** The sedating properties of this drug may help to calm the tremor down.

- **Inderal (propranolol):** This beta-blocker works for some people, but it's generally more useful with the other kinds of tremor that aren't seen in MS.

- **Zofran (ondansetron):** This antinausea medication works pretty well but costs a fortune.

- **Mysoline (primidone):** This highly sedating medication, which has some antiseizure properties, sometimes helps when nothing else does.

- **Topamax (topiramate):** This migraine medication, which is also used to treat certain non-MS tremors, may provide some benefit for intention tremor.

As you can see, the medication options aren't great, but they're all worth trying.

- **Mechanical options:** Such options—which use physical or behavioral strategies rather than medicinal ones—are offered by your occupational therapist (OT). Consider these tips:

- Stabilizing your forearm against your body, a table,

or a chair may be helpful because the tremor typically involves the entire arm.

- A brace may help reduce unwanted movements in your wrist during particular tasks such as writing or eating, but the brace should be removed after the activity is finished. Wearing the brace full-time would reduce mobility in your joints and lead to weakened muscles.

- *Weighting*, an option in which you attach light weights to your wrists or ankles, provides stability and cuts down on your tremor. You can also add weight to the object you're using. Weighted utensils, for example, can make eating easier, while a heavier pen can improve your writing. Additional weights, of course, are more tiring to use, so you need to balance your need for stability with your need to conserve energy.

Unfortunately, none of these options eliminate tremor. Instead, your goal is to find the strategies that minimize its impact on your daily activities.

For people with a severe tremor that hasn't been helped by any of these medications or mechanical strategies, a technique called *deep brain stimulation (DBS)* may be helpful. DBS involves brain surgery to implant wires deep into specific brain regions that control movement. The wires are attached to an internal pacemaker-like device that can be programmed according to the person's need. This device is currently approved by the FDA only for Parkinson's disease, but it has been used successfully in some people with MS.

202

Chapter 8

Handling Problems with Bladder and Bowel Function, Pain, Sex, and Speech and Swallowing

In This Chapter

▲ Taking charge of bladder and bowel changes
▲ Dealing with changes in sexual feelings and responses
▲ Controlling the sensory symptoms and pain that MS can cause
▲ Managing changes in speech and swallowing

*D*on't panic! Bladder and bowel, sex, pain, and speech and swallowing problems have nothing in common. We aren't suggesting that they go together or that you should expect to have all of them. However, if you happen to have problems in any of these areas, we want to make sure that you have the information you need to manage them effectively. And, because these types of symptoms can sometimes be difficult to talk about (particularly bowel, bladder, and sexual changes), we want you to feel prepared to discuss them with your doctor or nurse without too much embarrassment. So, in this chapter, we talk about all these symptoms and the best ways to manage them.

Eliminating Elimination Problems

In case you've been experiencing some changes with bladder or bowel function and haven't figured out why, here's the skinny: Approximately 80 to 90 percent of people with multiple sclerosis (MS) experience a problem with bladder function at one point or another. Bowel changes are less frequent, but they're still important to recognize and know how to manage. No one likes to feel out of control, and we're guessing that bladder and bowel control are at the top of most people's priority lists! Given how early toilet training happens in life, it isn't too surprising that problems in this area are so threatening to self-confidence and self-esteem. This section talks about the types of changes that can occur and suggests strategies to get you back in the driver's seat (and off the toilet seat).

Managing your bothersome bladder

Basically, you'll come across two types of bladder problems in MS: Keeping it in when you want to and getting it out when you want to. Sounds pretty basic, doesn't it?

Introducing the parts involved in the process

It turns out that there are some key players involved in peeing. For example:

- ✔ The *kidneys* remove waste products from your blood, producing approximately one ounce of urine per hour.

- ✔ The *bladder* (a muscular sac resembling a balloon) gradually stretches to hold the accumulating urine.

- ✔ The *urethral sphincter* is the gatekeeper for your bladder; it remains closed until your bladder needs

204

to empty, and then it opens to allow the urine to pass out of your body.

↳ The *urethra* is the hollow tube that that the urine passes through on its way out of your body.

When the plumbing is working . . .

When the urinary system is working without a hitch, here's what happens:

1. After six to eight ounces of fluid have accumulated in your bladder, nerve endings in the bladder wall send a signal—"It's getting full in here!"—to the area of the spinal cord that controls the *voiding reflex* (which is also known as the urination reflex).

2. The spinal cord shoots a signal to your brain—"Time to find a bathroom!"—and you head in that direction.

3. When you're ready, the brain talks back to the spinal cord, which, in turn, sends two important messages: It tells the bladder to contract (to push out the accumulated urine) and it tells the urethral sphincter

Other valuable resources for symptom management

Take a look at the National MS Society's List of Publications (www.nationalmssociety.org/pubcatalog) to find brochures about each of the symptoms in this chapter. You can download the publications from the Web site or request them by calling (800) FIGHT-MS (800-344-4867). Or check out *Multiple Sclerosis: A Self-Care Guide to Wellness*, 2nd edition, by Nancy Holland and June Halper (Demos Medical Publishing, 2005).

muscle (the gatekeeper) to relax and let the urine come out.

In other words, the nervous system circuitry needs to be in good working order so that the necessary messages get where they need to go. And, the bladder and the urethral sphincter need to work in complementary fashion. But, as you can imagine, when MS *lesions*—areas of inflammation, demyelination, or neuronal damage in the brain and spinal cord—mess up the works, various types of problems can occur.

When the plumbing isn't working . . .

Bladder problems in MS can be divided into the following two types:

- **Storage problems:** These problems happen when the bladder is small and overly active (spastic). Rather than expanding to hold the accumulating urine, the bladder begins to contract as soon as a small amount has been collected. And to top it off, the urinary sphincter keeps opening to let the urine out. So, instead of a nice, relaxing trip to the bathroom, you experience intense and frequent urges to pee—sometimes as often as every 15 to 20 minutes. You may also experience dribbling or even the occasional flood.

  If you're having this type of bladder problem, contact your neurologist, urologist, or nurse specialist. He or she can give you medication to calm the hyperactive bladder. Fortunately, you can choose from several medications, so you and your healthcare professional can experiment to find the one that provides the greatest benefit with the fewest side effects. The most commonly used medications include:

206

Ditropan (oxybutynin), Detrol (tolterodine), Sanctura (trospium chloride), and Vesicare (solifenacin succinate), among others. Each of these medications can reduce urinary frequency and the feelings of urgency so that you can get to the bathroom more comfortably.

Emptying problems: These problems happen when the bladder and the urinary sphincter are out of sync with one another. When the bladder contracts to push out the accumulated urine, the urinary sphincter contracts rather than relaxing, trapping the urine inside. With this kind of bladder, you may experience urinary frequency, urgency, dribbling, and perhaps incontinence. You may also feel as though you need to urinate but then find yourself sitting or standing there waiting (and waiting, and waiting) for something to happen.

Contact your doctor if you're having these emptying problems because (as with storage problems) medication may help you. If your bladder only retains a small amount of urine after your best efforts to empty it, the problem may respond to Lioresal (baclofen), an antispasticity medication that can help relax the sphincter.

Otherwise, the best strategy for emptying the bladder involves *intermittent self-catheterization* (ISC). Don't faint—it's really not as bad as it sounds. You insert a plastic tube (about the size of a thin straw) into your urethra (hint: for guys that's through the opening in your penis; for women, it's through an opening above the vagina) and empty your bladder at a convenient time and place—generally every 4 to 6 hours or so. It's painless (yes, we really mean painless) and quick, so you can do it anywhere you happen to be. ISC eliminates the unpleasant symptoms and may actually improve your bladder function to the point that you no longer need to do it. Your doctor may also prescribe a medication like Ditropan (oxybutynin) or Sanctura (trospium chloride) to stop symptoms of urgency and to extend the length of time between catheterizations. In case you're wondering, women have an easier time than men getting used to the idea of ISC, but men find the procedure easier to learn because they can actually see what they're doing.

Determining which problem you're suffering from

You may have noticed that storage problems and emptying problems cause very similar symptoms, which means that neither you nor the healthcare professional can tell what's going on just from the symptoms you're having.

The simplest procedure for diagnosing the problem is to measure the amount of urine left in your bladder after you urinate (this leftover urine is called *residual urine*). To do this, the physician or nurse either inserts a catheter to remove and measure the residual urine, or does a bladder ultrasound to measure it. If the residual is less than 100 cubic centimeters (about three ounces), the problem is generally with storage; if the residual is greater than that, the problem is probably with emptying.

Both storage and emptying problems can have you scurrying to the bathroom multiple times during the night. This problem is called *nocturia*. Because disrupted sleep is a major contributor to fatigue in MS, taking care of your bladder symptoms will actually help solve two problems at once.

208

Staying on the lookout for urinary tract infections

Urinary tract infection (UTI) is an infection in one or more of the structures in the urinary system. It's a common problem in MS—so common, in fact, that this is one of the first things your doctor will check any time your symptoms act up (see Chapter 6 for more information about the role that infections and fever can play in causing pseudoexacerbations of MS). Anyone with an emptying problem is at risk for a UTI because urine that sits around builds up bacteria. However, women are generally at greater risk for a UTI than men because their anal, urethral, and vaginal openings are so close together (which is why women are encouraged to wipe from front to back).

A mild UTI may cause nothing more than increased urgency and frequency of urination. With a more significant infection, though, you may experience burning or discomfort when urinating or foul-smelling urine. You may also see blood or mucous in the urine. Because so many of the symptoms of a UTI can also be caused by other bladder problems, the doctor will culture a urine specimen to look for bacteria. After the bacteria are identified, the doctor can prescribe the appropriate antibiotic.

If you get an antibiotic for your UTI, be sure to take it for the full number of days it has been prescribed because a UTI quickly recurs if it's not fully treated. Even worse is the fact that an untreated UTI can pose a serious threat to your health.

Preventing urinary tract infections

The best way to deal with UTIs is to prevent them in the first place. Here are some strategies you can try:

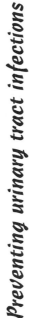

✔ **Empty your bladder completely—by urination if you can and by ISC if you can't.** *Double-voiding*

209

may also help. For example, after you've finished peeing, wait a few seconds, stand up if you've been sitting down or move a bit if you've been standing up, and then try again. The movement can restimulate the urination process.

🖎 **Drink plenty of fluids.** Many people with MS try to manage a misbehaving bladder by cutting down on fluids. This is called the "If I don't drink, I won't have an accident" philosophy. However, cutting back on fluids causes the urine to become overly concentrated, which significantly increases your risk of infection. Because liquids help flush wastes, mineral deposits, and bacteria from your system, we recommend drinking six to eight glasses of water per day. Other fluids are okay too, but keep in mind that caffeine, the aspartame in diet sodas, and alcohol are big-time bladder irritants that will increase urgency and frequency.

🖎 **Keep your urine as acidic as possible.** Acidic urine is less friendly to bacteria. You can maximize acidity by increasing your daily intake of protein, cranberries (or their juice), plums, and prunes, and by decreasing your intake of citrus fruits and juices, milk and milk products, beverages or antacids containing sodium carbonate or sodium bicarbonate, and potatoes.

If you're prone to recurrent UTIs, your doctor may prescribe a long-term, low-dose antibiotic, such as Septra (sulfamethoxazole), to reduce the amount of bacteria is your system.

Dealing with your bowel symptoms

Like bladder control, bowel control depends on a healthy

nervous system in which nerve signals flow smoothly between your gastrointestinal tract, spinal cord, and brain.

When the plumbing is working . . .

Here's how the system is supposed to work:

1. The stomach partially digests the food you eat and then sends it to the small intestine, which in turn sends it, with slow, propulsive movements, to the large intestine.

2. After it makes its way to the large intestine, the food passes through four sections, the last of which is called the *sigmoid colon*, where the fluids are absorbed and a solid mass is formed. When the mass moves from the sigmoid colon into the rectum, you feel the urge to have a bowel movement.

3. After the rectum has filled, nerve endings in the rectal wall send messages to the spinal cord, which signals the internal sphincter (which is normally closed) to open, allowing the mass to pass through the anal canal. The internal sphincter is controlled by the spinal cord, which means you don't have conscious control over it. The external sphincter (which is also part of the anal canal) is controlled jointly by the spinal cord and brain, which gives you the control to decide when and where to take care of business.

When the plumbing isn't working . . .

When your various parts can't "talk" to each other, normal bowel activities can get messed up, and that's when you need to contact your neurologist or nurse. The most common problem is constipation. Diarrhea and incontinence occur much less frequently.

Constipation, which is defined as infrequent (compared to

211

your usual habits) or difficult (painful or hard to pass) bowel movements, is caused by the following factors:

✔ **Demyelination in the areas of the brain and spinal cord that control bowel function.** This demyelination can slow the process to the point that too much fluid is withdrawn from the stool. The result is a hard, dry mass that's difficult and sometimes painful for you to pass.

✔ **Symptoms that limit your mobility.** Symptoms such as weakness, fatigue, or stiffness slow bowel activity, which results in a dry, hard stool.

✔ **Limited fluid intake.** When you stop drinking fluids in an effort to manage your bladder problems, you deprive your body of the fluids it needs to function properly. To make up for this, your body absorbs more fluid from the stool as it passes through your system. The result, again, is a hard stool that's difficult to pass.

✔ **Some medications.** Certain medications, particularly those used to treat bladder problems, may slow bowel activity and result in—you guessed it—a hard stool that's difficult to pass.

Diarrhea (loose watery stools) is actually uncommon in MS. If you experience this kind of change, you and your doctor should be looking for a different cause. What can happen in MS, however, is that moist stool from higher up in the colon can leak out around hardened stool that's trapped in your rectum. In other words, the real problem is constipation rather than diarrhea.

Loss of bowel control can also occur in MS when your brain doesn't receive the necessary signals telling you that

212

you need to go. Fortunately, this problem is pretty rare, and the same strategies that we talk about in the next section will also help your avoid unpleasant accidents.

Developing a regular bowel regimen

The keys to comfortable bowel management are preventing the problems in the first place and developing a regular bowel regimen. But, remember, "regular" doesn't necessarily mean "daily." Instead, it just means at an interval that's normal for you (probably every one to three days). The following strategies will help you keep things moving along:

✔ Drink six to eight glasses of liquid per day.

✔ Eat a diet that's high in fiber, such as raw fruits and vegetables, nuts, seeds, and whole grain cereals and breads. (See Chapter 11 for more info about healthy eating.)

✔ Pick a consistent time of day for a relaxed bowel movement. The ideal time is about 20 minutes after a meal (breakfast is generally best because you're at home before the start of your busy day), when your natural *gastro-colic reflex* is working to move contents through the bowel.

Using additional medications

Sometimes, even the best regimen in the world doesn't solve the problem. If this is the case for you, medications can be useful. But, the trick is to use the least potent one that does the job—you don't have to bring in the canons if a BB gun will do. Work closely with your doctor or nurse to find the program that works best for you. Some combination of the following over-the-counter strategies may be the most helpful:

213

- Daily use of a high-fiber product like Metamucil or Citrucel may be sufficient to promote regular bowel movements.

- Regular use of a stool softener like Colace can help with hard, dry stools.

- If the first two aren't sufficient, a mild laxative, such as Pericolace or Perdiem, can produce a bowel movement. Stronger laxatives should be avoided if possible because they're generally habit-forming.

- Glycerin suppositories may be sufficient to stimulate a bowel movement. If that isn't effective, a Dulcolax suppository may do the trick.

- Enemeez Mini-Enema is a lubricating suppository that safely stimulates bowel action.

You can occasionally use Fleet or other enemas to address a major blockage, but you shouldn't use them on a regular basis because your bowel may become dependent on them.

Sizing up Sexual Symptoms

Because MS can affect your sexuality in a variety of ways, it's an important subject for us to talk about in case you experience any changes along the way. In this section, we describe the kinds of problems that can occur and then show you the strategies for dealing with them.

Identifying the changes you may be experiencing

Sexual feelings and responses are pretty complicated, even without MS. Like the bladder and bowel functions we talk

214

about in the section "Eliminating Elimination Problems" earlier in this chapter, sexual feelings and responses depend on healthy, intact wiring between the brain and spinal cord. They're also sensitive to other factors. For example, consider these all-to-familiar statements: "I'm just not in the *mood* right now," "Not right now honey, I have a *headache*," "I'm too *tired* to even think about it," and "I *hate my body*." In other words, how you feel emotionally and physically, as well as how you feel about yourself, can affect how you feel and respond sexually. And because all of this is challenging even for people without MS, you can imagine how MS symptoms might make things even more complicated.

Sexual changes are actually pretty common in MS. Approximately 85 percent of men report at least occasional problems, with the most common being getting or maintaining an erection. And, approximately 50 to 75 percent of women report problems, the most common of which are loss of interest and changes in vaginal lubrication and sensation.

When MS lesions get in the way

So, first things first: When everything goes smoothly, sex can feel pretty easy and automatic—you don't have to do much work because your body basically takes over. For example, when your body or mind is stimulated in a sexual way, your body responds, and, if you're male, you get an erection, and if you're female, you get vaginal lubrication and engorgement. The sexual excitement builds to the point of orgasm and everything is hunky-dory.

However, when MS lesions damage the nerves that carry messages between your brain, spinal cord, and whatever parts you happen to consider your erogenous zones, the messages get short-circuited. And when the messages get short-circuited, the following changes can happen:

215

➤ Things that used to turn you on may not do it for you anymore.

➤ Your mind may have sexy thoughts and feelings, but your penis or vagina or nipples may not do their usual thing.

➤ You may not enjoy being touched or stroked on the same parts of your body that you used to.

➤ Your body may feel aroused and ready to go but peter out along the way.

➤ Everything may be just fine except that you can't seem to reach orgasm (very, very frustrating after all that excitement and effort).

When MS symptoms—or the medications used to treat them—get in the way

Other MS symptoms can get in the way of your sex life too. Here are some examples:

➤ If you're overwhelmed by MS fatigue, just getting through the day may be a chore and may leave you with little energy for sex.

➤ Stiffness in your legs may make all those kinky positions you used to love virtually impossible.

➤ Sensory changes may cause parts of your body to respond to touch differently than they used to so that something that used to feel good now feels irritating or painful.

➤ If your bladder is giving you a lot of grief, you (not to mention your partner) may be so worried about accidents that you're unable to relax and enjoy yourself.

216

➤ Depression can certainly put a damper on sexual feelings.

➤ Even cognitive changes can get in the way. If you're having trouble maintaining focus or you're easily distracted, you may find maintaining sexual arousal difficult (which is why guys are told to think about baseball scores when they're trying to postpone ejaculation as long as possible).

In addition to the MS symptoms themselves, some of the medications you may be taking to manage those symptoms can also get in the way. For example, consider the following:

➤ Antidepressant medications can interfere with arousal and orgasm.

➤ Antispasticity medications and medications to treat pain can make you too tired to care.

➤ Bladder medications can dry you up in more ways than one (dry mouth and vaginal dryness are common side effects).

➤ The beta-interferon medications can cause flu-like symptoms that make you just want to crawl into bed (alone) for a day or so.

When your own—or other people's—attitudes get in the way

Today's culture is filled with many loud and clear attitudes about sex. Everyone is supposed to be young, healthy, thin, and sexually alluring. No flab, blemishes, wrinkles, baldness, or infirmities of any kind are allowed. With these messages coming at you from all sides, you may wonder how it's possible to be sexual now that you have MS. Consider

217

these common reactions: "This doesn't even feel like my body any more. How can I be attractive to someone else if I don't feel attractive to me?" and "How can I feel sexy when I'm barely keeping my head above water?" Sexuality begins in your mind (even though it doesn't usually feel that way) so being sexual when you have MS begins with feeling comfortable with yourself and your body.

And chances are, you aren't the only one in your relationship having hang-ups about all this. Your sexual partner may be worried about hurting you or tiring you out. Or, he or she may feel guilty or selfish about wanting to have sex even though you're tired. If MS has interfered with your relationship in other ways—for example, by making it necessary for you to shift around your roles and responsibilities a bit—you both may be finding it difficult to sort out your feelings about each other and the relationship. All these feelings and attitudes can get in the way of sexual feelings and expression.

Silence isn't golden: Talking is the first step

The biggest roadblock to getting help with sexual problems is silence. Too often, people tend to clam up about issues like this that make them uncomfortable. The best way to get the big white elephant out of your bedroom is to begin talking about it with your doctor and your partner.

Talking with your doctor

Most MS specialists ask their patients about sexual symptoms because they know that the problems are common. However, other physicians don't. The fact is that no one is all that comfortable talking about sex (not even doctors!). And if you're single or gay or lesbian, the subject is even less likely to come up.

Because your doctor may be one of those who's uncomfortable talking about sex, it's probably going to be up to you to broach the subject in order to get the information and help you need. If the very thought of talking about sexual stuff with your doctor or nurse makes you cringe, you may want to take this book or one of the National MS Society brochures about sexuality and intimacy along with you to help the conversation along (you can find the brochures at www.nationalmssociety.org/sex).

When you visit your healthcare professional, he or she will either make treatment recommendations or refer you to a specialist for additional help. Some urologists specialize in male sexual problems. And women are most likely to receive the information and assistance they need from MS specialist nurses or mental health professionals, or from their gynecologist.

Talking with your partner

Although communicating with your healthcare professional is very important, talking with your partner should also be right up there on your priority list. After all, it takes two to tango, and even the most loving partners can't read each other's minds.

If you haven't talked much about sex before, this is the time to start, because changes in sexual feelings and responses can be easily misunderstood or misinterpreted. To illustrate our point, consider a common scenario:

Janice is incredibly exhausted. She finally gets the kids to sleep and can't wait to snuggle into bed and get some rest. Her husband, Phil, is looking forward to a little playtime with his beautiful wife. Janice can tell that Phil is feeling affectionate and starts to worry. She loves him a lot, and never wants to disappoint him, but the truth is, she hasn't been that interested in sex lately. She just hasn't felt

219

like herself—she's so tired all the time, and the last couple of times they had sex, she couldn't really get into it. It felt like someone had turned off the switch. She ended up just feeling let down and frustrated. Sex had always been really good for them so she's wondering what's wrong with her. Phil picks up on Janice's negative vibes (the fact that she's facing away from him gives a pretty good clue) and starts to worry. The sex wasn't so great the last couple of times—he could tell that Janice wasn't having her usual fun time. Maybe he doesn't turn her on anymore—he's not in as great of shape as he used to be. Or, maybe she finds him boring after all this time. Or, maybe she's having an affair. . . .

When worries and fears begin to build, it doesn't take long for couples to find themselves feeling pretty uncomfortable. For example, in this scenario, Phil may begin to pull away emotionally because he doesn't want to be rejected. Then Janice may start to worry that Phil doesn't love her or find her attractive any more. And the list goes on and on.

If you're facing a similar situation, remember that communication has a much higher chance of success than this type of attempted mind-reading, so find a comfortable time and start the conversation. Use brochures from the National MS Society to jump-start the process (you can find the brochures at www.nationalmssociety.org/sex). Knowing that sexual changes can be a part of MS may help clarify the situation and relieve you both about what's going on between the two of you.

Treating your sexual symptoms

Now that we've told you about all the sexual changes that can happen when you have MS, you're probably wondering

Resources to help boost your sex life

Here are some great books (with lots of pictures) to help you get your groove back:

✔ *Sex For Dummies,* 3rd Edition, by Dr. Ruth K. Westheimer with Pierre A. Lehu (Wiley, 2006).

✔ *The Ultimate Guide to Sex and Disability,* by Miriam Kaufman, Cory Silverberg, and Fran Odette (Cleis Press, 2003).

✔ *Enabling Romance: A Guide to Love, Sex, and Relationships for the Disabled (and the people who care about them)* by Ken Kroll and Erica Levy Klein (Woodbine House, 1995).

✔ *The Good Vibrations Guide to Sex,* 3rd edition, by Cathy Winks and Anne Semans (Cleis Press, 2002).

Also, take a look at www.goodvibes.com, which is the Web site for Good Vibrations, a company in California that specializes in sexual health and pleasure. Good Vibrations has three locations, a Web site, and a catalog. The Web site offers disability-related information and an online magazine that features a column about sex and disability.

what you can do to treat them. Well, you've come to the right place. In this section we describe the management strategies for each of the problems you may encounter. Because some of the strategies are unique to one sex or the other, we talk about those first, and then we describe the strategies that apply to everyone.

Ladies first

We'll go ahead and get the bad news out of the way first: There's no magic bullet. Although the manufacturers of Viagra (sildenafil) tried very hard to demonstrate its useful-

221

ness for women as well as for men, they stopped their clinical trials in women after concluding that women's sexual responses are much more "complex" than men's (surprise, surprise). Just remember that if MS affects your ability to get aroused or reach orgasm, this is, in fact, a huge loss—and this loss shouldn't be minimized by you, your partner, or your doctor. The good news is that many women find pleasure in closeness, cuddling, and sensual physical contact even if they can't reach orgasm.

In the meantime, here are a few tips to enhance your comfort and pleasure:

- ✔ **Get to know your own body very well from head to toe.** For example, figure out what feels good, what doesn't feel good, what you enjoy, and what's definitely off-limits, and then share that information with your partner. Through self-exploration, many women have discovered erogenous zones they didn't even know they had—like the crook of the elbow or behind the knee. Everyone's different, so whatever feels good for you is okay!

- ✔ **Use a water-soluble lubricant such as Astroglide, KY Jelly, or Replens to deal with vaginal dryness.** Don't scrimp—the more the better. But, avoid petroleum jelly products because they can promote infection.

- ✔ **If numbness or sensory changes are a problem, try getting some additional stimulation with a vibrator.** Vibrators now come in many different styles—surely one will be able to get you going. Don't be bashful, try one. Check out the sidebar for helpful resources.

If none of these tips work for you, you can try out some

of the symptom management strategies that we talk about in the section "For all you lovers out there" later in this chapter.

For the men

Erectile problems have recently hit prime-time television. Particularly if you watch sporting events, you'll be bombarded with commercials for the erection-enhancing medications Cialis (tadalafil), Levitra (vardenafil), and Viagra (sildenafil). If you have difficulty getting or maintaining an erection, talk to your doctor because one of these medications may be helpful for you. Clinical experience indicates that they're effective for about 50 percent of men with MS.

Here are a couple of important things to keep in mind about these oral medications:

✔ **These medications don't increase sexual desire or cause erections to happen.** Instead, they allow an erection to occur when your penis is stimulated. In other words, these medications increase blood flow to the penis only after a sufficient amount of physical stimulation has occurred.

✔ **Even though each of these medications is readily available over the Internet, we strongly recommend that you consult with your physician before taking any of them.** We say this because they can interact with other medications you may be taking. For example, if you take a nitrate medication such as Nitrostat or Transderm-Nitro to lower your blood pressure, Cialis, Levitra, and Viagra can cause your pressure to drop too far.

Injectable medications, such as Prostin-VR (alprostadil), papaverine, and Regitine (phentolamine), are another op-

223

tion for treating erectile dysfunction. When you want to have an erection, you inject the medication (with a very fine needle) into a point at the base of your penis that's relatively insensitive (we know what you're thinking, but it's really not that bad). Most guys describe the sensation as something like being flicked with a towel. Unlike the oral medications, the injectables produce an erection within a few minutes, whether or not you feel aroused or your penis has been stimulated, so many men prefer this option. The erection usually lasts an hour or until you ejaculate.

When using an injectable medication, keep the following cautionary facts in mind:

✔ *Priapism* (an erection that lasts too long) can occur with these medications. It's important to adhere to the prescribed dose of medication and use it only as your doctor recommends—in this case, more isn't better. An erection that lasts more than four hours can cause irreparable damage to your penis (so contact your physician immediately if you run into this problem).

✔ Approximately 7 to 10 percent of men develop scarring (in the form of a small bump or nodule) at the injection site. However, proper training in injection technique greatly reduces this risk. If you develop scarring of this type, it's important to discuss it with your doctor so that you can be appropriately treated, because progressive scarring can lead to a curvature of the penis. Luckily though, the nodule usually disappears after you stop using the injections.

Other options for managing erectile dysfunction include surgically-implanted penile prostheses that work mechanically rather than chemically, or a vacuum tube that creates a vacuum around the flaccid penis to produce an erection. For more information about all of these options, check out *Multiple Sclerosis: A Guide for Families*, 3rd edition, by Rosalind Kalb (Demos Medical Publishing, 2006).

For all you lovers out there

Keep in mind that arousal doesn't always have to come first. Sometimes, engaging in a little sensual cuddling is enough to get your juices going even when you think your arousal switch is in the off position.

Sometimes, however, arousal or performance isn't the problem. Instead, other MS symptoms may be getting in the way of your sex life. If this is the case, do what you need to do to take care of them. Consider the following problems (and solutions):

✔ **Fatigue can put sex on the bottom of your priority list.** However, managing your fatigue effectively will give you more energy to get it on. Try to plan sexual activity for times of the day when you have more energy—even if it means getting up a little earlier in the morning to make time before the busy day begins. (Check out Chapter 7 for more details on managing your fatigue.)

✔ **Stiffness or spasticity can interfere with comfortable positioning.** Flexibility is key to whatever acrobatics you might enjoy. You can do stretching exercises or use medications to relieve your spasticity and loosen up your limbs. (Flip to Chapter 7 for more tips to sidestep your spasticity.)

✔ **Bladder problems can put a damper on sexual activity.** To avoid embarrassing accidents (and to allow yourself to relax and be in the moment), empty your bladder or catheterize yourself before you have sex. Although some partners find the prospect of urinary accidents pretty uncomfortable, most take it in stride after they understand what the problem is and what you're doing to take care of it. (Refer to the section "Eliminating Elimination Problems" earlier in the chapter for more ways to manage your badly behaved bladder.)

➤ **Weakness can make sexual activity difficult and tiring.** For example, being on top may feel much more tiring than lying on your back, or lying on your side may be the most restful of all. It's a good idea to experiment with different positions to find out what puts the least strain on weakened muscles. This is one of those situations where it helps to think creatively—just because you've always had sex one way doesn't mean it's your only option. Who knows what you might discover!

➤ **Cognitive changes can cause you to be distracted, which in turn makes it difficult for you to become or stay aroused.** So, it's important to create a sensual, distraction-free environment for sex. Unless you're watching a great sexy movie that turns you on, shut off the TV. Do whatever feels most soothing and sensual with the lights, and make sure you aren't going to be interrupted or distracted by goings-on in the house.

If you think your medications are getting in the way, the best place to start is with a conversation with your doctor. Sometimes it's possible to change the dose or the timing of the dose in order to relieve a problem you've been having. If, for example, you're taking a bladder medication that causes vaginal dryness or pain, or if you're taking spasticity medication that makes you very tired, the doctor may

226

change the dosing schedule to make you more comfortable for sexual activity. If you're taking an antidepressant that interferes with sexual arousal or orgasm, you may be able to skip a dose before sex. While this is definitely *not* recommended at the beginning of a major depressive episode, it can work well for someone who has been comfortably stable on an antidepressant for several weeks or months. So it's possible to adjust your medications, but only after talking with your doctor.

If your head is getting in the way—you've lost your self-confidence, you don't feel attractive any more, you're too worried or preoccupied to think about sex these days, or your partnership is under so much strain that sex isn't high on the priority list—chatting with a mental health professional can be wonderfully helpful.

Sex is about more than just a few body parts, and intimacy is about more than just sex, so fixing those parts is only half of the solution to MS-related sexual changes. If you're having trouble communicating, trusting one another, or dealing with whatever changes the MS is causing in your relationship, chances are that all the Viagra or Astroglide in the world won't solve the problem. So, don't be too bashful about talking with a couple's therapist if things are dicey—he or she can help you get back on track. (Refer to Chapter 3 for more on dealing with the feelings and reactions you're having and to Chapter 15 for details on what your partner or family may be going through as well.)

Sidestepping Sensory Symptoms and Pain

MS can cause many different kinds of sensory changes, most of which are annoying and uncomfortable but not serious. In other words, you may hate them but they don't indicate big-time disease progression, and they generally aren't incapacitating. For example, numbness and pins and needles in the arms or legs are both very common. From the doctor's perspective, there's no need to treat these symptoms unless they're particularly bothersome, in which case a short course of high-dose corticosteroids may be helpful.

Pain deserves prompt attention because it can be distracting, debilitating, and depressing—and who needs that? For years, people were told that MS doesn't cause pain. Well, it does and it can have a significant impact on your quality of life. At least 50 percent of folks with MS experience pain at one time or another. Pain in MS can be divided into the following two main types:

➤ **Primary pain:** This pain, which is also called *neuropathic pain* is caused by inflammation and demyelination along the sensory pathways in the brain and spinal cord. In other words, this kind of pain has a neurologic basis.

➤ **Secondary pain:** This type of pain occurs as an indirect result of other problems. For example, if your posture has changed as a result of weakness or stiffness in your legs, you may begin to experience pain in your back or hips.

Primary pain

Several different types of pain can occur as a result of damage to the nerves:

➤ *Dysesthesias*, the most common pain in MS, are achy, burning sensations that generally occur in your arms, legs, or trunk. The "MS hug" is a tight, band-like sensation around your chest or mid-section.

228

✔ *Trigeminal neuralgia* is a severe, lancing or stabbing pain in the face (in the area of the trigeminal nerve).

✔ *Lhermitte's sign* is an electrical sensation that some people with MS experience. This sensation travels down their spine and into their legs when they bend their head forward.

Medications are the first-line treatment for neuropathic pain. The treatment process requires somewhat of a try-and-see approach because pain is an individual experience and people respond differently to the medications. The usual strategy is to start at a low dose of one medication and work up to an effective level. The key is to find a medication level that provides relief without causing too much sleepiness or any other unpleasant side effects. Your neurologist may recommend lower doses of more than one medication at a time in order to maximize effectiveness while minimizing side effects.

Even though no medications have been specifically approved for the treatment of MS pain, a wide variety has been used with some success:

✔ Antiseizure medications, including Tegretol (carbamazepine) and Neurontin (gabapentin) are commonly used to treat trigeminal neuralgia and dysesthesias.

✔ Lyrica (pregabalin) is FDA-approved to treat neuropathic pain from diabetes and is currently being studied in MS.

✔ Cymbalta (duloxetine hydrochloride) is FDA-approved for the treatment of depression and for neuropathic pain caused by diabetes. It has been used successfully for MS-related pain as well, partic-

229

ularly dysesthesias.

- Tricyclic antidepressants, including Elavil (amitriptyline), Norpramine (desipramine), and Pamelor (nortriptyline) are also helpful with disesthesias.

For trigeminal neuralgia that doesn't respond to any of the medications, the doctor may recommend a surgical procedure called a *percutaneous rhizotomy*. Although the procedure can be done in a variety of ways, the common goal is to deactivate the trigeminal nerve sufficiently to block the sensation of pain.

Significant pain may also accompany certain symptoms of your MS. For example, the muscle stiffness (spasticity) that's so common in MS (take a look at Chapter 7) can cause extremely painful spasms. These spasms can be managed with the antispasticity medications baclofen and Zanaflex (tizanidine). Valium (diazepam) can be particularly helpful for painful nighttime spasms in the legs and feet. Optic neuritis (also described in Chapter 7), may be accompanied by severe eye pain that generally responds to a short course of high-dose intravenous corticosteroids.

Primary pain doesn't respond to the standard pain medications used for injuries, such as aspirin, Tylenol (acetaminophen), or the various formulations of ibuprofen (Motrin or Advil), because the source of the pain is different. Primary pain also doesn't respond well to narcotics.

Although medications of various types can be extremely useful for managing your pain, you can also consider other alternative options. Acupuncture, for instance, may be helpful for some types of pain (however it hasn't be studied extensively in MS). Some people find meditation and other relaxation strategies to be beneficial as well. (Flip to Chapter 10 for more on the ups and downs of alternative medicine.)

Secondary pain

Secondary pain is pretty common in MS because weakness, spasticity, and other MS symptoms can affect your whole musculoskeletal system. Your neck, lower back, and knees are the usual suspects when it comes to problems. The best way to address this kind of pain is to try and prevent it in the first place with the right types of exercise, careful attention to your posture while walking and sitting, and optimal use of the correct mobility aids (when

Cannabinoids: Deriving benefits from marijuana

Cannabinoids are chemical derivatives of marijuana plants. Recent research efforts have focused on trying to capture the benefits of cannabinoids for various problems, including neuropathic pain, while minimizing the side effects and health risks associated with smoked marijuana. Health Canada, the drug regulatory agency for Canada, recently approved the use of Sativex, an *oromucosal* spray (which means that it's sprayed into the mouth and absorbed through the mucous membrane), developed from marijuana extracts by GW Pharmaceuticals, for the treatment of MS-related pain. The company hasn't yet applied to the U.S. Food and Drug administration for approval, but it has been given the go-ahead by the FDA to test the drug in the United States. The approval in Canada was based on data indicating that Sativex reduced *central pain* (pain induced by damage or dysfunction in the brain and spinal cord) and sleep disturbance in a small, short-term study involving 66 people with multiple sclerosis. A larger study is now underway in Canada. For more information about the issues surrounding the use of marijuana and its derivatives for treatment of MS symptoms, take a look at the National MS Society's statement on marijuana at www.nationalmssociety.org/marijuana.

needed). Your rehabilitation team (see Chapters 4 and 7) can recommend strategies to help maintain your comfort and flexibility.

If and when you develop secondary problems with your neck, back, or knees, it's important to make sure that the healthcare professional who's treating you is aware of your MS and its relationship to the problems you're having. This is definitely a time when it's helpful to get the professionals on your team to talk to one another. For example, an orthopedist consulted about a knee or back problem may recommend certain types of weight-bearing exercise on the assumption that your difficulties are the result of weak muscles when, in reality, the underlying problem has to do with impaired nerve conduction to those muscles.

Many people with neck or back pain consult a chiropractor. Even though the data from studies on chiropractic therapy suggest that it may benefit lower back pain, you need to consult with your neurologist before beginning treatment. Because of your MS, manipulations of your spine may not be in your best interest.

Sorting out Speech and Swallowing Problems

Lesions in the brain can affect speech and swallowing. Even though these types of problems are less common than many of the others we talk about in this book, it's important to be aware of them because they can have a big impact on your quality of life—slurring your speech can definitely give people around you the wrong impression, and nothing is more frightening than randomly choking on your dinner. We talk about these problems together because they're evaluated and treated by the same clinician—the speech/language pathologist (S/LP). Flip to Chapter 4 for more information about this important member of the rehab team.

Speech and voice problems: Articulating the facts

Like the other functions we talk about in this chapter, normal speech and voice quality depend on complex messaging in the central nervous system. When the nerve impulses can't travel where they need to go, speech and voice quality become impaired. Approximately 25 to 40 percent of people with MS experience these kinds of problems at one time or another. *Dysarthria* is the term used to describe problems relating to speech production, such as slurring, unclear articulation, and problems with volume control. *Dysphonia* is the term for problems with voice quality, such as harshness, poor pitch control, excessive nasality, increased breathiness, or hoarseness.

Problems with speech and voice quality can come and go during relapses or periods of extreme fatigue. If you begin to experience any changes that interfere with everyday communication, request a referral to an S/LP. Individualized therapy techniques can relieve many of these problems, and the sooner you start treatment, the better your outcome is likely to be. Your healthcare professional or the National MS Society (800-FIGHT-MS or 800-344-4867) can refer you to an S/LP with experience in MS.

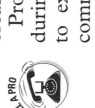

The S/LP will test the muscles in your mouth and throat that are necessary for speech and will evaluate your respiratory function and your ability to control pitch and loudness. He or she will also perform a *motor speech evaluation* to determine if your breathing, voice production, articulation of words, and flow of speech are working appropriately together. And lastly, the S/LP will complete a *communication profile* to figure out what your communication needs are at home and at work—for example, checking to see if you talk mostly in one-on-one situations with people who know you well or if you need to be able to communicate in large, noisy groups. Ultimately, the S/LP's goal is to ensure that you can communicate effectively with others whenever and wherever you want to.

After the S/LP has identified whatever problems you're having, he or she develops an individualized treatment program for you, typically consisting of a daily exercise routine for your lips, tongue, soft palate, vocal cords, and diaphragm. He or she may also give you some strategies to compensate for any problems you're having with speech clarity. If necessary, the S/LP may also recommend certain medications to help manage the problems. An antispasticity medication like Lioresal (baclofen) or Zanaflex (tizanidine) may help if your problems with voice quality and loudness are caused by spasticity. If tremor in your vocal cords, jaw, lips, or tongue is causing the problem, the doctor may recommend a medication such as Klonopin (clonazepam). And, finally, if fatigue is contributing to your problems with voice control and volume, you may find amantadine or Provigil (modafinil) useful.

For more detailed information about the assessment and treatment of speech problems, take a look at the book *Multiple Sclerosis: The Questions You Have; The Answers You Need*, 3rd edition, by Rosalind Kalb (Demos Medical Publishing, 2004).

Watching out for swallowing problems

Swallowing isn't as simple as it seems—in fact, the process involves about 30 muscles in your mouth and throat and eight of your cranial nerves. So, as you can imagine, MS lesions can interfere at any point in the process, from when

234

you put food in your mouth to when it arrives in your stomach.

When the nerve impulses that make swallowing possible aren't working correctly, you develop *dysphagia*, or difficulty swallowing. When this happens, food can pass into your airway and lungs, causing you to choke and cough. Over time, particles of food that remain in the lungs can cause *aspiration pneumonia*, (we talk about this serious complication in Chapter 13). Fortunately, most people with MS won't develop this kind of serious problem. But, if you notice that your eating has become much slower, you have difficulty swallowing different kinds of food (liquids, for example, may give you more problems than solids, or certain kinds of solid foods may cause you more difficulty than others), or you find yourself coughing a lot during or after meals, ask your doctor for a referral to an S/LP.

The S/LP will evaluate your swallow with a test called a *videofluoroscopy* (also referred to as a *modified barium swallow*), that tracks via X-ray a bolus of food as it travels from your mouth down to your stomach. Depending on the type of problem you're having, the S/LP can teach you safe swallowing exercises that improve muscle coordination during swallowing and recommend modifications in the way you eat or the consistency of the foods you eat.

For more detailed information about the management of swallowing problems, take a look at the book *Multiple Sclerosis: The Questions You Have, The Answers You Need*, 3rd edition, by Rosalind Kalb (Demos Medical Publishing, 2004).

235

Chapter 9

Getting Your Head around Problems with Thinking and Mood

In This Chapter

▼ Dealing with cognitive impairment

▼ Understanding how cognitive changes are evaluated and treated

▼ Keeping mood swings and other emotional changes in check

▼ Treating and overcoming depression

*T*alk about adding insult to injury! Not only can multiple sclerosis (MS) cause a wide variety of physical symptoms, it can also affect the way people think and feel emotionally. It's important to understand what these changes are, and how they may affect you because early recognition and treatment are key to managing these symptoms successfully.

In this chapter, we discuss the ways that MS can affect your cognition and describe how these problems are evaluated and treated. We also talk about the mood changes that are so common in MS, with particular emphasis on strategies for managing mood swings and depression.

Handling Problems with Thinking and Memory

For many people, the idea that MS can affect the way they think is the most frightening aspect of this disease. "I can handle the physical symptoms, just don't mess with my mind" is a pretty common refrain. Surprisingly enough, cognitive changes weren't even acknowledged or addressed by the medical community until about 25 years ago (which is somewhat perplexing given that Jean-Martin Charcot noted these symptoms in his early descriptions of MS in the late 1800s). For years, patients were told that MS couldn't affect the mind or that it did so only rarely. But fortunately, MS researchers and clinicians have finally begun to focus significant attention on this important problem.

As you read about cognition in the following sections, remember that cognitive dysfunction isn't an emotional disorder—a person can have problems with thinking and memory without having an emotional problem.

Defining cognition

The term *cognition* refers to the higher-level functions of the human brain, including:

✔ Processing incoming information (attention and concentration)

✔ Acquiring, storing, and retrieving new information (learning and memory)

✔ Organizing and manipulating information to prioritize and problem-solve, as well as plan and execute complex activities (executive functions)

✒ Acting on information and communicating it to others (expression)

Even though the list makes these functions sound separate and independent, remember that they're in fact interdependent. For example, you can't remember something without having paid attention to it in the first place; you can't organize information in an effective way if you can't remember it; nor can you deal with information effectively or communicate it to others without having learned and organized it in a meaningful way. Therefore, problems in any one of these functions can affect how you think and perform.

Understanding how MS can affect your cognition

Research studies on cognitive function in MS have demonstrated that as many as 50 to 66 percent of people will experience some cognitive changes over the course of the disease. Even though the severity of these changes can vary from mild to quite severe, we're happy to report that the majority of these changes are in the mild-to-moderate range. So, don't panic. The following sections give you the information you need to recognize any problems that you may be having and figure out what to do about them.

It's important to familiarize yourself with the kinds of changes that can occur because:

✒ **Cognitive changes can occur at any time, and their severity doesn't appear to correlate with either length of time since diagnosis or the level of a person's physical disability.** For example, a person with significant physical limitations, who has had MS for some time, can be totally free of cognitive symptoms, while a person with a recent diagnosis and few physical symptoms can have significant cognitive impairment.

✔ **Even relatively mild symptoms can have a pretty big impact on various activities of daily living.** For instance, people with MS are more likely to leave the workforce because of cognitive symptoms and fatigue than because of mobility problems! Early departure from the workforce is a critical issue for people with MS, but it can often be avoided with adequate symptom management (see Chapter 18 for details).

✔ **Cognitive fatigue can interfere with your ability to get things done.** Research has shown that people with MS who are concentrating very hard on a cognitively strenuous task can experience a kind of mental fatigue that feels like acute "brain drain." Fortunately a brief rest from the task will generally help you get back on track.

✔ **Cognitive changes tend to progress slowly over time.** Even though MS relapses can include a sudden worsening of cognitive symptoms as well as physical ones, which tend to improve as a relapse ends, problems with thinking and memory don't generally disappear completely.

✔ **The sooner these kinds of cognitive problems are identified, the easier it is to develop effective strategies to manage them.** Small problems are always easier to work around than bigger ones. When you're able to put your finger on a problem with thinking or memory early on, you can find ways to compensate for it before the problem begins to interfere significantly with your daily life.

239

Like the physical symptoms that can occur in MS, the cognitive changes are highly variable from one person to another. One person may experience a lot of problems while another person experiences none or very few. In other words, no two people experience the same changes in exactly the same way. However, the following types of problems are the most common in MS.

Memory

Memory is the function that seems to be most affected in MS. Even though memory is a complex process involving many different components, the major impairment in MS is in learning and retaining new information, which is why people complain that they can remember everything that happened 20 years ago but not what happened this morning.

Until fairly recently, experts believed that the primary memory problem for people with MS was with the retrieval of information that had been stored in memory. In other words, these experts believed that a person could learn new information and tuck it away in memory, but then be unable to recall or retrieve it from storage when needed.

More recent evidence suggests that the problem may involve the initial learning phase. People with MS may need longer time or a few more repetitions to learn and store new information successfully. After it has been stored, however, it can generally be recalled without difficulty. For example, if you have memory problems, it may take you longer than someone without memory problems to memorize a list of words. But once you have the words memorized, you'll remember them just as well as the other person does.

Information processing

Slowed processing is important because it may be the pri-

240

mary reason why a person with MS needs more time or repetitions to learn new information. When processing is impaired, the person has trouble keeping up with incoming information, whether it's from conversations, TV shows, or books. People describe this slowing by saying, "I can still do everything I used to be able to do, but it all seems much slower—like my brain needs to be oiled."

Attention and concentration

Attention and concentration, which form the basis for many other cognitive functions, can also be impaired by MS. For example, people who are used to being able to focus on many complex and competing tasks at the same time may notice some frustrating changes, such as being easily distracted by interruptions or competing stimuli, having difficulty moving smoothly from one task to another, or finding it more difficult to multi-task (an essential skill in any occupation, particularly parenthood).

Executive functions

Executive functions include the high-level processes of planning, prioritizing, and problem-solving. Research has shown that people with MS may find thinking through complex problems or projects more difficult because they lose the mental agility to shift from concept to concept along the way. People often describe this impairment as "feeling stuck" or "lost in a maze."

Visual perceptual skills

Visual perceptual skills, which include simple perception or recognition of objects, as well as sense of direction and orientation in space, can be affected in MS. These problems can interfere with activities ranging from reading a map or driving, to programming your VCR or dealing with those pesky "some assembly required" projects.

Verbal fluency

Verbal fluency includes the ability to find the word you're looking for quickly and easily. "It's on the tip of my tongue" is a particularly common complaint from those who have MS, as is "I'm talking to someone and all of a sudden I'm stuck without the word I need." People who experience these kinds of problems may feel less confident about their ability to talk smoothly and comfortably with others.

General intelligence

People with MS sometimes say they feel "dumber." The good news is that general intelligence is usually not affected in MS. However, individual functions that make up general intelligence, such as memory, reasoning, or perceptual skills, can be affected or slowed temporarily during a relapse or more permanently over the course of the disease. So, a person's *intelligence quotient* (IQ), which is a composite score made up of individual subtest scores on all these functions, can become lower over time. The fact that several of the subtests rely heavily on speed and dexterity also contributes to lower IQ scores in those individuals who are experiencing problems with manual dexterity. This impact on IQ scores is important to know about because a drop in IQ score is one of the factors that's used to determine eligibility for Social Security Disability Insurance, which is discussed in Chapter 18.

Deciding when an evaluation is in order

Taking a bunch of tests to see how your brain is working may not be your idea of fun, but consider some of the reasons why you may decide to go for it anyway:

- ✔ When the neurologist asks you to remember three words or count backwards by 7s (part of the brief

242

mental status exam that neurologists sometimes do to evaluate cognition, which picks up only very severe problems), you do just fine. But you've been experiencing some worrisome changes, and you want to understand what's going on.

✔ You've received some feedback from family members or colleagues that you aren't quite up to snuff these days.

✔ Your job has become more difficult and you want to figure out what's going on and address the problem before your boss addresses it for you.

✔ You're considering a career change because of difficulties you've begun to experience in your current work. An assessment of your strengths and weaknesses can help you identify other potential career paths.

✔ You're considering applying for Social Security Disability Insurance (SSDI) and you know that cognitive dysfunction is one of the four factors that determine eligibility for a person with MS (check out Chapter 18 for more information on SSDI).

✔ You aren't experiencing any problems at the moment but you know that MS can affect a person's cognition and you want to establish a baseline against which to compare future evaluations.

The most important thing to know about a comprehensive cognitive evaluation is that it gives you valuable information about your strengths as well as any areas of difficulty. This information comes in handy as you begin to develop strategies to compensate for any problems you're experiencing.

Knowing what to expect during an evaluation

The *cognitive evaluation* is a series of tests (generally referred to as a *test battery*, which includes paper-and-pencil items and puzzles of various types) that's designed to evaluate the full range of cognitive functions. Evaluations are performed by neuropsychologists as well as some occupational therapists (OTs) and speech/language pathologists (S/LPs). Even though the three disciplines approach the evaluation process a bit differently, and use somewhat different tests, all are interested in evaluating how and to what degree cognitive changes are affecting your ability to function at home and at work. (Flip to Chapter 4 to read more about these professionals.)

A full cognitive evaluation can take six to eight hours to complete, but it's generally spread out over a couple of days to minimize the effects of fatigue. Also, shorter test batteries can be used to determine whether the more extensive battery is warranted. Your neurologist may be able to refer you to a local clinician for the evaluation. Otherwise, the National MS Society can provide a list of neuropsychologists, OTs, or S/LPs in your area who have experience in MS (call 800-FIGHT-MS or 800-344-4867). If no one in your area is familiar with MS, you can also see a brain injury specialist because some of the symptoms are similar and the test battery is virtually the same. Full evaluations can be quite expensive, so make sure you discuss cost, payment options, and insurance coverage ahead of time.

The test items are designed to tap your abilities and limitations. You'll likely find that some are easy for you and others much more difficult—just like the mix you had on your standardized tests in grade school and the SATs later on. You may also find—if you're in fact experiencing cogni-

244

tive changes—that some tasks that you once found easy now seem more difficult.

The clinician doing the testing will carefully study your test results and compare them to data from the general population of people in your age bracket. He or she will also use your school and work history, as well as the results of the certain tests to determine what your abilities were prior to MS, and which, if any, seem to have changed from that baseline. Most importantly, the clinician will use your scores to determine your cognitive strengths—because these strengths will be your most powerful tools to compensate for any deficits you may have.

Let's say, for example, that you have a lot of trouble remembering stuff from telephone conversations or meetings (auditory memory), but you have a phenomenal memory for stuff you see or read (visual memory). In this case, notes, pictures, or other visual cues could be helpful memory aids for you. Or, maybe you have memory problems but you're a whiz at organization. You can figure out ways to substitute organization for memory in many areas of daily living. (See the section "Employing practical strategies for managing daily cognitive challenges" later in the chapter for more details.)

Identifying treatment options

So you're probably wondering what you do with all this evaluation info once you have it. You'll work with your doctor as well as the clinician who evaluated you to decide on a treatment plan that works for you.

The treatment of cognitive symptoms falls into three categories:

◣ **Symptomatic treatments:** Even though a variety of medications have been evaluated, only the drug

Finding additional information about cognition

If you want to read more about MS-related cognitive changes, check out the following resources for some firsthand accounts of personal experiences, info about the research that's being done, and a variety of strategies to help you compensate for any changes you're experiencing:

✔ The National MS Society's Web Spotlight on Cognition at www.nationalmssociety.org/cognition.

✔ *Multiple Sclerosis: Understanding the Cognitive Challenges* by Nicholas LaRocca and Rosalind Kalb (Demos Medical Publishing, 2006). This book is a guide to symptoms, assessment, treatment, and management strategies.

✔ *Improving Your Memory For Dummies* by John Arden (Wiley Publishing, 2002).

Aricept (donepezil), which is FDA-approved for treatment in Alzheimer's disease, has shown some modest (but not spectacular) benefit for MS-related memory problems.

Because the cognitive problems that occur in MS are completely unrelated to Alzheimer's disease, there's no particular reason to expect great things from Aricept, but some neurologists are happy for their MS patients to give it a try.

✔ **Disease-modifying therapies:** These therapies—the interferons (Avonex, Betaseron, Rebif) and Copaxone (glatiramer acetate)—have all been shown to reduce the number and severity of attacks and to reduce central nervous system lesions as shown on MRI scans.

Because there's fairly extensive evidence to show that cognitive problems correlate to the total amount of lesion area in the brain (referred to as *lesion load*), it's reasonable to assume that starting a disease-modifying therapy early in the disease would be a good strategy for reducing the risk and progression of cognitive symptoms. So, if you don't already have reason enough to start treatment with one of the disease-modifying therapies, this could be the powerful incentive you need. (Check out Chapter 6 for more details on these therapies.)

✔ **Cognitive remediation:** This type of treatment, which is also called *cognitive rehabilitation*, is a practical, solution-oriented approach to managing cognitive changes. Offered by neuropsychologists, OTs, and S/LPs, cognitive rehabilitation consists of the following interventions:

- Restorative interventions: These interventions are like physical therapy for the brain. The clinician uses your test results to identify areas of deficit and then gives you exercises that may help strengthen the impaired functions.

  The best examples of this kind of intervention are computerized exercises to improve attention and memory. Even though the research has shown that people's performance on certain types of tasks improves with these exercises, the improvements don't carry over very well to everyday life. After all, how many people live their lives in front of a computer screen in a quiet room with no distractions?

- Compensatory interventions: These seem, by all accounts, to be the most useful. They consist of finding *workarounds*, or strategies to compensate

247

for whatever cognitive ability has been compromised. In the same way that people use calendars to help themselves remember dates, address books to help keep track of contact information, and computers to make it easier and faster to process information, the cognitive rehabilitation specialist can help you identify tools and strategies to compensate for whatever problems you're having.

Although there are an unlimited variety of workaround possibilities, the most common ones involve substituting organization for memory—for example, lists, filing systems, work and family calendars, and "tickler" mechanisms, such as alarms on your watch or computer to remind you to take a medication or go to an appointment. The remediation specialist can also recommend strategies to improve attention, reading comprehension, executive functions, and others.

Other factors like depression and stress also can affect cognition, so be sure to talk with your doctor if you're concerned that either of these problems may be interfering with your thinking or memory. You can read about ways to manage depression later in this chapter. (Flip to Chapter 12 for information about stress management.)

Employing practical strategies for managing daily cognitive challenges

Even though there's no substitute for working with a specialist to identify and design effective compensatory strategies, here are some common sense suggestions that you can use to begin managing any difficulties you may be having. Your first step is to get comfortable with the idea that it's okay to do things differently—creative flexibility is your key to success. From there:

✔ Develop a personal organizer (paper or electronic) that has your important information in one place, including appointments, contact information, to-do lists, a tickler system for birthdays and anniversaries, and whatever else you need.

✔ Create a family calendar to track everyone's activities, and make each family member responsible for writing down the important stuff.

✔ Set up a filing system to organize important papers so that everything has its place.

✔ Deal with the mail on a daily basis to avoid unnecessary accumulation (sort out the junk and put the important stuff in a safe place).

✔ Create a system to process incoming bills, including a tickler system to ensure that they're paid on time.

✔ Establish a consistent "home" for glasses, keys, and wallets to avoid endless hunting expeditions.

✔ Create a computerized master checklist for repetitive tasks such as grocery shopping or packing for a trip.

✔ Establish a file of driving directions to carry with you in your car.

✔ Create a distraction-free zone in the house for tasks or conversations requiring concentration.

✔ Schedule your day so that the activities requiring the most cognitive effort can happen when you're at your best, which is often earlier in the day.

Letting loose on the unsuspecting

This brief story shows that even the most pleasant people can become moody and irritable: One of our patients was standing in a grocery aisle trying to decide between two brands of laundry detergent. Because of problems with attention and distractibility, his efforts were hampered by the hustle and bustle in the store and by two women who were talking loudly several feet away from him. Finally, overcome with frustration, he loudly shouted, "Shut up!" This very polite, generally mild-mannered man was extremely surprised and embarrassed by his own behavior. He said of himself that he no longer had the same control over his emotions — he felt as though the nuts and bolts had been loosened a bit. Others have described themselves as feeling raw, or super-sensitive to irritants around them. If you're experiencing increased irritability or uncomfortable bouts of temper, be sure to let your doctor know.

➤ Make sure that each telephone in the house has a pen and pad of paper near it.

➤ Create step-by-step project templates to help you stay on track with multistep tasks such as preparing a meal, balancing your checkbook, preparing your income taxes, and planning a vacation.

Managing the Emotional Ups and Downs

In addition to the array of emotional *reactions* that people can have to a challenging disease like MS (take a look at Chapter 3 for a rundown of the most common), some important kinds of emotional *changes* seem to be part of the disease itself. The distinction between reactions and changes is an important one because many people find it easier to seek help for emotional issues that they know are part and parcel of their MS.

The kinds of changes we talk about in this section don't have anything to do with being a sissy or with being crazy or weak. Instead, they're emotional symptoms that can often be caused by the same changes in the central nervous system that cause the physical and cognitive symptoms we talk about earlier in this chapter and in Chapters 7 and 8.

Controlling mood swings

Mood swings are by far the most common emotional change seen in people with MS. Even though these moods are much less intense than the mood variations seen in *bipolar disorder* (formerly called manic-depressive disorder), they can be very uncomfortable for people with MS and their family members. People describe themselves (and their partners and children are happy to verify it) as unusually moody, irritable, cranky, and quick-to-anger. (By the way, bipolar disorder is more common in MS than in the general population.)

Even though it's certainly true that a person with MS can have a lot to feel cranky about, particularly if it's been a bad day, many of the mood swings in MS seem to bear little relationship to the severity of the disease or to day-to-day symptom activity. In other words, these mood swings sometimes seem to happen out of the blue—as if they have a mind of their own.

Here are some strategies that people with MS have found useful for dealing with mood swings:

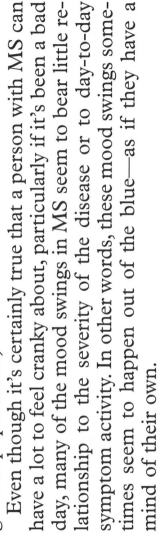

✔ **Talk it up:** Even though your mood swings may be neurologic in origin, they can still be relieved somewhat by talking about them. In support groups, for

251

example, people share their stories, discover how other people have dealt with their mood issues, and generally get more comfortable with the idea that mood swings are just one more aspect of MS that they need to come to terms with. So, talking about your mood swings actually gives you more of a sense of control over them.

- **Identify your triggers:** It's also important to pay attention to the things that seem to trigger your mood swings. For example, if particular situations make you tense or irritable, it's a good idea to try to create a buffer for yourself—remove yourself from the situation, practice some deep breathing or meditation, or speak up about what's bothering you.

- **Get moving:** Exercise can be very beneficial. A significant body of research in MS points to the benefits on mood of both cardiovascular exercise (which is of course geared to a person's abilities and limitations) and yoga. And, in the end, almost everyone feels better when they're getting sufficient exercise.

- **Discuss meds with your doc:** When the mood swings don't respond to any of the other interventions, a low dose of Depakote (depakene) can be very effective. This medication, which is primarily used to treat seizures, seems to make the swings less dramatic and helps people feel more like themselves again. An antidepressant medication may help as well. So, if you're experiencing uncomfortable mood swings, don't hesitate to tell your physician.

252

Getting a handle on uncontrolled laughing or crying

Uncontrolled laughing or crying, which is a relatively uncommon phenomenon, has been given many different names over the years, including *emotional incontinence* (but no one liked that term very much), *pathological laughing and crying* (they didn't like that too much either), *pseudobulbar affect* (because of the area of the brain that's thought to be involved), and most recently, *involuntary emotional expression disorder* (IEED).

This kind of uncontrolled laughing or crying is thought to result from damage in the prefrontal cortex of the brain that interferes with the corticobulbar tracts (which control emotions), and it occurs in about 10 percent of people with MS. Even though it's generally (but not always) found in those with more progressive disease and significant cognitive changes, it's equally common in both women and men.

When a person experiences this kind of uncontrolled laughing or crying, he or she cries without feeling sad or upset or laughs without feeling amused or happy. And once started, the laughing or crying can't be stopped voluntarily. For obvious reasons, this involuntary behavior can be extremely upsetting and embarrassing for the person with MS (and for anyone else who happens to be in the room). Imagine for a moment how it would feel to burst out laughing at your mother-in-law's funeral or your boss's retirement party, or to cry in the middle of a business meeting or blind date.

As with the mood swings that are so common, it's important to remember that uncontrolled laughing or crying isn't a sign of craziness or stupidity or any of the other labels that may come to mind. And people with this problem are no more depressed than other people with MS.

253

Crying when there's nothing to cry about

One of our patients found herself crying whenever she was in an emotionally charged situation. Whether trying to have a conversation with her boss, a small disagreement with her husband, or a motherly conversation with the teenagers, she always seemed to break out into tears. This bright, articulate, and capable woman became extremely self-conscious in any situation that might elicit the unwanted response.

After we determined that she wasn't depressed or otherwise distressed, we suggested that she focus on identifying and heading off the emotional build-up that seemed to precipitate the tears. With this suggestion, she became adept at sensing the increase in emotional tension, and would subsequently take a timeout to breathe deeply. Even though it was a tad embarrassing to have to say to people, "Just give me a minute here to gather my thoughts," it was a lot less embarrassing than bursting into uncontrolled tears.

Over the years, doctors have tried a variety of medications to control these uncontrolled episodes of laughing and crying. Even though people who experience them aren't clinically depressed, the medications that have been most effective were the antidepressants Elavil (amitriptyline) and Prozac (fluoxetine). Sinemet (levodopa), a drug used in Parkinson's disease, has also been used. Most recently, an experimental drug that's a combination of dextromethorphan and an enzyme inhibitor to sustain an effective level of the dextromethorphan is being studied for the treatment of uncontrolled laughing and crying. So, if you (or a family member) are experiencing this problem, be sure to consult a physician.

Dealing with severe depression

We're going to spend a lot of time talking about depression here—not to depress or upset you—but to get your attention and clarify what's meant by the term.

Defining depression

Severe depression is common in MS—significantly more common, in fact, than in the general population or with other chronic diseases. More than 50 percent of people with MS will experience a major depressive episode at some point during the illness. Did that get your attention? Depression is generally unrelated to the time since diagnosis or to the level of disability. In other words, it can occur early in the disease in people with little or no disability. This means that it isn't just a reaction to the challenges of living with a chronic, unpredictable disease, but also a symptom of the disease itself.

What do we mean by depression? For starters, remember this: Many people use the term casually in everyday conversation—"I'm so *depressed*," "This job is really *depressing* me," or "This book is so *depressing*"—that they tend to lose sight of what depression really is.

So, we're not talking about having a down day or feeling discouraged or blue about a lousy date, a disappointment at work, a bad exam grade, or even a chronic disease. What we're talking about is a serious medical condition, referred to as *clinical depression* or *major depression*, which can have significant consequences on your health and well-being. People who are depressed carry an additional, unnecessary emotional burden. They can't enjoy life, participate actively in their own care, or plan or problem-solve effectively. And they're difficult to live with.

255

When left untreated, severe depression can even lead to death. Studies have indicated that the rate of suicide in MS is over seven times higher than in the general population. In fact, it's one of the leading causes of death in MS after cancer, heart disease, and stroke.

Recognizing the signs

Depression differs from the normal grieving we talk about in Chapter 3, but it can be difficult to differentiate on a day-to-day basis because some of the feelings are so similar. Depression also differs from the mood swings we talk about in this chapter. But, again, it may be difficult to distinguish between the two because depression can manifest itself in ways other than sadness or melancholy (for example, it can be shown through irritability and sullenness). The key element that distinguishes depression from these other mood states is its persistence over an extended period of time.

For the doctor to diagnose a major depressive episode, a person must have experienced at least five of the following nine symptoms (one of which must be either depressed mood or decreased interest) for most of the day every day for a minimum of two weeks:

- ✔ Depressed mood (feeling blue, down-in-the-dumps, hopeless)

- ✔ A significantly reduced level of interest or pleasure in most or all activities

- ✔ A considerable weight loss or gain (5 percent or more change of weight in a month when not dieting) or change in appetite

- ✔ Frequent thoughts of death or suicide (with or without a specific plan), or attempt of suicide

256

✔ Difficulty falling or staying asleep (insomnia), or sleeping more than usual (hypersomnia)

✔ Behavior that's agitated or slowed down, which is readily observable by others

✔ Feeling fatigued or very low in energy

✔ Having thoughts of worthlessness or extreme guilt

✔ A diminished ability to think, concentrate, or make decisions

A quick review of this symptom list tells you why depression can be tricky to diagnose in people with MS. Each of the last five items on the list can also occur in MS, even in the absence of depression. So, a consultation with a mental health specialist with experience and expertise in MS may be required to make the diagnosis.

Unfortunately, physicians still don't routinely ask about patients' moods. If you notice any significant changes in your mood (or your family members or friends do), it's important to bring these changes to your physician's attention. You have no need to feel embarrassed or awkward—mood changes are as much attributable to your MS as any other symptom, and are among the most treatable.

Discovering the causes of depression in MS

Even though it seems clear that depression is as much a symptom of MS as a reaction to it, the cause for the depression isn't clear. Like mood swings and IEED, depression seems to be caused, at least in part, by neurologic changes in the mood control centers of the brain.

It's also important to mention here that some of the medications currently used to treat MS may increase the risk of depression, or worsen existing depression, in some people.

257

The Goldman Consensus Statement on Depression in Multiple Sclerosis

Following review and approval by the National Multiple Sclerosis Society's Medical Advisory Board, the "Goldman Consensus Statement on Depression in MS" was published in 2005 in the journal *Multiple Sclerosis* (volume 11, pp. 328–337). This document grew out of a concern among MS specialists about the lack of recognition and inadequate treatment of this serious condition. The Goldman Consensus Group, made up of experts in the field of MS and psychiatry, has provided recommendations for the recognition, diagnosis, and management of depression. One recommendation is that people with MS be routinely screened for depression during their visits to the neurologist so that those who indicate possible symptoms of depression can be referred for a thorough evaluation. Because this recommendation may never be implemented as widely as it should be, we strongly urge you to share the Goldman Statement with your physician and discuss any changes in your mood. Your doctor or the National MS Society (800-FIGHT-MS or 800-344-4867) can refer you to mental health specialists with expertise in MS.

For example, the following medications have the potential to affect mood:

➤ **Corticosteroids:** When taking high doses of these medications to treat an MS relapse (see Chapter 6) some people feel energized—almost giddy—but then find themselves going into a real funk as they come off of them. If you have a history of depression, make sure that your physician is aware of this when corticosteroids are prescribed.

258

✔ **Interferon medications:** These medications, which are approved to treat relapsing forms of MS, each carry warnings about depression (check out Chapter 6 for a rundown of these medications). Even though there was some initial concern from the clinical trial of Betaseron (that the medication may increase a person's risk of depression and suicide), subsequent studies with the medication and the other interferons haven't borne this out. The individuals who experienced the depressive episodes while on these medications usually had histories of depression that preceded the trials.

The bottom line is that the labeling of each of these medications contains a warning about depression, causing some patients and doctors to be reluctant to use them. The expert consensus seems to be that the medications are safe, but if you're taking an interferon medication and experience a significant change in your mood—with or without a history of depression—you should talk about it with your doctor.

Neither Copaxone (glatiramer acetate) nor Tysabri (natalizumab), two other approved disease-modifying therapies in MS, has been associated with any mood problems.

Treating your depression

Depression is a treatable condition, but there are challenges. The biggest challenges to treatment are the reluctance of people to seek help for it and the failure of clinicians to diagnose it accurately and manage it aggressively. Just as people don't like the idea that MS can mess with their thinking as well as their bodies, they don't like the idea that it can wreak havoc on their emotions either. This dislike is certainly understandable, but it isn't a good reason to deprive yourself of the means to feel better and get on with your life.

Seeking help for depression doesn't mean that you're giving in to it. Instead, it means you're strong enough to take charge of your well-being. Because the research shows that depression doesn't just clear up by itself, the sooner you begin to take care of it, the sooner you're going to feel better.

The consensus among mental health specialists is that the best treatment for severe depression is a combination of antidepressant medication and psychotherapy. Even though each has been shown to provide some benefit, the combination is thought to be the most beneficial.

Here are a few key things to remember about antidepressant medication:

✔ Antidepressant medication can take up to four to six weeks to have a noticeable effect.

✔ If you stop taking your medication as soon as you feel better, the depression is likely to return. It's important, then, to stay on your medication until your doctor recommends otherwise.

✔ The antidepressant medications currently on the market (and there are about a zillion) have different modes of action and different side effects. So, be patient—it may take some time to find the medication and dosage that work best for you.

✔ Even though neurologists, internists, family practice doctors, and some nurses can prescribe antidepressant medications, they usually aren't specially trained in this area. Psychiatrists are familiar with all the available antidepressants and have the expertise to identify the best medication or combination of med-

260

ications to meet your needs. They'll monitor your depression on an ongoing basis to ensure that it's treated adequately. It's not enough to feel *better*; the goal is to feel *good*.

➤ Psychiatrists who are familiar with MS are ideal if you need a prescription for an antidepressant. Second best is the psychiatrist who's willing to learn about your MS and talk to your neurologist. It doesn't help much to get good treatment for your depression if the side effects of the medication make your MS symptoms worse (for example, some medications may increase your fatigue).

➤ Because you may be taking several other medications for your MS, it's critically important that the person treating your depression is aware of these medications and their potential interactions.

➤ Virtually all of the available antidepressant medications have sexual side effects, with Wellbutrin (bupropion) being the least problematic in this regard. If you're severely depressed, you may not care much about sex right now. Or, if your MS is interfering with your sexual function (see Chapter 7), you may figure that one more hit in that area doesn't really matter. But, if sexual activity is important in your life, be sure to discuss this with the person who's prescribing antidepressant medication for you. After your mood is stabilized, the doctor can recommend strategies—such as changing the timing of your medication or skipping a dose every now and then—to minimize the impact on your sexual activities.

Chapter 10

Considering Complementary and Alternative Medicine

In This Chapter

▼ Recognizing CAM and its allure

▼ Separating fiction from fact

▼ Understanding the potentially useful therapies

▼ Being an educated consumer

These days, people are looking for ways to take charge of their own health and wellness. In the United States, a huge industry has developed around this need to go beyond what traditional medicine can offer. The appeal of nontraditional therapies and treatments seems to be particularly strong for anyone who has a chronic illness that mainstream science hasn't been able to cure. So, it isn't surprising that the use of nontraditional interventions is high among people with multiple sclerosis (MS). In fact, most people with MS have used some form of complementary and alternative medicine (CAM) at one time or another.

To help you be a knowledgeable CAM consumer, in this chapter, we define CAM and explain how it differs from mainstream medicine. We also emphasize the importance of placebo-controlled clinical trials to evaluate the safety and effectiveness of any treatment, and we let you know which types of CAM have been shown to benefit people with MS. We stress the importance of talking with your doctor about all aspects of your treatment plan and of finding safe and effective ways to combine CAM strategies with your standard MS care. And, most importantly, we give you strategies for evaluating the various types of substances and practices that are touted as "cures" for MS. Our goal is for you to be an educated consumer.

Defining CAM

CAM, short for *complementary and alternative medicine*, includes those substances or therapies that a person chooses to use along with the treatments prescribed by his or her physician (complementary), as well as those that a person uses instead of prescribed treatments (alternative). We're happy to report that most people with MS are choosing to use the nontraditional therapies as a complement to their regular MS treatment.

Over the years, CAM has been defined in several different ways, with the defining characteristic being that the practices fell outside of traditional medicine. Today, more and more researchers are trying to evaluate these interventions with the same rigorous studies that have traditionally been used to evaluate standard treatments. As any CAM therapy or substance demonstrates its safety and effectiveness in clinical trials, it makes its way into mainstream medicine. Exercise, for example, is now recognized as an important component of regular healthcare.

The National Institutes of Health divides CAM into the following categories:

- **Biologically based therapies:** This category includes special diets, herbal medicine, vitamin and mineral supplements, and pharmacologic, biological, and instrumental therapies (for example, bee venom therapy, candida treatment, chelation therapy, cooling therapy, removal of dental amalgams, enzyme therapy, and hyperbaric oxygen therapy).

- **Alternative medical systems:** These systems include acupuncture and traditional Chinese medicine, Ayurveda, and homeopathy.

- **Lifestyle and disease prevention:** In this category, the main approach considered is exercise.

- **Mind-body medicine:** This group includes treatments such as biofeedback, hypnosis and guided imagery, meditation, music therapy, pets, prayer and spirituality, T'ai Chi, and yoga.

- **Manipulative and body-based systems:** Massage body work (for example, chiropractic, Feldenkrais, Pilates, reflexology, and Tragerwork) and unconventional physical therapies (colon therapy and hippotherapy) make up the treatments in this category.

- **Biofield medicine:** Therapeutic touch is in this category.

- **Bioelectromagnetics:** This category includes magnets and electromagnetic therapy.

Understanding the Allure

CAM is a huge industry in the United States, encompassing a wide variety of practitioners and products. The first step to becoming an educated consumer of CAM products and services is to understand their allure. For example, consider the following reasons why people are attracted to CAM:

✔ **People like the idea of taking control of their bodies, their lives, and their health.** Products that claim to offer that kind of control have wide appeal.

✔ **Safe, *healthy*, and *natural* are all buzzwords these days.** They're used to promote a lot of products, including some that are safe and healthy, and some that aren't. Because of the way they're advertised, many consumers believe that the products they can buy without a prescription—in a grocery store, pharmacy, or health food store—are somehow safer and healthier than the ones their doctors prescribe. The simple fact is that we know less about many of them than we know about prescription medications that have been evaluated by medical experts.

✔ **People living with MS and other chronic diseases are understandably frustrated by the long wait for a cure.** The available MS medications (check out Chapter 6 for a description of the approved disease-modifying therapies) are only partially effective, and folks are impatient for something better. To these people, anything that promises to "cure MS" or "strengthen the immune system" sounds like the silver bullet.

Putting CAM to the Test

CAM is a mixed bag of goodies: Some treatments are beneficial, some won't hurt you but won't do much good either, and some are out-and-out dangerous. In the face of all the ads and testimonials (for example, "I threw away my cane!" and "I was totally cured!"), here are some key points to keep in mind:

▶ If a cure for MS had already been found, the National MS Society and other MS organizations would have broadcast it far and wide.

▶ Because not all products and services are equally regulated in this country, you need to know how to evaluate what's out there.

▶ What you see (on a package, in an ad, and on the Internet) isn't necessarily what you get.

In the following sections we explain why you can't believe everything you hear about a CAM treatment, and we give you some tips on how to sort through the CAM bag of goodies to find what's right for you.

Your MS doctor and your pharmacist are your best sources of information about which CAM strategies may be helpful for you without interfering with your prescription medications.

Understanding the role of the FDA

The U.S. Food and Drug Administration (FDA) is responsible for ensuring the safety and effectiveness of a whole host of things, including prescription drugs, medical devices, such as pacemakers or MRI machines, the nation's food supply, and cosmetics. Even though that may sound like a lot, just remember that the list doesn't include any of the supplements sold in stores or the treatment strategies prescribed by nonmedical practitioners.

Because CAM interventions aren't regulated, manufacturers and practitioners are free to say whatever they want about them. Unlike the pharmaceutical companies, for example, who can't print or say anything about their products that the FDA hasn't approved, the manufacturers of supplements are free to do as they please. When you pick up a supplement such as echinacea or St. John's Wort at the store, you can't even be sure that the labeling on the box matches the contents of the bottle, let alone that the claims made about the products are true. The situation is the same with bee venom therapy, magnet therapy, or any other nontraditional therapy. So you, as the consumer, need a way to sort out the claims (check out the section "Becoming a Cautious CAM Consumer" later in the chapter for details).

Sorting out the wheat from the chaff

We bet it's music to your ears when you hear someone say "You've got to try this! My MS got so much better. It was like a miracle!" Who doesn't want to feel better? Just remember that one person's experience with a therapy or supplement can be very different from someone else's. So, one guy's blog may be filled with reports of success while your buddy from the support group didn't feel any better and had some really unpleasant side effects.

Given the natural ups and downs in the disease course and the fact that MS symptoms tend to come and go unpredictably, it's impossible to tell if a treatment works without testing it on a whole lot of people.

Appreciating the power of the placebo response

Physicians and researchers have repeatedly found that people with a variety of diseases will improve any time they're given a new treatment—even if the treatment used is a placebo (a fake pill, injection, or other substance that looks

267

and feels just like a the real thing). And the evidence suggests that it's not all in their heads. Even though the response may be partially psychological ("I really, really want this to work."), some studies have shown that certain chemical changes in the body also contribute to the effect. Unlike the benefits provided by a true treatment, however, the placebo benefits don't last long.

Understanding the role of the double-blind, placebo-controlled clinical trial

Given the powerful nature of the placebo response, it isn't all that surprising that many people feel better—at least temporarily—any time they try something new. So, the only way to sort out the placebo response from a true treatment response is to test the treatment in a *double-blind placebo-controlled clinical trial*, which sounds a lot more complicated than it is.

Researchers rely on clinical trials to evaluate a potential treatment. *Placebo-controlled trials* are designed to demonstrate a potential treatment's superiority to placebo. These trials typically involve two matched groups—one that receives the study drug and one that receives a placebo. All of the study participants—patients, doctors, and research staff—are *blinded*, meaning that they're kept from knowing who's getting the real drug and who's getting a placebo. The placebo effect is so strong that a hefty percentage of the placebo group will show some improvement in their condition—sometimes as high as 70 percent. In order for the study drug to "prove" itself the better candidate, the treatment group needs to show greater benefit than the placebo group over the full length of the study. And it needs to provide this benefit without significant side effects.

The disease-modifying therapies that have been approved for use in MS (check out Chapter 6) have all been tested successfully using large, blinded, placebo-controlled trials.

Because most CAM interventions have never been put through this kind of rigorous evaluation, there's no way to know how safe and effective they really are.

The placebo-effect isn't a *bad thing*—feeling better is always a reasonable goal. For instance, even though physicians rely on controlled trials to tell them which treatments offer more than a placebo response, many CAM practitioners try to harness the power of the placebo response to give their patients relief. The goal of treatment in MS, however, is to control the disease and its symptoms safely over the long haul.

Identifying CAM Interventions That May Be Useful in Managing MS Symptoms

Although few CAM treatments have been studied in large controlled trials, enough small studies have been done with some of the treatments to indicate which may prove useful and which may not. In the following sections we fill you in on what's been found so far.

If after reading this book you want to do some more reading on CAM interventions used by people with MS, take a look at the book, *Alternative Medicine and Multiple Sclerosis*, 2nd edition, by Allen Bowling, MD, PhD (Demos Medical Publishing, 2006).

Herbs, vitamins, and other CAM options that go into the body

CAM treatments come in many varieties, including those that are swallowed, injected, infused, or inhaled. For example, take a look at the following:

Bee venom therapy: Bee venom contains proteins that affect the immune system. However, the exact mechanism isn't known. This therapy can produce rare, but potentially serious adverse effects, including severe allergic reactions and death. A recent clinical trial demonstrated that bee venom is no better than a placebo for treating MS.

Diets and fatty acid supplements: Although many types of diets have been proposed to treat MS over the years, study results regarding diets and fatty acid supplements aren't conclusive at this time.

Most MS specialist neurologists recommend a balanced diet that's low in saturated fats and high in fiber and polyunsaturated fatty acids. Some evidence suggests that supplements of omega-6, omega-3, and vitamin E may also be beneficial.

Herbs: Herbs should be used with caution by people with MS because there are some that may actually worsen MS or interact with MS medications. The message concerning herbs and MS is similar to that for unconventional medicine and MS as a whole: Some of them may be beneficial, some may be harmful, and nearly all have yet to be fully understood. Having said that, consider the following:

- Herbs that may be of benefit for certain MS-specific symptoms include kava kava for anxiety, valerian for insomnia, cranberry for preventing urinary tract infections, and psyllium for constipation.

- Herbs to avoid because they stimulate the immune system (which is already overactive in MS) include alfalfa, arnica, astragalus, boneset, calendula, cat's claw, celandine, drosera, echinacea,

270

garlic, Asian and Siberian ginseng, licorice, mistletoe, reishi mushroom, saw palmetto, shiitake mushroom, and stinging nettle.

🖒 **Homeopathy:** *Homeopathy*, a system of medicine that was developed in the 1800s, is a low-risk, low-to-moderate-cost therapy with unproven effectiveness in MS. It shouldn't be used in place of conventional medications for controlling disease activity.

🖒 **Hyperbaric oxygen:** This form of oxygen therapy increases the oxygen content of the blood and tissues of the body. Studies have repeatedly demonstrated that hyperbaric oxygen isn't an effective treatment for MS.

🖒 **Low-dose naltrexone (LDN):** Naltrexone is approved in the United States for the treatment of alcohol and opioid addictions. At much lower doses it's being prescribed by some doctors for the treatment of several diseases, including MS and other autoimmune conditions. A very small uncontrolled trial was recently completed in Crohn's disease, but LDN hasn't yet been studied in MS.

🖒 **Marijuana:** The use of marijuana, in addition to being illegal in the United States, is associated with significant side effects. And, the possible interactions of marijuana with prescription medications aren't well-understood. Research is underway on marijuana-related chemicals to see if they can safely reduce pain, spasticity, and bladder symptoms in MS.

🖒 **Prokarin (formerly called Procarin):** Limited information is available about the safety and effectiveness of this expensive skin patch treatment that contains histamines, caffeine, and other undisclosed ingredients. Although a clinical trial indicated that it may be useful for the treatment of MS-related fatigue, the opinion of the National MS Society's Medical Advisory Board is that its limited benefits don't justify its costs.

✔ **Vitamins and other supplements:** People with MS should be cautious with vitamin supplements because they, like other forms of CAM, are a mixed bag of goodies. For example, consider the following findings:

- Antioxidant vitamins (A, C, and E) offer possible benefits (by decreasing the harmful effects of free radicals that are involved in the damage to your myelin and axons) and pose possible risks (by stimulating the already overactive immune system).

- Vitamin C doesn't appear to be effective for the prevention or treatment of urinary tract infections.

- Vitamin B6 is tricky; too little B6 can interfere with normal nervous system functioning whereas too much B6 harms the nervous system and can actually cause MS-like symptoms.

- A small subgroup of people with MS may have a vitamin B12 deficiency and should be treated with vitamin B12 supplements.

- People who take higher amounts of vitamin D may have a reduced risk of developing MS. However, vitamin D doesn't alter the disease course in people who already have the disease. Taking too much vitamin D can damage your liver.

- Vitamin D helps to maintain healthy bones by increasing the body's absorption of calcium. Suf-

272

ficient quantities of vitamin D and calcium are essential for preventing *osteoporosis* (bone loss). (Check out Chapter 11 for information about the risk of osteoporosis in MS and recommendations for keeping your bones healthy.)

- Calcium EAP (calcium-2-aminoethylphosphate—also known as calcium orotate) is a compound developed by Dr. Hans Nieper in the 1960s. It's very expensive and its safety and efficacy in MS have never been evaluated in a controlled clinical trial.

- Selenium, zinc, DHEA (dehydroepiandrosterone), and melatonin may all activate the immune system and should therefore be used in low doses or not at all.

Exercise, prayer, and other CAM options done independently or in a class

Some forms of CAM involve activities that you can do on you own or in groups. For example, consider these activities:

- **Aromatherapy:** Aromatherapy, in which the essential oils from certain kinds of plants are inhaled or applied by massage, has a low risk and a reasonable cost. Several small clinical studies suggest it's beneficial for anxiety and depression, but further research is needed.

- **Cooling:** Reducing a person's body temperature slightly (with a cooling vest or other cooling strategy) may help speed nerve conduction in people with MS. Limited research studies have found that cooling produces improvement in many MS-associated

273

symptoms, including weakness, fatigue, spasticity, walking difficulties, urinary difficulties, speech disorders, visual difficulties, sexual problems, incoordination, and cognitive difficulties. Cooling therapy may soon make the transition to standard medical practice in MS.

➤ **Exercise:** Exercise that's geared to a person's abilities and limitations not only promotes general health but may also have beneficial effects on MS symptoms, including weakness, walking difficulties, muscle stiffness, osteoporosis, low back pain, bladder difficulties, bowel problems, fatigue, insomnia, depression, anxiety, and anger. People with MS who are heat-sensitive should avoid becoming overheated (check out Chapter 11 for tips on how to exercise comfortably).

➤ **Prayer and spirituality:** These are being evaluated to determine whether they can improve overall health or improve the course of a disease. Research is underway to evaluate their effectiveness in MS.

➤ **T'ai Chi:** This low-risk therapy is a component of traditional Chinese medicine that combines the physical benefits of exercise with the relaxing effects of meditation. T'ai Chi may improve walking ability and decrease stiffness in people with MS.

➤ **Yoga:** Yoga is relatively inexpensive and safe. Even though it hasn't been rigorously investigated, it may relieve anxiety, pain, and spasticity. Many chapters of the National MS Society offer yoga programs (call 800-FIGHT-MS or 800-344-4867).

Acupuncture, massage, and other CAM options performed by a practitioner

The following CAM interventions are provided by a clinician or practitioner with specialized training or expertise:

✔ **Acupuncture:** Acupuncture, a component of traditional Chinese medicine, involves inserting thin needles into specified acupuncture points on the body to alter the body's energy flow. In small and preliminary studies in MS, acupuncture has provided some relief of anxiety, depression, dizziness, pain, bladder difficulties, and weakness.

✔ **Biofeedback:** Biofeedback uses monitoring equipment to make a person's bodily functions (for example, heart rate) visible so that the person can learn to modify or control the function. It may be beneficial for some MS-associated conditions, including anxiety, insomnia, pain, bladder and bowel incontinence, and muscle stiffness.

✔ **Chelation therapy:** This type of therapy involves intravenous infusions of chemicals that bind to *chelates* (harmful metals) in blood. Although it's effective for treating cases of heavy-metal toxicity such as lead poisoning, there's no scientific evidence that chelation therapy is effective in MS. It's very expensive, and serious side effects (including kidney injury, bone marrow damage, and even death) may result.

✔ **Chiropractic:** This therapy involves manipulations of the spine to correct mild bone abnormalities that are thought to exert pressure on the nerves. There's no strong published evidence that chiropractic therapy is beneficial for MS attacks or for altering the course of the disease. Users of chiropractic should be aware of the rare side effects, including stroke.

➤ **Dental amalgam removal:** The removal of *dental amalgams* (the silver-colored fillings dentists use to repair cavities) is based on the idea that the mercury contained in them is toxic to the body's nervous and immune systems. In spite of the hype this treatment has received over the years, there's no evidence that removing dental amalgams and replacing them with other materials has a beneficial effect on MS.

➤ **Hippotherapy:** Therapeutic horseback riding offers possible benefits for walking difficulties, spasticity, weakness, bladder and bowel problems, and depression.

➤ **Hypnosis and guided imagery:** Neither hypnosis nor guided imagery has been fully investigated. Both are well-tolerated, low-to-moderate-cost therapies that may relieve anxiety and pain in people with MS.

➤ **Magnets and electromagnetic therapy:** Low-intensity magnets and pulsing electromagnetic fields have been used in medicine for hundreds of years in an effort to correct what are thought to be electrical imbalances in the body. A few small studies have suggested that pulsing electromagnetic fields may improve spasticity and bladder problems in MS, but further studies are needed to evaluate their efficacy and safety.

➤ **Massage:** Massage, which involves many different techniques, helps to relax muscles and relieve stress. Even though it hasn't been extensively studied in MS, limited studies in other conditions suggest that it may improve mood and reduce spasticity and certain types of pain.

Becoming a Cautious CAM Consumer

You and your family members are likely to be bombarded with sound-bites and advertising regarding various types of CAM. In your eagerness to get a grip on your MS and feel better, you may be persuaded to try a little bit of this and a little bit of that, without carefully considering the pros and cons. Here are some suggestions to help you become a savvier consumer:

➤ **Be cautiously skeptical:** Take every claim with a grain of salt until you see solid evidence from a controlled clinical trial.

➤ **Always ask the following questions, and don't give up until you have the answers:** What does the treatment involve? How and why is it supposed to work? How effective is it? What are the risks? How much does it cost?

➤ **Talk with your doctor and pharmacist about any CAM intervention that you're considering:** These professionals are your best sources of information about possible risks and interactions with your prescribed medications. When you don't mention the CAM you're using, it's like asking your doctor to treat your MS with a blindfold on.

➤ **Watch out for the following red flags:**

- Advertisements that rely heavily on testimonials or anecdotal evidence rather than objective data on efficacy, safety, and cost
- Marketing hype that makes exaggerated claims of

"miraculous" results for a variety of different diseases

- Promises of relief from lots of different symptoms (products that claim to fix everything probably don't fix much of anything)
- Claims to strengthen your immune system (The MS immune system is already overactive, so additional boosts may be harmful.)
- Products with secret ingredients
- An antimedical emphasis that berates conventional medicine
- Expensive, highly invasive treatments with no supporting data or scientific rationale

✔ **Don't trip over the following misconceptions:**

- "Natural" doesn't necessarily mean "safe." Even though some natural compounds are safe and beneficial, others can be toxic.
- Even supplements that are beneficial can contain chemicals that are potentially harmful.
- More isn't necessarily better. As with prescription medications, higher supplement doses aren't necessarily more effective than lower doses, and the additive effects of multiple supplements may actually be harmful.

278

Additional resources to help guide your CAM detective work

The world of CAM can be as confusing as it is alluring. Check out these other resources for more of the information you need to be an informed consumer of CAM products and services:

Books

✔ *Alternative Medicine and Multiple Sclerosis*, 2nd edition, by Allen C. Bowling (Demos Medical Publishing, 2006).

✔ *The Alternative Medicine Handbook: The Complete Reference Guide to Alternative and Complementary Therapies* by Barrie Cassileth (W.W. Norton & Company, 1999).

✔ *Tyler's Honest Herbal: A Sensible Guide to the Use of Herbs and Related Remedies* by Steven Foster and Varro Tyler (Haworth Press, 1999).

✔ *PDR for Nutritional Supplements* (Thomson Healthcare, 2001).

✔ *PDR for Herbal Medicines*, 3rd edition (Thomson Healthcare, 2004).

Web sites

✔ The Rocky Mountain MS Center (www.ms-cam.org): This site aims to create a worldwide community of people interested in CAM and MS, provide unbiased, up-to-date information about CAM and MS, and measure people's experiences with CAM therapies.

✔ Oregon Center for Complementary and Alternative Medication in Neurological Disorders (www.ohsu.edu/orccamind/): This collaboration between the conventional and alternative medicine communities is committed to CAM research in neurological disorders.

➤ Quackwatch (www.quackwatch.com): Quackwatch is a non-profit corporation that was founded by Dr. Stephen Barrett, whose purpose is to combat health-related frauds, myths, fads, and fallacies.

Agencies

➤ Federal Trade Commission, Consumer Response Center, CRC-240, Washington, DC 20580; phone: 877-FTC-HELP (877-382-4357); Web site: www.ftc.gov.

The Federal Trade Commission investigates false advertising.

➤ National Center for Complementary and Alternative Medicine, P.O. Box 7923, Gaithersburg, MD 20898; phone: 888-644-6226; TTY: 866-464-3615; Web site: nccam.nih.gov; e-mail: info@nccam.nih.gov.

The Center, which is one of the 27 institutes and centers that make up the National Institutes of Health (NIH) in the U.S. Department of Health and Human Services, is the Federal Government's lead agency for scientific research on CAM.

➤ National Council Against Health Fraud, 119 Foster Street, Peabody, MA 01960; phone: 978-532-9383; Web site: ncahf.org.

The National Council Against Health Fraud is a private non-profit, voluntary health agency that focuses on health misinformation, fraud, and quackery.

Part III

Staying Healthy and Feeling Well

The 5th Wave   By Rich Tennant

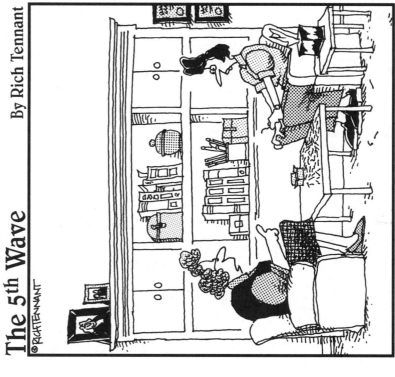

"Straightening paper clips is one way to deal with stress, but have you considered exercise or meditation instead?"

In this part . . .

An important strategy for living comfortably with multiple sclerosis (MS) is knowing how to take care of the whole you—so that you're primed to meet whatever challenges MS brings your way. To help you take the best possible care of yourself, we provide info on preventive healthcare, and we show you how to handle your stress. This part also gives the lowdown on how you and your care partner can maintain your health and quality of life if and when the disease progresses in spite of everyone's best efforts.

Chapter 11

Paying Attention to Your Health— It's Not *All* about MS

In This Chapter

▲ Making wellness a comprehensive plan

▲ Protecting your health with routine checkups

▲ Eating the right stuff

▲ Understanding the importance of exercise

▲ Setting yourself up for success

---

*M*ultiple sclerosis (MS) can really grab your attention. Matter of fact, it may take so much of your time and energy that you don't have any left to think about other important health issues (for example, dental care and routine physical checkups). And if you and your doctor are focusing exclusively on your MS care, neither of you may take the time to think about preventive healthcare strategies or wellness. Besides, no one who's been "blessed" with MS should have to worry about anything else, right?

Unfortunately, the fact is, the healthier you are, the more comfortable you'll be and the better able to deal with whatever challenges MS brings your way. So, in this chapter, we talk about important strategies for feeling and functioning at your best, including timely checkups, routine screenings for other health problems, healthy eating, a regular exercise regimen, good dental care, and adequate rest.

Enhancing Your Wellness by Paying Attention to the Whole You

Wellness is all about feeling the best you possibly can. And remember that you can most definitely be well even though you have MS. You can achieve wellness by paying attention to the whole you and by making sure that you have the following:

- ✔ Adequate rest (Check out Chapter 7 for tips on how to deal with MS fatigue and maximize your energy.)

- ✔ Good stress management strategies (Chapter 12 is all about managing the stresses of everyday life.)

- ✔ Whatever form of spiritual sustenance you want and need

- ✔ A healthy diet

- ✔ The right kind of exercise program

A feeling of balance (and we don't mean the walking-on-a-tightrope kind) is also important. For instance, a healthy life includes time for work and recreation, togetherness and solitude, and busy times and vegging out. Balance also comes from making sure that MS doesn't steal the show. The goal is for MS to take up no more of you and your family's time, energy, and resources than it actually requires (flip to Chapter 15 for more on these family matters).

For a comprehensive, step-by-step guide to wellness, take a look at these resources:

✔ *The Art of Getting Well: A Five-Step Plan for Maximizing Health When You Have a Chronic Illness*, by David Spero (Hunter House, 2002).

✔ *Multiple Sclerosis: A Self-Care Guide to Wellness*, 2nd edition, edited by Nancy Holland and June Halper (Demos Medical Publishing, 2005).

Scheduling Routine Checkups to Protect Your Health

Even though MS is definitely enough for any one person to have to handle, it doesn't protect you from other health problems. Although some people with MS report that they get fewer colds than they used to (maybe that overactive immune system is good for something after all!), you can expect to deal with all the usual things—colds, flu, and stomach bugs—along the way. And most people with MS die from all the same stuff as everyone else—cancer, heart disease, and stroke. So, remember, you're not off the hook when it comes to taking care of your health.

In addition to whatever care you're getting for your MS, it's important that you have a primary care physician or nurse on your team who can give you a general tuneup on a periodic basis and refer you for the health screens that are recommended for your age group. Few neurologists provide this kind of care on a routine basis because they're focusing their attention on your MS needs.

For ideas about what type of preventive care you personally need, check out the National MS Society's brochures, *Preventive Care Recommendations for Adults with MS: The Basic Facts* (www.nationalmssociety.org/preventive) and

285

Dental Health: The Basic Facts (www.nationalmssociety .org/dental). You can also request these brochures by calling (800) FIGHT-MS (800-344-4867). If you want friendly e-mail reminders about your health screening tests, check out www.myhealthtestreminder.com. (For more information about the safety of various types of vaccinations for people with MS, take a look at Chapter 23.)

Gynecological exams, mammograms, chest X-rays, colonoscopies, routine dental care, and other procedures may pose an accessibility challenge if you have mobility issues or use a mobility aid, such as a motorized scooter or wheelchair. So, when you make your appointment, check to make sure that the facility and testing equipment are fully accessible and that someone will be available to provide assistance if you need it. Nothing is more frustrating than arriving for a scheduled appointment only to discover that you can't get through a doorway, onto an examining table, or close to an X-ray machine. If you have trouble locating accessible facilities, call the National MS Society at (800) FIGHT-MS for recommendations in your area.

Making Healthy Eating a Priority

Unfortunately, you can't eat your way around MS. Even though a variety of special diets have been promoted as MS cures, none have been shown in controlled trials to alter the course or severity of MS (check out Chapter 10 for more information on the role of clinical trials in evaluating alternative and complementary therapies). Like everyone else, you'll benefit most from a healthy diet that provides the recommended nutrients for a person your age and that promotes good cardiovascular health.

The U.S. Department of Agriculture (USDA) has recently created a new, more personalized version of the familiar Food Pyramid (mypyramid.gov). When you type in information about your age, sex, and activity level, it tells you how much of each food group you need to eat on a daily basis, as well as tips on what foods offer the best bang for your buck. The bottom line, no matter what your individual needs are, is that you get the most benefit from a diet that

✔ Contains a balance of grains, fruits, vegetables, lean meats (or meat substitutes), and low-fat dairy products

✔ Provides you with only as many calories as you need

Taking MS into account when planning your menu

In addition to a balanced, low-fat, high-fiber diet (and a daily multivitamin), MS specialist neurologists and nutritionists recommend that you keep the following important points in mind:

✔ **Calories count.** If you eat more calories than you burn, your weight will go up—it's as simple as that. Along with its other benefits, exercise burns calories. So, if you're less mobile or active than you used to be because of your MS, to maintain the same weight, you need to reduce the number of calories you're taking in.

And, in order to make all your calories count, the best strategy is to get them from nutritious foods rather than from those yummy but not-so-nutritious desserts and junk foods that do nothing for your waistline or your well-being.

✔ **Calcium protects your bones.** Everyone needs hefty amounts of calcium for strong bones and teeth.

However, a person with MS—particularly women at or near menopause—may be at increased risk for osteoporosis (bone loss) for a couple of reasons:

- Mobility problems, fatigue, weakness, and *spasticity* (stiffness) can all contribute to a reduction in physical activity, including weight-bearing exercise, which, in turn, can lead to bone loss.

- The corticosteroids that are used to treat MS *relapses* (exacerbations) can increase the risk of bone loss.

- Heat sensitivity, fatigue, and reduced mobility may decrease the amount of time spent in the sun, which affects your exposure to vitamin D (which is necessary for calcium absorption).

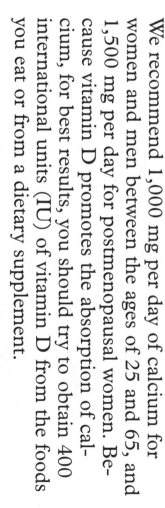

We recommend 1,000 mg per day of calcium for women and men between the ages of 25 and 65, and 1,500 mg per day for postmenopausal women. Because vitamin D promotes the absorption of calcium, for best results, you should try to obtain 400 international units (IU) of vitamin D from the foods you eat or from a dietary supplement.

✔ **Fluids help fight urinary tract infections.** People who are experiencing bladder problems tend to cut back on liquids in order to avoid having to pee all the time. However, reduced fluid intake can worsen fatigue and constipation, and can increase the risk of urinary tract infections. So, do your best to drink eight glasses of liquid per day (and take a look at Chapter 8 for additional bladder management strategies).

Water is hands-down the best, but low-calorie sodas (without aspartame if you have an ornery bladder), skim milk, seltzer, and plain tea or coffee (decaffeinated for that same ornery bladder) come in second. And finally, high-calorie sodas and fruit juices take a definite third. Ice cream, yogurt, sorbet, gelatin-based desserts, and soups are also good sources of fluid.

✔ **With enough fiber, all systems are a go.** Constipation is a common problem in MS (flip to Chapter 8 for some good management strategies). So, if you're less physically active and don't drink enough fluids, the problem is likely to be even worse. And some of the medications used to treat common MS symptoms—such as amantadine for fatigue, baclofen for spasticity, and the medications for overactive bladder—may also contribute to the problem. But, adequate fiber intake can help a lot. You should aim for about 25-30 grams a day, from foods such as whole grain breads and cereals, brown rice and whole wheat pasta, dried beans, lentils, and peas, and vegetables, fruits, and nuts.

Battling the barriers to healthy eating

Even with the best of intentions, maintaining good eating habits can be difficult. But, being alert to some of the ways that MS symptoms can interfere with healthy eating can help you stay on track. For example, consider these troublesome symptoms:

✔ **Fatigue:** If just getting through the day takes all your energy, putting time and effort into healthy meals can seem overwhelming (take a look at Chapter 7 for suggestions on how to manage MS fatigue). So, rather than eating balanced meals, you may find yourself grabbing the nearest (unhealthy) snacks. Or you may reach for the quick fix—a blast of some-

289

thing sugary that gives you a momentary boost but then leaves you feeling tired and hungry—rather than protein, which reduces fatigue and helps you maintain a more consistent blood sugar level. Pretty soon you have a vicious cycle going, with fatigue contributing to poor nutrition and poor nutrition fueling your fatigue.

A nutritionist can recommend healthy dishes that are easy to prepare. An occupational therapist (OT) can give you lots of energy-saving tips, including recommendations for helpful cooking gadgets and tools, ideas on how to arrange your cooking space, and strategies for simplifying your shopping trips. Check out Chapter 5 for more information about these members of your rehab team, and call the National MS Society for referrals to specialists who are experienced in MS (800-FIGHT-MS).

✔ **Depression:** Like fatigue, depression is common in MS. And, unfortunately, people who are depressed may experience significant changes in their appetites—either eating a lot less or a lot more than they used to. Neither extreme is particularly healthy.

If you've lost interest in food or don't seem to enjoy eating the way you used to, or if you find yourself eating a lot of not-so-healthy comfort food to boost your spirits, be sure to let your doctor know. Other things, like fatigue and certain medications, can cause appetite changes, but it's still important to find out if depression is the culprit. (Flip to Chapter 9 for more on mood changes and MS.)

✔ **Accessibility or mobility issues:** Sometimes people have difficulty putting together healthy meals because they can't navigate the stores or their kitchens the way they used to. For example, foods may be on inaccessible shelves, pots and pans may be stuck in out-of-the-way places, the kitchen may be too small to accommodate a scooter, and the counters may be too high. So, when things get more challenging, you may find yourself skipping meals or relying more heavily on prepared foods or take-out. We're not big fans of either of these strategies. If you find yourself eating more prepared foods, be sure to check out the ingredients because many frozen foods are high in sodium or fat, which can raise blood pressure and cause you to put on the pounds.

A nutritionist can point you in the direction of some healthier products and can also suggest some simple menus that you can fix in a jiffy. Also, an OT can help you figure out how to make your cooking space more organized and accessible so that the items you need are within your reach.

For detailed information about MS and nutrition, and practical strategies for food selection and preparation, check out the National MS Society's booklet, *Food for Thought: MS and Nutrition,* at www.nationalms society.org/food or by calling (800) FIGHT-MS.

Improving Your MS and Overall Wellness with Exercise

Here's the basic message: Exercise is good for you. Even though it wasn't all that long ago that people with MS were told *not* to exercise, we now know that physical activity geared to your abilities and limitations provides many benefits, including

✔ Reducing your fatigue (difficult to believe but absolutely true)

291

- Maintaining and increasing your endurance and the flexibility of your joints and muscles

- Improving your cardiovascular health

- Improving bowel and bladder functions

- Strengthening your bones

- Improving your mood

Overcoming the hurdles

In spite of all the good reasons to get out there and move around, people with MS often find it challenging. Here are the most common hurdles and some strategies for getting over them:

- **"I'm too tired to even think about exercise."** Exercising to increase your energy level doesn't sound logical, but it works because it improves cardiovascular function and tones your muscles. The trick is to start small and build up gradually. Pick a time of day when your energy is pretty good and do something physical, even if it's only a little—swim a half a lap, walk to the next driveway and back, spend one minute on the treadmill, or make one trip up the stairs.

  Set your goals within reach so that every step is a victory, and don't raise the bar until you're comfortable. If it takes a few days or a week to go to the next level, so be it. Allowing yourself to do things differently—or at a different pace—than you used to, is your key to success (see Chapter 3 for details). Your physician or physical therapist (PT) can help you design an exercise regimen that's just right for you.

✔ **"I hated exercising before I had MS and I don't like it any better now."** Okay, so you don't enjoy jogging, swimming, aerobics, or anything else that makes you think of sweat. But keep in mind that physical activity doesn't have to be competitive and you don't have to go to the gym. Instead, you can work in your garden, walk in the mall, join a yoga class, or take a walk with your best friend. If you love to watch movies, set up a TV in front of your treadmill or recumbent bicycle, and exercise with your favorite stars—you can see them but they can't see you, so it all works out. Chances are that you'll add a few more minutes to your routine just to see what happens in the next scene.

✔ **"The competition was what I loved, and if I can't do it competitively, I don't want to do it at all."** All you competitive folks out there probably have the toughest challenge of all. When being the best or the fastest or the toughest isn't possible, you need to redefine your goals. Perhaps you can level the playing field a bit by getting into adaptive sports of some kind—adaptive skiing, wheelchair basketball, or disability-friendly ropes courses (the National MS Society can fill you in on opportunities in your area). Or, maybe you can decide to compete with yourself rather than with others—by challenging yourself to swim one more lap or speed up your walk around the block.

You may need to experiment with a few different activities to find something that satisfies your competitive urges. And believe it or not, you may even find yourself enjoying non-competitive activities that you never took the time to try before.

293

✔ **"If I can't do it as well as I did before, I'm not interested."** In Chapter 3, we talk about how important it is to grieve over the old stuff so you can get on with the new—and this is a case in point. If you pride yourself on your fabulous tennis serve or glorious golf swing, and MS suddenly gets in the way, you're going to have to grieve over that loss before you can start thinking about what's next. After you get your head around the idea of doing your sport differently or less gracefully, you may find that there's still a lot to enjoy about it—the essence of the game, the companionship, or the time spent out-of-doors.

If you become unable to pursue the sport at all, it will take you a while to find satisfying substitutes. You'll probably have to try a few different things before you find something you like, but the chances are great that you'll find something to enjoy.

✔ **"It takes me so much longer to do stuff that I never have time to exercise any more."** Time is one of your most valuable resources, especially when you have MS. So, the more demands you have on your time and the longer it takes you to do the things that are important to you, the more important it is to think through your priorities. If physical activity improves your mood and helps you feel more mobile and energetic, you may want to put it pretty high on your priority list. You don't need to carve out a lot of time either—just 15 to 20 minutes a day will do the trick (and you don't even have to do it all at once!). Choose an activity that's close by and convenient so you don't have to spend a lot of extra time getting there and back.

294

Exercising your options

You don't have to be a great athlete to get physical. People with MS can enjoy a wide variety of activities. Here are some that you may want to try:

✔ **Water activities in a cool pool:** These are ideal if your MS is heat-sensitive. Most people do well in water that's no warmer than 80 to 84 degrees. The buoyancy of the water makes swimming and water aerobics safe and comfortable even if you have weakness or balance problems. The National MS Society can give you information about MS aquatics programs in your area.

✔ **Aerobic exercise:** Aerobic exercise is any activity that raises your pulse and respiration rates. Running or walking outside or on a treadmill, cycling outside or on a stationary bike, and rowing are the activities that people generally think of as aerobic exercise. But, you can actually raise your heart rate by simply sitting in a chair and doing windmills with your arms. You only need to do 15 minutes a day to get the aerobic benefits, and research has shown that you can get the same benefits even if you divide the time into three five-minute periods over the course of the day.

✔ **Yoga:** This is an excellent, noncompetitive form of exercise that combines healthy breathing techniques with movements that improve flexibility and balance. Yoga is also a wonderful stress-reliever. Many chapters of the National MS Society offer yoga programs that are geared toward your abilities and limitations, so call (800) FIGHT-MS to find out about programs in your area.

✔ **T'ai Chi:** This gentle martial art that's made up of slow-motion movements can maintain or improve balance, flexibility, and strength. Like yoga, T'ai Chi is an excellent activity for reducing feelings of stress.

✔ **Stretching exercises:** These types of exercises are important for maintaining comfort and flexibility, particularly if you're experiencing spasticity. Stretching helps you loosen up tight muscles and maintain full range of motion in your joints.

Take a look at *Stretching for People with MS* (www .nationalmssociety.org/stretching) and *Stretching with a Helper for People with MS* (www.nationalmssociety .org/stretchinghelp). You can also request hard copies of these brochures by calling (800) FIGHT-MS.

✔ **Weight training with free weights or exercise machines:** This can help you tone your muscles and increase your flexibility and endurance. Remember, however, that lifting weights can't strengthen muscles that have been weakened by poor nerve conduction. After the nerves that stimulate the muscles have been damaged by MS, those muscles aren't likely to become stronger with exercise. Weight-training will, however, help to strengthen the surrounding muscles that you use to compensate for those that are no longer working up to snuff.

✔ **Therapeutic horseback riding:** This activity promotes balance and strength (just think of all the effort it takes to keep yourself upright on the back of a moving horse!), and it's great for stretching out leg muscles tightened by spasticity.

Clearly you have a lot of options. But be sure to talk to your doctor or physical therapist before starting any new exercise program, just to make sure that you're opting for an activity that's appropriate and safe given whatever your current symptoms are. Experiment with various activities until you find one that's right for you. Remember that the best exercise program is one that you enjoy enough to do on a regular basis.

Maximizing your comfort and safety during exercise

The goal of exercise is to feel and function better. But, the old "no pain, no gain" philosophy doesn't apply here—there's no need to push yourself to the limit. Here are some tips to help you be comfortable and safe while getting the greatest possible benefit out of your physical activities:

✔ **Try to plan your exercise during peak energy times.** There's no point in starting when you're already exhausted. If you begin to exercise and quickly get very tired, take a short break. Sometimes it only takes a few minutes to feel ready to go again.

✔ **Take a few minutes to warm up before (and cool down after) any vigorous activity.** For instance, it's a good idea to drink a glass of cold water or juice before you start to help keep your body temperature down. And loosen up your joints with gentle stretches or rotations to avoid strain. After you finish exercising, gently stretch out the muscles you've been using to avoid cramping and stiffness, and take another drink to cool yourself off.

✔ **Don't push yourself beyond your limits.** It's much healthier and more effective to get moderate

297

exercise on a regular basis than to push yourself to exhaustion once and then be too worn out to do anything for the rest of the week.

✔ **Exercise in a cool environment.** Even a slight elevation in your core body temperature—as little as half a degree—can cause your symptoms to act up. These little flare-ups, which are called *pseudoexacerbations*, are nothing to worry about; they'll disappear after your body has cooled down again (see Chapter 6 for more details). If your MS is particularly sensitive to the heat, you can protect yourself by sipping cold water during your workout, wearing a commercially-available cooling garment, such as a vest, bandanna, or headband, and staying close to a fan or air conditioner.

✔ **If you're balance-challenged, be sure to stand near a wall or chair when you exercise, or ask someone to spot you.** If you don't feel sure-footed enough to balance standing up, your physical therapist can recommend exercises for you to do while seated on a chair or mat.

✔ **Watch out for slippery floors in exercise facilities and around pools.** So that you don't slip and fall, it's a good idea to wear non-skid shoes any time you're going to be maneuvering on a wet floor.

✔ **Before engaging the services of a personal trainer, make sure that he or she has some experience with people with MS.** Trainers who are unfamiliar with MS generally don't understand the limitations imposed by MS fatigue or by muscles that have been weakened by lack of nerve conduction. Your physician or physical therapist can recommend an exercise regimen for you to do with your

298

trainer. Be sure you work with your trainer to set realistic goals given your level of ability.

For more information about exercise and MS, check out the National MS Society's booklet, *Exercise as Part of Everyday Life*, at www.nationalmssociety.org/exercise or by calling (800) FIGHT-MS.

Increasing Your Chances of Success

Turning over a new leaf is never easy. Anyone who has made a New Year's resolution knows how challenging it can be to change behavior—and this whole chapter is about changing your behavior in ways that will enhance your health and wellness. So, whether you're trying to be more vigilant about your medical or dental checkups, improve your diet, or increase your level of physical activity, the best strategy is to come up with a plan that you can live with. Follow these guidelines to set yourself up for success:

- **Set reasonable goals.** Unreasonable expectations only set you up for failure.

- **Focus on the things you can change rather than on those you can't.** Even though MS is here to stay—at least for the time being—you can do a lot to take care of yourself and feel well.

- **Don't get caught up in your "failures."** If you have a momentary lapse from your new diet or exercise regimen, don't beat yourself up about it. Instead, try to put that energy into getting back on track tomorrow. An occasional day off is good for the soul.

- **Work with a buddy to make things easier and**

299

more pleasant. Partners, neighbors from down the street, or friends from your support group are all good candidates for an exercise partner. And chowing down with a diet buddy can make those low-cal meals taste better too.

✔ **Every time you do something good for yourself—whether it's eating something healthy, getting some good exercise, or getting a mammogram or chest X-ray—pat yourself on the back.** Recognizing the things you do to take care of yourself is an important step toward feeling more in control of your body and your health in spite of MS.

Chapter 12

Handling Stress without Giving Up Your Life

Imagine this all-too-familiar scene: A young woman goes to her neurologist in a tizzy. She has two young kids and has recently gone back to work because her husband is worried about getting laid off. The babysitter is moving away, the basement flooded during the last storm, and her parents need help moving into their new retirement home. Not to mention that she was recently diagnosed with multiple sclerosis (MS), a chronic illness that seems to do whatever it wants to do whenever it wants to do it. People are telling her that stress isn't good for her MS and she's panicked that she's going to get worse. She's trying to rid her life of stress, but somehow it's not working.

Chances are that your life feels just as stressful at times

Understanding the Relationship between Stress and MS

Not all stresses are alike. Even though people use the term stress a lot—"I'm so stressed." or "The stress is really getting to me."—they're actually referring to many different kinds of experiences. These experiences run the gamut from the hassles of daily life, such as traffic jams, bickering children, and misplaced keys, to sudden crises, such as the death of a loved one or the loss of one's home, to ongoing stresses like financial worries or marital problems. And research suggests that the various types of stress may interact with MS in different and sometimes contradictory ways. For example, consider the following facts:

- ✔ *Sudden acute stresses*, such as car accidents or missile attacks (yes, that's actually been studied!), seem to have no impact on either the onset or progression of MS. In fact, some evidence suggests that brief traumatic stresses may even reduce a person's risk of MS relapses.

- ✔ A large study found that the death of a person's child significantly increased his or her risk of developing MS.

- ✔ Ongoing, chronic trauma or stress seems to increase the risk of MS relapses.

302

In other words, the relationship between stress and MS isn't at all clear. To make it even more complicated, the research in this area also suggests that the impact of a person's life stresses depends in large part on his or her coping and problem-solving skills and support system. Because MS varies so much from one person to another, and no two people have the same coping mechanisms or resources, no one can really predict how life's stresses are going to affect you or anyone else. So, rather than worrying about how the unavoidable stresses of daily life are going to affect your MS, your best bet is to figure out how to manage those stresses more comfortably.

Recognizing Your Own Signs of Stress

Because everyone's situations and coping skills are different, you can safely assume that no one's stresses are exactly like anyone else's—and neither are their strategies for dealing with those stresses. So, your best bet is to identify the things in your life that stress you out. Then you can figure out the strategies that are most helpful to you in dealing with them. A good place to start is by learning to recognize how you feel when you're stressed. Sounds easy, right? Not so fast! Because everyone reacts differently to different stressors, it's impossible to create a master list. But, in this section, we go over the most common physical and emotional responses.

From sweaty palms to pounding hearts: Knowing your physical signs of stress

The human body is programmed to respond to life-threatening events. You may remember the old *fight-or-flight response* you learned about in high school biology. This response, which is leftover from the days when the earliest humans had to scramble for survival, is built into

303

everyone's physiological makeup. When confronted with a threat, your body, including the immune system, goes into high gear in preparation to protect itself. Fortunately, modern life doesn't generally involve imminent physical danger, but the physiological processes are still active in everyone. So, because of these processes that affect your body, some of the most obvious responses to stress are physical ones. For example, you may

➤ Develop a rapid heart beat

➤ Have sweaty palms

➤ Get knots in your stomach

➤ Find your mouth going dry

➤ Feel worn out

➤ Develop a pounding headache

Some of the physical responses to stress may be difficult to distinguish from your MS—such as feeling worn out or getting a dry mouth (which is a common side effect of the medications used to treat bladder problems). With all this stress-related physiological activity going on, it's not all that surprising that MS symptoms may kick in a bit more as well. You may experience blurry vision or you may feel more tingly, for example. These changes are generally short-lived and calm down when you do.

Anxiety and irritability: Knowing your emotional signs of stress

Not only does the body react to stress, but the mind does too. Some common emotional reactions to stress include feeling

304

- Anxious or worried about a lot of things

- Irritable or grumpy much of the time

- Down in the dumps

- Overwhelmed and overcommitted

- Pessimistic and gloomy

You may also find yourself anticipating the worst all the time, or you may be having a lot of nightmares. All of these thoughts and experiences may make it difficult for you to get a good night's sleep, concentrate, make decisions, or enjoy what you're doing. (Because problems with concentration and decision making can also be symptoms of MS, be sure to check out Chapter 9 for more information about cognition.)

Many of these feelings and experiences can also occur with depression. If "you find yourself feeling down pretty consistently for more than a couple of weeks, be sure to consult your physician. Depression is common in MS and deserves to be treated promptly. (Flip to Chapter 9 for more information about how to recognize and treat depression.)

Identifying the Major Stresses in Your Life

When you're feeling stressed out and overwhelmed, it's important that you try to sort out the good, the bad, and the ugly. By that we mean figuring out what the sources of your stress may be, deciding whether they give you more pleasure than pain, and differentiating between those you can do something about and those you can't.

To help you get the sorting process started, you may want to keep a stress diary for a couple of weeks to see what your stresses are all about. This diary doesn't need to be anything elaborate, just some brief notes about what's going on when you notice yourself feeling stressed. A small pad or pocket calendar works well because you can keep it handy for those stressful moments on the go.

The following sections show you some real-life examples of how to sort out various stressful situations. Even though these examples may not be specific to you, you can still use our advice to handle your specific situation.

Dealing with the devil: Job stress 101

Whether anyone likes it or not, stress is an inevitable product of having a job. Unfortunately, though, MS can cause you to have even more stress than the average worker. Just remember that even if your job is incredibly stressful, it still provides you with income, interesting challenges, enjoyable relationships with co-workers, and health insurance. Not a bad trade-off.

So, if you decide that keeping your job is a good thing, you have to identify the particular things about your job that cause you stress (and then determine whether you can actually control the stress and how). Perhaps your boss is a pain, the nine-to-five schedule is grueling given your fatigue level, and your office is about a zillion miles from the nearest bathroom.

Chances are you can't do a whole lot about your boss, so it's not worth spending a lot of time and energy thinking about him or her. On the other hand, you know that some people in the office are taking advantage of flextime and even working from home some days. And you think that one of the offices closer to the bathroom may be opening up soon. So, you could talk to your boss (charmingly, of

TIP

course) about accommodations that may make your work life a little less stressful (check out Chapter 18 for more information about on-the-job accommodations). In other words, the goal is to zero in on the things that you may actually be able to change instead of wasting energy on those that you can't.

Handling family stress with grace and composure

As with job stress, it's important that you deal with your family stress by determining the stressors and deciding whether they're controllable or not (is your Aunt Frieda really controllable?). So, suppose that your family comes to your house for the holidays every year. This is a tradition that you and the family really enjoy. You love decorating the house, feeding everyone a delicious meal, and having lots of presents for everyone to open. For you, family time is what the holidays are all about. But this year, you're exhausted and your symptoms are acting up, the kids have been a real pain lately, and your husband is so busy at work that he's virtually no help at all.

Even though asking your sister-in-law to host the family this year is definitely an option, it's important to think about what you'd gain and what you'd lose by turning the event over to her. In other words, don't throw the baby out with the bath water. If having the family at your house gives you pleasure, figure out how to do it with less stress. You can, for example, do the following:

✔ Order presents online instead of going to the mall.

✔ Order food from a restaurant instead of cooking (or start cooking now and put stuff in the freezer so you don't have to do all of it at the last minute).

307

- Hire someone to clean the house, or have a family powwow to talk about how to divvy up the chores.

- Let your husband know that the decorating job is his—even if he has to do it at 3 a.m.

As we talk about in Chapter 3, one of the most important strategies for coping with MS (and reducing your stress) is getting comfortable with the idea that it's okay to do things differently.

Controlling the uncontrollable: *Managing your MS stress*

So, you say you're incredibly stressed out about your MS. You worry all the time about getting worse, losing your job, and ending up in a wheelchair. Clearly, your first choice for getting rid of this stress in your life would be to dump the disease—but that's not exactly possible. The next best choice is to focus on the things you can do something about rather than the things you can't.

For example, you can talk with your doctor to make sure you're doing all the right things to slow the progression of your MS. You can also make an appointment with a vocational rehabilitation counselor to talk about your job situation and career options in case you become unable to do your current job (Chapter 18 covers all of your employment woes). The next step is trying to figure out what frightens you most about a wheelchair. Even though most people never need one, it doesn't hurt—and it generally helps—to visualize how you would manage at home, at work, and in the world if you were using a scooter or chair. You may even want to talk with some people with MS who use mobility aids to see how they've managed with them. The National MS Society can put you in touch with folks who'd be happy to talk with you. You can contact the Society by calling (800) FIGHT-MS (800-344-4867).

You can deal with the stress of MS by taking on the individual fears and challenges one by one. You'll be surprised how much more confident and prepared you'll feel after you go head-to-head with each boogeyman.

Developing Your Stress Management Plan

Given all the hoopla about stress, you're probably wondering how to get a handle on the stresses in your own life (see the "Recognizing Your Own Signs of Stress" section to figure out how to identify your stressful triggers). The first step in your stress management plan is to remind yourself (repeatedly, if necessary) that stressing yourself out about stress is pointless. Here's why:

▶ **Trying to eliminate stress is impossible.** It simply can't be done because stress is inherent in everyday living. When people try to get rid of stress in their lives, they end up feeling anxious and inadequate when it doesn't work. And even if they partially succeed, they're often dissatisfied with the results.

▶ **Giving up activities that are important to you—like your job—because they're stressful is a lose-lose strategy.** You may lose some of the stress in your life, but you also lose income and a major source of satisfaction and self-esteem. And, it turns out that unemployment is pretty stressful, too.

▶ **Happy events are also stressful—and you certainly don't want to rid your life of those.** Marriage, a new baby, the holidays, buying a new house, and planning a vacation are all examples of events that cause stress even though they're pleasurable and exciting. If all of these stresses were eliminated, life would be pretty bland.

When people try to control their MS by ridding their lives of stress, they may feel guilty when their symptoms act up or the disease progresses anyway. In other words, they blame themselves when their MS misbehaves. Just remember that it's difficult enough to deal with a chronic, unpredictable disease without also taking blame for it. It makes a lot more sense to follow your neurologist's recommendations for managing your MS (check out Part II for lots of information about managing MS and its symptoms) while also figuring out how to manage the stresses of your everyday life. Together, these strategies will help you feel and function at your best.

Like managing your MS, managing stress is an ongoing process—it isn't something you can do once and then forget about. In this section, we give you some pointers for how to begin dealing with the MS-related stresses you're experiencing now and those that may crop up in the future. You can also check out *Stress Management For Dummies* by Allen Elkin (Wiley, 1999) for a much more detailed overview of general stress management strategies.

Figuring out your priorities

Part of adapting to life with MS is adapting to the unpredictability of your symptoms and their potential impact on your everyday life. As you probably know, MS symptoms can make it more difficult for you to do all the things your want to do. So, if you're feeling stressed out about keeping up with stuff, and you're worried about how to meet every-

310

one else's needs and expectations, it's time to set some priorities for yourself.

Keeping in mind that you can't be much good to anyone else if you aren't taking adequate care of your own needs, you need to make sure that you're making time for yourself and setting clear limits with others about what you can and can't do for them. Identifying your personal priorities can help you figure out how to put your time and energy to the best possible use (take a look at Chapter 7 for other ideas on managing your energy supply).

To start sorting out where your priorities lie, take a look at your work and personal calendars for the last month. Put a smiley face next to each activity that was meaningful, enjoyable, or productive, and a frowning face next to each activity that was unnecessary, a waste of time, or unproductive. It's amazing how much time people spend doing things that are actually unimportant to them.

Setting realistic goals

If you overcommit, overplan, and overpromise, you're setting yourself up for stress. On the flip side, if you set realistic goals you're setting yourself up for success. So, if you find that it's taking you longer to do things, take your productivity into account when you plan your day. For example, if your fatigue is overwhelming later in the day, plan the big stuff for the mornings. You'll feel a lot less stressed if you can look back at the end of a day and feel good about what you've accomplished. In the end, you have to pick and choose the things that are most important to you and give yourself enough time to succeed at them.

Here's something to try: For the next week, write out your planned schedule for each day, guesstimating how long each activity is going to take. Then, after you're finished with that particular activity, make a note of how long each one actually takes. This kind of information can help you plan a lot more realistically in the future.

Cutting yourself some slack

Sometimes people are their own worst enemies and they beat up on themselves for not doing things well enough or fast enough. For example, are you harder on yourself than you are on everyone else? Do you beat yourself up when you don't do everything just right? Are you always doing the "should-a, would-a, could-a" thing? If you answered yes to any of these questions, you have to remember this: Chances are high that you're going to have days when you just can't do everything on your list, or that you won't be able to do things exactly the way you want to. Instead, it's important to be proud of what you can do and forgiving of what you can't.

If you're experiencing a lot of pressure from the people around you, they need to cut you some slack as well. So talk to them about what's going on with you. (Chapter 14 is all about how to talk about your MS with other people.)

Taking some practical steps

Daily life is filled with small stresses that can quickly add up to be bigger ones. In other words, it isn't any one thing—such as struggling with the buttons on your blouse, getting stuck in traffic, or misplacing the folder that you need for your first meeting—that wears you down. Instead, it's the fact that they all happened before your first cup of coffee and you're behind schedule before the day has even started. So that you don't get bogged down by the small stuff, here are a few suggestions for eliminating some of those pesky problems:

312

✔ **Give yourself extra time to get where you need to go.** Feeling rushed all the time is uncomfortable for everyone, but it's even worse when you're dealing with a bunch of MS symptoms that slow you down.

✔ **Organize your living and work spaces so that everyday items have a regular home.** Nothing is more stressful than spending half your time looking for the stuff you need (and the other half trying to maneuver around the many piles littering the floors).

✔ **Do things the easy way rather than the hard way.** Take shortcuts whenever you can, use the best tools that assistive technology (AT) has to offer, and call in the troops when you need help (Chapter 7 has more information on AT).

✔ **Build rest times into your day.** Once you're exhausted, everything feels more stressful. Taking the time to refresh your body and your mind will help keep stress at bay.

✔ **Every day, think of one thing you want to do just for yourself, and then make sure you do it.** It's easy to spend all your time doing things for other people—your partner, kids, boss, and colleagues are all lined up with demands on your time and energy. Taking the time to do something for yourself isn't selfish—it's essential to your health and well-being.

✔ **Plan ahead.** Feeling more prepared for various tasks always makes you feel less stressed. Here are some tips to help you plan:

- Organize your tasks (household chores, errands, work activities) in chunks that make sense. Rather than running all over the place helter-skelter, figure out all the activities that need to be done in a certain part of town, in the basement, or on the floor where your boss's office is, and then do those things all at the same time. Doing things systematically is a lot less stressful than running yourself ragged by going back and forth.

- If going to the supermarket freaks you out or wears you out, plan your trip ahead of time. Use a standardized grocery list that's organized according to the aisles in the store (your store may actually have one of these). Check off the items you need that week and go only to the aisles where they are. Besides taking less energy, this strategy cuts way down on impulse buying, which can save you money!

- If you're traveling, do an accessibility check well ahead of time. Be specific about what your needs are so that you get the appropriate accommodations when you arrive. (Take a look at Chapter 23 for ten tips for traveling with MS.)

- If you're getting lost more while driving, plan your route ahead of time and carry a set of directions in your car. If you do this for every trip, you'll have a handy file of directions in your glove compartment. Just be sure to write or type them in large size print so you can see them easily while you're driving. (Check out Chapter 9 for more information on cognitive symptoms.)

- If you have bladder issues, don't wait until you have to pee to figure out where the nearest bathroom is. Scope out the bathrooms as soon as you arrive at a new place so you won't have to stress about getting there on time.

- If you're stressed out about an upcoming event, take time to plan it out in your head (or write it down if that makes you feel better). Try to sort

314

out what you're worried about and rehearse your strategy for dealing with it. Mastering something successfully in your head is the first step to mastering it in real time.

- Keep a firm hold on your sense of humor. Your humor can get you through a lot of tough times and can help you defuse stress along the way.

The examples are endless. What they all have in common is the fact that they give you a greater feeling of control, which means you feel less stressed.

For many more ideas, take a look at the book, *300 Tips for Making Life with Multiple Sclerosis Easier*, 2nd edition, by Shelley Peterman Schwarz (Demos Medical Publishing, 2006).

Tapping available resources

Another good way to relieve some of the pressure on yourself is to make the best possible use of your available resources. No matter what problem you're trying to solve, you can bet that someone or something out there can help. It may be a person with the expertise that you don't have, a tool or mobility aid that you've never considered before, or just a ready source of good information.

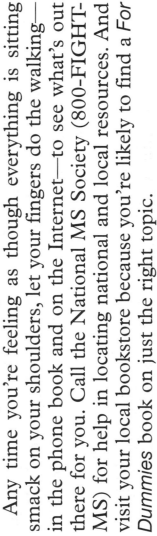

Any time you're feeling as though everything is sitting smack on your shoulders, let your fingers do the walking—in the phone book and on the Internet—to see what's out there for you. Call the National MS Society (800-FIGHT-MS) for help in locating national and local resources. And visit your local bookstore because you're likely to find a *For Dummies* book on just the right topic.

Zoning in on your "MS-free zone"

When you find that keeping up with your old pace becomes difficult, it's easy to begin feeling as though MS is taking over your life and is hogging the whole show. The bigger the MS looms, the more stressed and out of control you feel. This overwhelming feeling tends to happen with advanced disease, but it can be just as valid an issue for people with a recent diagnosis.

One good way to confront these feelings and lessen your stress is to spend some time in your *MS-free zone (MSFZ)*. While the MSFZ isn't a magical kingdom, it's almost as good. Your MSFZ is the place where your MS can't reach you. Whether it's reading a good book, listening to music, praying, giggling with a friend over lunch, working with clay, or whatever, it's your place to take a timeout and re-group. Your MSFZ is by invitation-only, and your MS isn't invited. Time in your MSFZ can feel as restful as a nap, as refreshing as a minivacation, and as satisfying and relaxing as a warm cuddle.

Practicing stress management techniques

Because stress management isn't a one-size-fits-all proposi-tion, the menu of techniques is extensive. We outline some of the basic types here, but you can check out *Stress Man-agement For Dummies* for all the details on how to apply these strategies and others to the wide variety of stresses (MS-related and not) in your life. The key is figuring out what works best for you and sticking with it. But, be ready to tweak the technique if your needs change. Here are the basics:

➤ Exercise is a known stress reliever, and believe it or not, with all the different kinds of exercise out there you're sure to find something you enjoy—team sports, aerobics, weight machines, T'ai Chi, yoga, swimming, cycling, and the list goes on and on.

The National MS Society can refer you to Society-sponsored exercise programs in your area (800-FIGHT-MS), or to a physical therapist who can design an exercise regimen that meets your specific needs and limitations. (Take a look at Chapter 11 for more information about exercise and MS.)

Relaxation strategies don't burn up a lot of calories, but they're great for relieving stress. You may need to try a few before you find the one that works best for you. Keep in mind that learning to relax takes practice, so it generally takes a month or so to really get the benefits. Here are some strategies you can try:

- **Deep breathing exercises:** The great thing about deep breathing is that it can be done anywhere, any time. We recommend that you start and end your day with some relaxed, comfortable deep breathing. Also, spend a few extra minutes breathing deeply any time you're feeling particularly stressed out.

- **Visualization:** This exercise involves clearing your mind of everything except for the one scene you want to focus on. Pick a scene that's filled with pleasurable stimuli—your favorite beach, a beautiful park, mountains covered with snow—and enjoy your "visit." You need to be able carve out several minutes in a quiet place for this relaxation exercise to work properly.

  When practicing visualization, we suggest starting with a few cycles of deep breathing. Then spend five to ten minutes experiencing as many details of your scene as you possibly can—the sights, sounds, smells, and anything else that your imagination can conjure up.

- **Meditation:** For those of you who find visualization to be a piece of cake, meditation is the next

317

step. The goal of meditation is to concentrate on a particular word, phrase, or sound (called a *mantra*), which you repeat silently or aloud over and over again. To meditate properly, you need a good 15 to 20 minutes a couple of times a day (preferably on a consistent schedule).

With practice, you can use the focused repetition of meditation to block out other thoughts, sights, and sounds. The word or sound you choose to repeat doesn't matter as long as it's something soothing and comforting. Being able to remain focused for more than a couple of minutes takes quite a bit of practice, but the payoff is a real sense of calm.

- **Progressive muscle relaxation:** Relaxing each of your 17 muscle groups in sequence is a great way to get your whole body into a comfortable and relaxed state. You can do this exercise sitting in a chair or lying on your bed. Either way, the process involves tensing and relaxing individual parts of your body and taking the time to notice how the changes feel. You can start from the top and work your way down or you can start from your fingers and toes and move inward toward the center of your body. Whatever you do, don't forget the small parts, such as your eyes, tongue, and jaw. Progressive relaxation makes for a relaxing start to the day and a peaceful way to prepare your body for sleep.

  If you have significant *spasticity* (stiffness) in certain muscles, tensing them may cause a spasm. Ask your neurologist or physical therapist for recommendations on how to best exercise those muscle groups. (Take a look at Chapter 7 for more information about spasticity.)

Developing effective stress management techniques takes time, practice, and patience. If you find it difficult to get into any of the techniques, or if you continue to feel stressed out in spite of your best efforts, you may want to consult an expert. The National MS Society (800-FIGHT-MS) can refer you to a mental health professional (such as a psychologist, social worker, or counselor) in your area who can help you find ways to manage your stresses more comfortably. Also, check out the National MS Society booklet, *Taming Stress in MS* for detailed instructions (www.nationalmssociety.org/brochures-tamingstress1.asp).

319

Chapter 13

Coping with Advanced MS

*Y*ou may be wondering whether you should read this chapter. If that's the case for you, check out the following pointers: If your multiple sclerosis (MS) is galloping along at a rapid clip and causing you a lot of problems, you definitely want to spend some time on this chapter. If, however, you're an MS "beginner," don't feel like you have to read this chapter right now. In fact, you may never need to read it. It's simply here for those folks—and their family members—who need and want to explore the grittier side of MS. When we say gritty, we mean when the disease progresses in spite of everyone's best efforts and when symptoms are tougher to manage. Even though we're happy to say that the majority of people with MS don't ever become severely disabled, we also know very well that saying so is little comfort for those who do.

So, if your MS is feeling too hot to handle, this chapter is specifically for you. We talk about the options you have in terms of treatment, and we provide ideas for making your environment as MS-friendly as possible. We also give you tips for avoiding uncomfortable and potentially dangerous complications. Finally, we spend some time talking about support and care options for those of you who are having difficulty managing things at home. In case you're a family member or friend who's providing care for someone you love, we end this chapter with some important tips for you.

Scouting Out the Treatment Scene

Chances are high that the first question on your mind is about the treatment options for your progressive MS. Before we get to your answer, though, we want to remind you that four disease types or "courses" have been identified in MS (you can read about them in Chapter 1). The vast majority of people are initially diagnosed with a *relapsing-remitting* course that's characterized by periodic attacks (relapses) followed by periods of remission. Other people experience a more steadily progressive course from the very beginning.

But, whether you were diagnosed with relapsing-remitting MS that eventually became more steadily progressive, or your MS has been progressive from the outset, the treatment scene is nowhere near as crowded as we would like it to be. We're optimistic, however, that some of the drugs currently under study will turn out to be safe and effective options.

Understanding your disease-management options

Here's the deal: All six disease-modifying medications that are approved by the U.S. Food and Drug Administration (FDA) to treat MS have been shown to be effective for people who experience relapses (flip to Chapter 6 for a description of these medications). So, as long as you continue to have relapses, you're still a good candidate for most, if not all, of these medications. However, the evidence is pretty strong that these medications have their greatest impact early in the disease, primarily by reducing the number and severity of relapses. The following sections show you your options if you aren't a candidate for the disease-modifying medications.

Options for people who don't have relapses

If you don't have relapses—that is if you have *primary-progressive MS* (and have never had relapses) or *secondary-progressive MS* (and used to have relapses but no longer do)—your options are much more limited. Novantrone (mitoxantrone) is the only one of the six medications that has been approved for people with secondary-progressive MS whether or not they continue to have relapses. And to date, no medication has been found to be effective for primary-progressive MS. That doesn't mean that those of you with progressive disease are out in the cold, however.

If your MS appears to be progressing significantly in spite of whatever treatments have already been tried, your neurologist may recommend a chemotherapy drug, such as Imuran (azathioprine), Cytoxan (cyclophosphamide), or methotrexate. Even though none of these medications has been specifically approved for use in MS, doctors have found that they may help to slow the disease course

322

Other valuable resources for dealing with your progressive MS

Here are some books that can help you decide how to best handle your progressive disease:

✔ *Meeting the Challenge of Progressive Multiple Sclerosis* by Patricia K. Coyle and June Halper (Demos Medical Publishing, 2001).

✔ *Multiple Sclerosis: A Self-Care Guide to Wellness,* 2nd edition, edited by Nancy Holland and June Halper (Demos Medical Publishing, 2005).

✔ *Multiple Sclerosis: The Questions You Have; The Answers You Need,* 3rd edition, edited by Rosalind Kalb (Demos Medical Publishing, 2004).

In addition, the National MS Society offers several brochures that deal with progressive disease. You can download the publications from www.nationalmssociety.org/majorchanges or you can request them by calling (800) FIGHT-MS (800-344-4867).

for some people.

These medications—like Novantrone—are *immunosuppressants* that are also used to treat various forms of cancer. Because these meds work by suppressing the entire immune system (rather than selected parts of the immune system as occurs with the five *immunomodulating therapies*), they all carry a certain degree of risk. The risks include infection, impaired fertility, and heightened risk of certain types of cancer.

Another strategy recommended by some MS neurologists is *pulse steroid treatment,* which involves intravenous infusion of 1,000 mg of methylprednisolone once a month for

323

a period of 6 to 24 months.

Because the research evidence for the chemotherapy drugs and for pulse steroids isn't conclusive, and none have been specifically approved by the FDA for use in MS, your insurance company may not be willing to cover them.

Experimental options for very active MS

You may also hear or read about a couple of experimental treatments that are being used to control very active, progressive MS, so we want to give you a heads-up about what they are. One option is *bone marrow transplantation*. This is a procedure in which your immune cells—including those that are thought to be causing damage in your central nervous system—are destroyed and then replaced using immune stem cells from your bone marrow. Another option is a process called *plasmapheresis*. In this procedure, the plasma in your blood, which is thought to contain certain immune factors that are stimulating your MS, is replaced with healthy plasma.

Each of these highly invasive treatments has been studied in small numbers of people with mixed results. Because they both pose significant risks and are still considered experimental, they may not be reimbursable by most insurance policies.

The fact that the available medications aren't particularly helpful for progressive MS doesn't mean that you have no other options. On the contrary, this is the time to call in the troops. A healthcare team—particularly one at an MS care center that's staffed by specialists—has a great deal to offer people like you who have more advanced disease. In the following sections we give you lots of tips for taking the best possible care of yourself.

324

Exploring ways to feel and function at your best

The goal of treating MS is to help you feel and function well. So, together, you and your healthcare team can identify and implement strategies to manage your symptoms and keep you active, comfortable, and safe.

Managing your symptoms

Comprehensive symptom management is essential to feeling and functioning well. So, if your doctor says that nothing more can be done to control your symptoms, find a different doctor—pronto. There are medications and management strategies to address virtually every symptom of MS (check out Chapters 7, 8, and 9 for full discussions of the symptoms and the ways to manage them). Even though you can't totally eliminate your symptoms, you and your healthcare providers can work together to identify the strategy (or combination of strategies) that provides you with the greatest relief and comfort. The right strategy (or combination of strategies) also helps to prevent problems like infection, bone loss, and joint problems (see the section "Taking steps to prevent unnecessary complications" a little later in the chapter for more).

Working with the rehabilitation specialists

Rehabilitation is particularly valuable if and when your disease starts to progress significantly. Depending on the level of intervention you need, you may receive rehabilitative services on an outpatient or inpatient basis. For example, your neurologist may refer you to a physical therapist (PT) or an occupational therapist (OT) for a certain number of outpatient sessions, which are followed up by a personalized program for you to implement at home. Or, you may be referred for a 10- to 14-day inpatient stay at a rehabilitation facility. At a rehab facility, you'll receive a thorough assessment by each member of the rehabilitation team, and then you'll go through intensive therapy in each area. The program is typically followed up with a personalized at-home regimen.

All of the members of the rehabilitation team are working together to help you maintain the highest possible level of function and comfort, given whatever limitations you may have. (Flip to Chapter 4 for a complete look at the members of the rehabilitation team.)

Staying healthy

When your MS starts taking a lot of your time, energy, and focus, you may find that you have a tendency to neglect other aspects of your health. You may find that because you see your MS doctor fairly frequently, you begin to rely on the neurologist or nurse for your general healthcare as well. But, we know from published research data that this strategy doesn't work very well. People who see MS specialist neurologists for all of their care have been found to be in less good health than their peers who also see their internist or family physician in addition to their MS docs.

So, remember that even though your neurologist will be paying close attention to your MS needs, he or she will probably not be checking your weight, blood pressure, cholesterol, blood sugar, and other health parameters. Nor will your neurologist be reminding you about the health screening measures recommended for your age group (for example, chest x-rays, ECGs, mammograms, prostate exams, and colonoscopies).

Having MS doesn't protect you from developing other health problems. Like the general population, most people with MS die of cancer, heart disease, and stroke. Because of this similarity to the general population, you need to take

326

the same care of your health as anyone else (see Chapter 11 for more on taking care of your general health).

Taking steps to prevent unnecessary complications

By now, one of your friends or family members has probably mentioned to you that he or she knew someone who died of MS. Don't let that scare you. Even though in rare cases death can result from a virulent, rapidly progressive form of MS or from severe complications in people with advanced MS, most people who have the disease die from cancer, heart disease, and stroke like everyone else.

The primary MS health risks are caused by preventable complications including

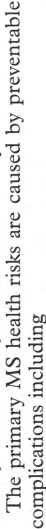
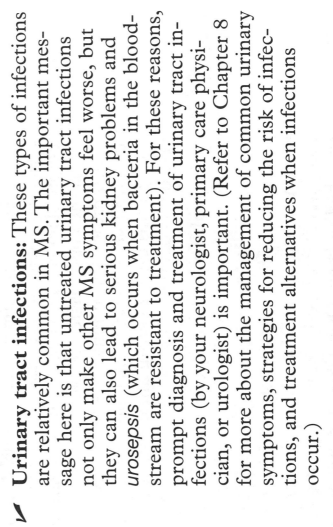

✔ **Urinary tract infections:** These types of infections are relatively common in MS. The important message here is that untreated urinary tract infections not only make other MS symptoms feel worse, but they can also lead to serious kidney problems and *urosepsis* (which occurs when bacteria in the bloodstream are resistant to treatment). For these reasons, prompt diagnosis and treatment of urinary tract infections (by your neurologist, primary care physician, or urologist) is important. (Refer to Chapter 8 for more about the management of common urinary symptoms, strategies for reducing the risk of infections, and treatment alternatives when infections occur.)

✔ **Spasticity (stiffness):** This symptom is a common one in MS (see Chapter 7). When left untreated, spasticity can lead to *contracture*, or "freezing" of the joints, which is a painful and debilitating problem.

327

The best way to avoid contracture is to use a regimen of stretching (and medication, if needed) to keep your joints flexible. Your neurologist and physical therapist can recommend the appropriate treatment strategies for you.

✔ **Dysphagia:** Some people with MS develop *dysphagia* (problems with swallowing). Coughing or choking while eating may be a sign that you're developing a swallowing problem. It's important to report these kinds of changes to your physician promptly because when left untreated, swallowing problems can lead to *aspiration pneumonia*, which is caused when food particles travel into the lungs rather than through the esophagus and into the stomach where they belong. This, like all types of pneumonia, can be serious, debilitating, and potentially dangerous. A speech/language pathologist can assess the type and severity of the problem you're having, and he or she can recommend the appropriate interventions.

Also important to remember is that people who have trouble swallowing may not get adequate nutrition. In this case, a consultation with a nutritionist may be recommended.

✔ **Skin problems:** If you spend extended periods of time in a scooter, wheelchair, or bed, you need to take particularly good care of your skin because you're at risk for *pressure sores* (which are also known as bed sores). These sores appear when various parts of your body are in constant contact with your bed or chair. Over time, this pressure restricts blood flow, resulting in damage to the skin in those areas. The buttocks and heels are particularly vulnerable to pressure sores, as are any bony areas, such as hips, elbows, and ankles.

328

So, if you're experiencing significant mobility impairment, it's important to check your skin carefully every day for signs of redness or irritation. Report any changes to your doctor immediately. The best way to deal with pressure sores is to prevent them from happening in the first place by making sure you lift your butt (or other part of your body) off the bed or chair every hour or so. Keeping your skin dry, but moisturized can also help. Just remember that after sores develop, they can be difficult to heal and threatening to your health.

- **Osteoporosis:** The risk of osteoporosis (the thinning of your bones) is increased for anyone with limited mobility who gets insufficient amounts of weight-bearing exercise. Frequent use of corticosteroids is also known to increase the risk of osteoporosis. So, if you spend significant amounts of time in a wheelchair or scooter (or if you take corticosteroids often), it's a good idea to get a baseline bone density evaluation, which is generally done by a radiologist, and you should have periodic screenings thereafter. Also make sure that you're taking in the recommended amount of calcium (Chapter 11 has the information you need about calcium intake and dietary recommendations).

- **Depression:** Keep in mind that the primary cause of suicide in MS is untreated or undertreated depression. So, given that depression is very common in MS, and that the suicide rate in MS is significantly higher than in the general population, it's important for you to remember that depression is one of the disease's most treatable symptoms. Don't hesitate to get whatever help you need. (Take a look at Chapter 9 for a discussion of depression and mood swings.)

While the risk of these complications is real, the good news is that doctors now have the know-how to prevent many unnecessary complications of MS. And with the advent of antibiotics, the infections (for example, urinary tract and kidney infections, as well as pneumonia) that once were fatal for many people are now much more easily treated.

Maintaining Your Quality of Life

The phrase "quality of life" means different things to different people. For example, what's important in your life may differ from what's important in someone else's life. The challenge, however, is the same for everyone who's dealing with the more advanced symptoms of MS: Find ways to keep life full, active, and satisfying despite whatever symptoms you may have. So, in this section, we offer some strategies for doing just that.

Holding on to what's important to you

Unfortunately, some people have a tendency to give up activities when they can no longer do them the way they used to. You may, for example, give up skiing because your balance and energy aren't what they used to be. Then, you may find that long walks with your partner are a lot more difficult and tiring than they used to be. And then you may decide that you can't really take your kids to the zoo anymore. Finally, one day, you realize you've given up a whole lot of things that made your life fun, full, and interesting.

Even though you may think you have to give up all the good stuff, we propose a different strategy: Figure out ways to do your favorite activities differently by using *assistive technology* (AT), or try out some alternative activities that may be just as satisfying. We know doing things differently is tough—so that's why we spend so much time talking about grieving in Chapter 3.

If you already have a "tool chest" of gadgets to help you do the things you want to do—congratulations—just keep adding to it. But, if you don't have that tool chest yet, your rehab team can help you figure out exactly what kinds of tools would work best for you (check out Chapter 7 for more on AT and Chapter 4 for more on the rehab team). We knew a man who kept his "tool chest" in the trunk of his car. Each day he'd think about the activities on his schedule, and he'd use whichever tool—cane, crutches, walker—that best fit the bill. In other words, he let the activities determine the tools instead of trying to make any one tool meet all of his needs.

The fact is that people with MS *do* enjoy adaptive skiing and other modified sports. Moms and dads *can* enjoy watching a soccer game or going to the zoo in a motorized scooter. A cruise *can* be just as much fun as trekking in Tibet. The key is recognizing that, even though the activities may be different or you may have to do them differently, they can still be part of a full and rewarding life.

Stay in touch: Preserving your connections with other people

Most social interactions are built around shared activities and interests. For example, you may go out to dinner with certain friends and play golf or go on trips with others. So, as you can imagine, when the activities are challenged, the relationships with these people may be challenged as well. When you find yourself in a situation like this, you may be worried about slowing everyone else down, being a nuisance, or feeling uncomfortable (even though you shouldn't!). Your friends may also feel awkward, or they may even shy away from you when the usual basis for the relationship is altered.

When your activity-level changes, you need to take the lead: Reach out to your friends and suggest alternative plans. Most often, when you do this, you'll find that your friends care more about you than they do about the activity, and they're usually happy to do things differently or a bit more slowly if they know it helps you. You may also find that they're perfectly willing to participate in another activity altogether. In the case of those people who care more about the activity than they do about you and your well-being—well, they probably weren't such good friends to begin with.

Establishing goals and enjoying the satisfaction of meeting them

Everyone needs to have goals. The satisfying process of setting achievable goals and meeting them is what allows you to feel productive, useful, and successful. If your MS progresses, you may find that some of your original life goals need to be tweaked or even changed entirely. You may, for example, need to alter your career ambitions (perhaps by becoming a school administrator rather than a classroom teacher or a music teacher rather than a performer) or trade competitive team sports for individual sports. The first step in making these kinds of transitions is healthy grieving. In other words, before you can identify and work toward new goals, you need to allow yourself to feel sad about the old ones (see Chapter 3 for more details on grieving). After you've dealt with your losses, you can begin to think about and experiment with some new possibilities. The key is to always have something to strive for—something that energizes you and taps your talents and creativity.

332

If you find yourself running out of ideas for goal-setting, think about speaking with a mental health professional to help you get started.

Keeping your self-image well-polished

People with more advanced MS can sometimes lose sight of who they are when the disease begins to affect them in so many different ways. They may begin to question their value to themselves and others.

If you find yourself starting to have these kinds of thoughts, take a careful look at that jigsaw puzzle picture of yourself that we talk about in Chapter 3. You're made up of many pieces—you have qualities, interests, abilities, and quirks that you've acquired over a lifetime. Even though MS may have affected many areas of your life, chances are high that those unique parts of you are still there. Your challenge, then, lies in figuring out new ways to engage those special parts of you.

If you're having trouble getting started, have a heart-to-heart with a few of your close family members, friends, and colleagues. They'll be happy to remind you what they love about you, what qualities and talents you share with them every day, and how you can still provide them with help and support in their daily lives. And if you need some suggestions about how to get these conversations started, consider doing a little prep work with a therapist or counselor (check out Chapter 4 for more info on mental health professionals).

Finding your "MS-free zone"

If and when you start to feel as though MS is affecting every part of your life, you need to go on a treasure hunt. The prize is your MS-free zone—that part of you that MS just can't touch. This part is different for every person: It may be your love of music, sense of humor, spirituality, passion for soap operas, or any one of the zillion other things that tend to make people happy. Your MS-free zone is simply a refuge from the demands of MS—a place where you can go to regroup when life feels overwhelming. Your zone is a valuable resource because it can give you the emotional energy you need to tackle the difficult stuff that goes along with the disease.

So, think about what moments in your day or week give you the greatest sense of freedom and relief. You'll know when you've found your MS-free zone because you won't be able to wait to go there periodically for a "breather," and you'll feel energized by your time there.

 If you're having trouble getting in touch with your MS-free zone, your friends and family may be able to help you figure out what it is. If they can't, contact a good mental health professional for assistance.

Helping yourself by helping someone else

Sometimes helping someone else is the best way to take your mind off of what ails you. Many people with MS have told us how much better they feel when they know they're doing something that makes a difference to other people, whether at home or at their jobs, in a support group of some kind, or doing volunteer work. Volunteer opportunities come in all shapes and sizes. You can, among so many others, help out at your kid's school, support a political candidate, visit the elderly in nursing homes, provide rides for someone who can no longer drive, read to someone with a visual impairment, or serve meals in a homeless shelter.

If you're interested in doing some kind of volunteer work but haven't found what you're looking for, think about contacting VolunteerMatch (www.volunteermatch.org), which is a national nonprofit organization that's dedicated to

How much of you is your MS?

If you want to know how much space MS takes up in your life, here's an exercise to try: Draw a large circle that represents you and your life. Now shade in the area of the circle that is your MS. Is it just a tiny wedge of your pie or is it a giant-sized portion? Is it a bigger part of you and your life than you want it to be? Can you think of any ways to turn it into a more manageable piece? Do you think it's the disease itself or your feelings and attitudes about it that are taking up so much space? If you're having difficulty answering these questions, you may want to consider talking them over with family members, other people with MS, or a mental health counselor. These folks may be able to help you get back in touch with those non-MS parts of yourself.

helping people find a great place to volunteer. Volunteer-Match offers an online searchable database of volunteer opportunities to help you find an organization to volunteer with. This site also provides other features and services, such as personalized alert e-mails that list new opportunities in your area.

You can also call the National MS Society at (800) FIGHT-MS (800-344-4867) to find out what volunteer opportunities your National MS Society chapter may offer. The Society is a volunteer-driven organization that thrives on the talents of people just like you.

Discovering Long-Term Care Services (Just In Case)

Like many people, you probably find the idea of long-term care to be really scary. Over the years, many, many people with MS have asked each one of us, "Am I going to end up in a nursing home?" The short answer is that the vast majority of people don't. However, a person with MS may need assistance—sometimes more than their family members can handle alone. So, in this section, we talk about some of the options that people have for getting the services they need at home and elsewhere. We urge you to plow ahead even though reading about this topic may be uncomfortable.

Knowing the types of long-term care available can help you and your family members figure out what works best for all of you now, and in the future should your needs change. Knowing your options helps you feel more in control and more prepared. The last thing you want to do is make a difficult long-term care decision during a crisis, when you don't have your wits about you. And, remember, if your situation stabilizes and you find that your care needs don't increase, you haven't lost anything except the time it took you to have these discussions. (Chapter 20 gives you financial planning tips to help you feel more prepared for whatever comes down the pike).

We strongly urge you to work as a team with your family members when making long-term plans and decisions so that no one feels left out of the process. This helps to ensure that everyone's questions, feelings, and concerns can be heard and dealt with. If you find it difficult to begin the conversation, get some help: Your neurologist, nurse, or the National MS Society (call 800-FIGHT-MS) can help you think through the options and identify good facilities in your area. A mental health professional can help your family talk with each other more comfortably, ensuring that each person's feelings and ideas get to be heard. This shouldn't be a conversation about who's doing what to whom—it should be about what options work best for all of you.

Defining long-term care

The term *long-term care* refers to a wide range of services designed to help you or a family member carry out daily life activities. These services run the gamut from housekeeping help, personal assistance in your home, adult day health programs, and respite care to community assisted living options and nursing home care. The number of options available may seem a bit mind-blowing, so keep in mind that you can use the expertise of professionals called *care managers* (also referred to as care coordinators or case managers). These professionals can help you sort it all out, generally on a fee-for-service basis. Care managers specialize in information and referral, patient advocacy, and coordination of health and social services. In other words, they can be your eyes and ears in the search for community resources and your navigator as you sort out options and make decisions. For information about local care manager options, contact the National MS Society at (800) FIGHT-MS.

Most of the services we talk about here have traditionally been geared toward the elderly. Not too surprisingly, younger adults with disabilities want opportunities to socialize with people their own age, to participate in age-appropriate activities, to have access to the most up-to-date computer technology, and to be able to choose from the kinds of menus that appeal to them. The good news is that a lot of progress has been made toward identifying the unique needs of younger folks with disabilities. You can call the National MS Society at (800) FIGHT-MS for help in identifying whatever resources in your area may be more suited to your needs.

Getting help in your home

When looking for help in your home, the two primary op-

337

tions are hiring someone from a community home care agency or finding someone on your own. Although each option has advantages and disadvantages as well as different cost implications, a home helper generally offers the following services:

☛ Companionship and supervision

☛ Assistance with basic housekeeping tasks, including light cleaning, cooking, and errands

☛ Personal care, including assistance with dressing, bathing, going to the bathroom, and grooming

☛ Nursing care, including help with medications and certain kinds of medical procedures

☛ Rehabilitation services, including physical therapy, occupational therapy, speech/language therapy, and social work services

For some great tips on how to hire help at home, check out *Hiring Help at Home: The Basic Facts* at www .nationalmssociety.org/hiringhelp as well as the information for family caregivers provided by the National Association for Home Care & Hospice at www.nahc.org/famcare giver.html.

Looking into adult day care

Adult day programs, which are sponsored by various community agencies, provide a range of social and wellness programs, as well as some personal care. The services available in adult day programs generally include:

☛ Meals

☛ Social activities

Long-term care resources

It wasn't too many years ago that people facing long-term care decisions had no resources to help them. Rest assured that the National MS Society (800-FIGHT-MS or 800-344-4867) is aware of community resources and is happy to help you and your family members with any decisions you have to make. You can also get valuable information from the following resources:

Agencies

✔ The National Association of Professional Geriatric Care Managers (phone: 520-881- 8008; Web site: www.caremanager .org)

✔ The National Adult Day Services Association (NADSA) (phone: 800-558-5301; Web site: www.nadsa.org)

✔ The National Center for Assisted Living (NCAL) (phone: 202-842-4444; Web site: www.ncal.org)

✔ The American Association of Homes & Services for the Aging (AAHSA) (phone: 202- 783-2242; Web site: www.aahsa.org)

Books

✔ In *Multiple Sclerosis: The Questions You Have; The Answers You Need*, 3rd edition, edited by Rosalind Kalb (Demos Medical Publishing, 2004), you can find a section on long-term care by D. Frankel on pp. 407–425.

✔ In *Multiple Sclerosis: A Guide for Families*, 3rd edition, edited by Rosalind Kalb (Demos Medical Publishing, 2006), you can find a section on planning wisely for possible care needs on pp.169–180.

- Rehabilitation therapies

- Counseling

- Personal care

- Nursing assistance

To check out the National MS Society's Guidelines on adult day care services, call (800) FIGHT-MS or go to www.nationalmssociety.org/prcpublications.

Identifying assisted living options

Many communities have assisted living residences where a person who needs help with daily activities can receive individualized support and healthcare services. The goal of these facilities is to provide people with the assistance they need while at the same time ensuring them safety and as much independence as possible. Assisted living residences typically provide the following services:

- A call system for emergencies

- Meals in a common area, if needed or wanted

- Housekeeping

- Transportation to doctor appointments and social events

- Medication management

- Health promotion programs

- Social programs

Assisted living residences may offer single rooms, studio apartments, or larger apartments, and they may stand alone or be part of a larger healthcare facility that offers various

340

types of living and care options. You can get the National MS Society's guidelines on assisted living by calling (800) FIGHT-MS or on the Web site at www.nationalmssociety.org/prcpublications.

Considering nursing home care

Nursing home care is an option when you feel that you've exhausted all other possibilities. Even though no one wants to think about moving into a nursing facility, you may find it comforting to know that they exist if safe care at home is simply no longer possible. As difficult as it may be to believe, a good nursing home can sometimes enhance the quality of life for someone with severe disabilities. Some of the benefits of nursing home care include

✔ Twenty-four hour care by qualified staff members

✔ Opportunities to participate in social and recreational programs

✔ A sense of safety and security that's no longer possible at home

✔ Assistance for a family member whose health and well-being are being severely affected by caregiving activities

The National MS Society's guidelines for nursing home care are available by calling (800) FIGHT-MS or at www.nationalmssociety.org/prcpublications.

Important Tips for Caregivers

This section is for those of you who are caring for a loved one with MS. Particularly as a person's MS progresses, the medical team's focus will increasingly be on his or her med-

341

ical, psychological, and social needs. So, you may find yourself feeling "out in the cold"—and rightly so. MS literature sometimes refers to caregivers, particularly partners in the caregiving role, as "the invisible patient" because their needs tend to go unnoticed. Because you may be the sole supporter of your own cause, here are some important things that you can do to ensure your own health and well-being:

- ✔ **Remember that your physical and emotional health are just as important as your partner's.** The caregiving role is both demanding and draining, and we know that caregivers tend to neglect their own health while caring for the other person. If you have trouble remembering to take care of yourself, keep in mind the flight attendant's message on every flight: "If you're traveling with a child or someone needing assistance, put your own oxygen mask on first and then assist the other person." In others words, you can't be of much help to someone else if you don't first take care of yourself. So, make sure you

  - Follow the recommended health prevention and screening measures for your age group.

  - Carve out time for your own relaxation and recreation.

  - Seek out support for yourself as needed.

- ✔ **Speak up on your own behalf.** Particularly if your partner's MS becomes more advanced, the physician may recommend a treatment or strategy that involves you, without spending a lot of time thinking about the treatment's impact on your life, health, or comfort. For example, the doctor may recommend that you assist with a stretching regimen or with the

342

other person's medications. Or, he or she may suggest that you help with the activities of daily living, such as bathing, dressing, or going to the bathroom.

If, because of your own work schedule, health needs, or other issues, you feel that you can't follow the doctor's recommendations, it's important to say so. It doesn't do anyone any good when the doctor recommends an intervention that isn't workable. Either the doctor or the National MS Society (800-FIGHT-MS) can work with you to figure out what resources you can tap for assistance.

➤ **Learn how to ask for help from others.** The best strategy when asking for help is to be specific. Instead of saying to your relative, friend, or neighbor, "I really need some help," you'll get far better results by being more specific. No one can read your mind, and most people don't want to risk offending you by guessing. So, instead, try "I'd like to get out to do some errands on Friday—could you stay with Jim from 2 p.m. to 4 p.m. so I don't have to worry about leaving him alone?" Or, "Jane needs to get to the doctor next Monday at 3 p.m. and I have to be out of town. Could you possibly take her?" Most people are happy to help when they know what you need and when.

➤ **Don't assume you can do it all alone.** Depending on your partner's needs, you may need to consider hiring some additional assistance. You can choose from a variety of types and levels of assistance that are available from outside agencies (check out the section "Discovering Long-Term Care Services" earlier in the chapter for details). The members of your healthcare team or the National MS Society can help you identify assistance options in your area.

343

➤ **Let others know that this is about you too.** You may get awfully tired of hearing "Oh, how's Mary doing?" or "What's the doctor saying about Hank's MS these days?" People tend to forget that MS involves the whole family, not just the person who has it. It may not be worth it for those who ask in passing, but it's important to let the people closest to you know that you'd like them to ask about you too. You can generally get the ball rolling by putting a word in here and there about yourself. Or, you can just be dead honest and say something like, "You know, it would really make me feel good if you could ask me how I'm doing too, because even though Steve is the one with MS, I'm living with it too!"

B.

For some great additional resources, check out Appendix

344

Part IV
Managing Lifestyle Issues

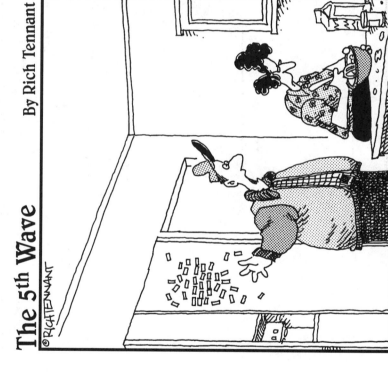

The 5th Wave   By Rich Tennant

"It's been two months since your diagnosis, and I know you're reluctant to talk about it. But we've got to start discussing it in some way other than messages left on the refrigerator with these tiny word magnets."

In this part . . .

This part is all about the important relationships in your life. You may be the one with the diagnosis and the symptoms, but there are people at home and at work who care about you and are affected by what's going on with you. Most folks will take their cue from you, so in this part we give you lots of suggestions about how to talk with others about your multiple sclerosis. We also guide you through some of the family and parenting issues that are likely to come up along the way.

Chapter 14

Presenting Your MS Face to the World

In This Chapter

▲ Educating others about your MS

▲ Talking about your MS in a dating situation

▲ Communicating the amount of help you need

You probably thought that dealing with your own feelings about being diagnosed with multiple sclerosis (MS) was hard enough. Well, guess what? You have to deal with everyone else's feelings as well. This task wouldn't be so difficult if all the people in your life reacted in the same way, or if you could predict what the various responses might be. But, the reality is that each person's response reflects his or her personality, communication style, emotional reactions to the news, and—most importantly—knowledge about MS. So, you need to be prepared to educate, explain, comfort, and reassure (or whatever else is called for). The bottom line, however, is that people will take their cues from you: The way you see your MS and present it to the world is the way they'll tend to see it too.

Explaining Your MS to Others

The first step in preparing yourself to deal with the reactions of others is to put on your teaching hat. If you want others to understand you and your MS, you're the one who's going to have to educate them.

Providing the basics

A person's knowledge of MS can range from nothing at all ("What's that? Oh, it's that telethon disease, right?") to know-it-all ("You really need to go to Timbuktu for that cure I read about last week on the Internet—it's a miracle!" or "Oh, I know what that is. My aunt has had it for 50 years and you could never tell it to look at her!" or "My friend's mother has that and she's in a nursing home."). So, you need to be ready to tell people what MS is and isn't, and how it's affecting you and your life.

Like any other teacher, you need to start by learning your subject. Educating yourself—with this book and the other helpful resources that are out there (see Appendix B)—prepares you to answer questions and correct misinformation.

The National Multiple Sclerosis Society, as you may already know, is one valuable resource. Brochures describing virtually every aspect of life with multiple sclerosis are available from the Society's Web site at www.nationalms

---

In this chapter, we talk about tricky stuff, such as how to deal with the person who starts crying about your MS, the one who tells you all about what happened to her best friend's cousin, or the friend who doesn't say anything at all. We also suggest ways to ask for help and how to politely turn it down, and we discuss when and how to talk about MS with someone you're dating. (Check out Chapter 17 for advice on how to talk about MS with your children.)

348

society.org/brochures or by calling (800) FIGHT-MS (800-344-4867). *What Everyone Should Know About Multiple Sclerosis* (suitable for the whole family), *What Is Multiple Sclerosis?*, and *Living with MS* are great brochures to give to anyone who has a lot of questions or gives you that "deer-in-headlights" look.

One of the most important pieces of information to share with others is that MS is a variable and unpredictable disease that affects each person differently. So, after you've given them the basic information about MS (which you can either describe in your own words or provide via print materials), the next task is to tell them about *your* MS. Here are some tips:

- ➤ **Clarify for people that you're not one of "Jerry's Kids."** The Jerry Lewis Telethon is for muscular dystrophy, which is a neuromuscular disease that primarily affects children. Instead, remind them that multiple sclerosis is thought to be an autoimmune disease that affects the central nervous system, primarily in adults.

- ➤ **Explain that MS affects different people in different ways.** Tell them that although some people with MS become severely disabled, most don't. Emphasize that your MS is your own and that nobody else's will be exactly the same.

- ➤ **Reassure those who burst into tears.** People may burst into tears just when you're feeling a bit in need of comfort yourself. Reassure them that several effective medications are available to treat MS and that you're doing all the recommended things to take care of yourself. You can also tell them that it's okay to spend the next five minutes feeling sad together, but then you'd much prefer to talk about the other stuff that's going on in your life and theirs. This is particularly helpful when you just don't have the emotional energy to cheer someone else up about your disease.

✔ **Depending on how much information you're looking to share, you can describe the ways that MS affects you.** This is a good opportunity to explain how variable symptoms can be from morning to evening or from one day to the next. You also want to give people a feel for some of those symptoms they can't readily see, such as severe fatigue, numbness or tingling, pain, or problems with attention or memory.

If they're interested in finding out more about any of the symptoms you have, or other symptoms that a person with MS might have, you can offer them a booklet from the National MS Society (for example, *Fatigue: What You Should Know, Gait or Walking Problems: The Basic Facts,* or *Vision Problems: The Basic Facts*).

✔ **Dodge fad "cures" and "miracle" drugs.** In response to well-meaning advice about what medications to take, cures to try, or foods to eat or not eat, the best strategy is usually to explain that you and your neurologist are working together to choose the best management strategies for your particular disease course and symptoms.

Dealing with common reactions

Even though you can't predict exactly how the people in your life are likely to respond to your MS diagnosis, you're likely to encounter some fairly common reactions at one time or another from family, friends, and colleagues. Here are some suggestions for how to deal with them.

350

Handling "How are you?"

People ask the question "How are you?" many times a day, often without even thinking about it. However, now when you hear it, it may not feel like such a simple question any more. When someone asks you how you are, it will be up to you to decide how much they really want to know and how much you want to say. Read on for some clues.

The fact is that most people who ask don't really care—they're just being polite and making small talk. So, we recommend not wasting your energy trying to tell them the truth if it's going to take a while. If you suddenly launch into a detailed account of what does and doesn't feel good that day, most people will be pretty startled. So, for the folks who are just making polite conversation, a simple "fine, thanks" should do the trick.

For the people close to you, who really do want to know how things are going, you have some options: If there's time, and you're in the mood, you can fill them in. If you're busy doing or thinking about other things and don't want to be distracted by your MS at the moment, you can say something like, "Let's get a cup of coffee later and I'll fill you in on all the gritty details." Or, a simple "Pretty much the same" works, too.

But what about those people who gaze at you mournfully and say "How are you?" as though you're at death's door? You need to decide whether the person who's asking is someone who really cares about you and how you're doing or just likes hearing about someone else's problems. Many people find it easiest to just say (with a surprised, quizzical look) "Why fine, thanks! How about yourself?"

Fielding the "But you look so good!" comment

Just when you're hoping that the important people in your life get what you're saying about your MS, you're likely to

351

hear this very common response from family members, friends, and colleagues: "But you look so good!" Figuring out how to respond to this double-edged sword can pose quite a challenge. On the one hand, it's always nice to know that others think you look good. On the other hand, this is a tough comment to hear when you're feeling really crummy—exhausted, numb and tingly, or weak as a wet noodle. Interpreting the underlying message of this comment is even tougher. Is the person trying to reassure and encourage you? Or is the real message a bit of a dig: "You look too good to be sick, so why aren't you doing all the things I need you to do for me?"

Your best strategy for responding to this comment is probably to try and sort out the underlying message before giving a response. If the person is an acquaintance or someone with whom you don't have a close family or working relationship, you may just want to say "thank you" and move on. If, however, it's someone close to you, who needs to understand that there's more to MS than meets the eye, you may want to consider the following options:

- ✔ "I'm afraid that what you see isn't always what you get! I wish I felt as good on the inside as I seem to look on the outside. Unfortunately, MS has a lot of symptoms that don't show."

- ✔ "Thanks—but today's not one of my better days. Could I have rain check, please? This MS fatigue is really killing me. Maybe we could postpone our dinner for another night."

- ✔ "I know I promised to take you to the mall today, but my vision is too blurry to drive right now. Let's see whether it's better tomorrow after I've had a chance to rest, and we can try then."

✔ "The heat and humidity are really getting to me—I feel like I can hardly move. Would you mind if we had the meeting in my office where it's cooler? Plus, that saves me from having to walk all the way to the conference room."

The key here is that you're the teacher, so decide how much information you want to share, and be prepared to explain some of the less visible ways MS can affect you.

Responding to unsolicited advice

Whether you want it or not, you're likely to get a lot of advice from people about how to take care of yourself and manage your life. Our patients tell us that they're always being sent little newspaper and magazine clippings filled with information about the latest "MS cure" or health fad. Family members, friends, and colleagues may weigh in on everything from treatment decisions (take something—don't take something) and employment decisions (quit—don't quit), to family-planning decisions (have children—don't have children), and dietary decisions (eat this—don't eat that). When you're first diagnosed and still trying to figure out what's what, the advice may feel great. But then you discover that what one person says is the complete opposite of what someone else says. Even when you talk to other people with MS, you get contradictory suggestions for managing the disease.

Most people who give advice are doing so out of care and concern for you. The upside of this is that they're reaching out to provide help and support. The downside is that some people get really cranky when you don't do what they suggest. The best strategy with the cranky folks is just to say "thank you" and let them know that you (and your partner) will be thinking carefully about all these decisions with the help of your healthcare team. You can read more about get-

353

ting comfortable with treatment and lifestyle decisions in Chapter 3.

Understanding that silence doesn't always mean someone doesn't care

Sometimes it happens that people clam up when faced with an uncomfortable situation. For example, say you tell a good friend or colleague that you've been diagnosed with MS and you hear nothing from him or her but silence. Or, maybe you're having a really bad day and no one seems to be offering any help with that heavy door or that stack of papers you dropped. Or, perhaps you come back to work with a new cane after being treated for a relapse and people look uncomfortable but don't say anything.

You wonder what's going on, right? Okay, so some people aren't very nice and they don't care, but generally that's not the case. Here are some other possibilities to consider:

✔ **An MS diagnosis is a shock for them as well as for you.** When people don't know what to say or how to say it, they sometimes say nothing at all. They may need a little time—and a little help from you—to know how to respond.

✔ **When people don't offer help, it's often because they don't know whether you want it.** We talk more about this in the "Communicating Your Needs" section later in this chapter, but, for now, keep in mind that no one can read your mind. People who want to help but don't want to embarrass you or hurt your feelings may hold back until you give the signal—by asking for assistance or taking their arm, for example.

✔ **When you show up with a new mobility device or helpful gadget, people may wait to see**

354

whether you're going to talk about it. They may be curious, concerned, or even excited to see you using a helpful new tool, but they may also be reluctant to ask a question or make a comment. Again, you need to lead the way. If you're willing or even eager to talk about it, an introductory comment from you will inevitably lead to questions and comments from others.

Remembering that MS is part of you but not all of you

You—as well as the family members, friends, and colleagues you decide to talk to about your MS—may sometimes need a reminder that you're still you in spite of whatever changes the MS brings along.

Showing off your equipment

No, we don't mean *that* kind of equipment. People's reactions to mobility aids, such as canes and electric scooters will vary tremendously, so be careful not to jump to conclusions. One of our patients waited months before deciding to use her new scooter in public. She was very embarrassed and sure that people would stare and feel sorry for her. During her public "debut," a man ran up and said, "What a great gadget — where did you get it? I want to get one for my wife. Do they come in blue?" Maybe the fact that her scooter was scarlet red and looked pretty spiffy made it easier for this man to break the ice. So, keep in mind that most types of mobility equipment now come in designer colors and some, like canes, for example, can be decorated in a variety of ways. Believe it or not, mobility aids can make a fashion statement. Refer to Chapter 7 for more info on assistive technology.

If you become so preoccupied with your MS that it's all you think or talk about, other people will follow your lead. They may happily talk about nothing but MS for awhile, but eventually most will get bored with the subject and start to distance themselves from you. Even though MS is probably the biggest thing on your mind, it's important to remember that the people close to you still want to connect with the you they knew before. Just like before you were diagnosed, your ideas, interests, opinions, and sense of humor are still important to them.

On the other hand, if you avoid the subject and people

Thanks, but I can speak for myself

In today's high-style, high-speed, youth/health-oriented culture, many people aren't all that comfortable with illness or disability. When meeting you for the first time, some people may assume that because you have difficulty walking, for example, you can't hear, think, or talk either. Or they may assume that you won't have much to offer them. Even though your patience may be stretched to the limit, this is an opportunity to educate people and help them feel more comfortable. Give them a chance to get to know you and pretty soon they'll see you and begin to forget about the mobility aid. As an example, consider the following situation: Sarah and John were out for dinner to celebrate their anniversary. They picked a handicapped accessible restaurant so that John wouldn't have any difficulty maneuvering around the tables in his motorized scooter. When the server approached the table to take their order, she turned to Sarah and said, "What would he like for dinner?" Sarah smiled at the server and said, "He'll be happy to let you know what he wants." John, recognizing that the world has a lot to learn about MS, and disability in general, simply said, "Thanks — I'll have the steak, medium-rare, please."

still insist on treating you like a sick person—talking only about your health, your symptoms, or your medications—it's time to help them shift the focus. You can remind them that your life is full of things besides MS. Here are some strategies to try:

✔ Introduce other subjects to let them know that you like to think and talk about other things.

✔ Ask about them—their life, loves, kids, work, and health—to show how important they are to you.

✔ Make a date for an outing or activity to let them know that you're still up for fun and excitement.

✔ If they don't take the hint, tell them that you like to get on with your life and keep your MS on the back burner whenever possible.

✔ If you get really desperate, tell them that talking about MS all the time is really boring.

✔ Go the extra mile to help people get to know you and see what's behind your mobility equipment.

Disclosing Your Diagnosis to a Prospective Partner

Multiple sclerosis is typically diagnosed in the 20s, 30s, and 40s, when many people are looking for their significant others. Dating isn't all that easy under the best of circumstances, so getting diagnosed with a chronic illness obviously adds another challenge. No one likes rejection, and everyone tries to find ways to avoid it. So, it may be tempting at times to leave the playing field in order to avoid the risk of being hurt or rejected by someone who's turned off by your MS. However, the result of that strategy isn't so

357

comfy either. This section gives you some ideas of how to present your MS in the dating world.

Say you're about to go out on a date with this incredibly attractive person you've been eyeing for a long time. Your MS is behaving pretty well at the moment and you're wondering whether you should talk about it. Or, perhaps a friend has fixed you up with someone she "knows you'll just love." Now you're trying to figure out whether to bring your cane so you'll feel steadier on your feet or whether you should tough it out and hope for the best in the two-inch heels you've been dying to wear. Or, maybe you want to ask someone out but you're just not sure whether you have an obligation to talk about your MS.

You may even be wondering whether the dating part of your life is over—because, after all, who would want to get into a relationship with a person who has MS? The truth of the matter is that people with MS do go on dates, fall in love, and find partners for life. However, in addition to the challenges described endlessly in popular magazines, there are a few added ones for those living with an unpredictable illness. The starting point for dealing with these challenges is communication.

Here are some helpful hints for making dating a little easier:

- **Reaching out to a new person always involves some risk and nobody ever knows what the final outcome will be until they try.** Even though it's true that some people may be put off by your MS, others won't be, particularly if you remember to show off your whole self, of which MS is only a part.

- **A first date doesn't have to be a show-all, tell-all event (although that can be fun too!).** Don't feel like you have to start with a "Hello, my name is

358

Harry and I have MS" declaration. Your goal the first time you're out with someone is to figure out whether it was worth your time and effort and if you ever want to see that person again.

If you have any visible symptoms—your leg drags or you use a cane to help with balance—you have the option to explain it, but you don't have to. The bottom line is that you don't owe any information on a first date that you're not comfortable sharing.

↙ **After you know that the other person is someone you want to spend more time with, get to know better, and develop more of a relationship with, start sharing more information.** A very good rule of thumb is to ask yourself when you would want to know similar information about the other person.

Most people have issues in their lives—health-, family-, or work-related issues—that they have some concerns about sharing. Generally when people with MS begin talking about their health issues, they find that other people have one thing or another to share as well.

↙ **When you decide that it's time to talk about your MS, you need to be prepared to let the person react in his or her own way.** This may be difficult. One person may come back at you with a lot of questions, while another may dismiss it with "Oh, that's no big deal." Or, another person may clam up.

It's a good idea to plan ahead a bit: Consider your personal style: Do you tend to use a lot of humor or are you more comfortable with facts and figures? Also consider the other person's style and try to anticipate possible reactions, questions, or concerns.

359

This is where you need to don your teaching hat (refer to the "Explaining Your MS to Others" section earlier in this chapter for more info on how to teach others about your MS). And then you need to sit back and give the person time and space to react.

You may think that the best strategy is to put off talking about your MS until the relationship is really solid. Even though this may be tempting, the better strategy is to take the risk early on—before you've invested your heart and soul.

Long-term relationships are full of challenges, with or without MS thrown in. Just think—no matter what the situation, a relationship requires you to be able to communi-

Don't wait: Last minute disclosures are risky

We heard a story recently about a young man who told his fiancée about his MS on the eve of their wedding. When asked why she cancelled the wedding, she responded that it had nothing to do with his having MS — *that* she could handle. The reason was that he hadn't trusted her enough with this important part of his life. For her, honesty and trust were far more important than MS. Had the young man taken the risk of disclosing his diagnosis early on, he would have saved himself a lot of worry and discovered something pretty nice about the woman he loved. This story underlines that having, or not having, MS is seldom the most important factor in a relationship.

So, even though talking about your MS with someone you really like is difficult, it's far better to get it out in the open early on. Everyone needs to find out how a prospective life partner feels about important life issues and you may be pleasantly surprised to discover that MS isn't the most important thing you bring to the table.

360

cate comfortably, problem-solve together, and work effectively as a team. Even though it may be scary to think about discussing your diagnosis, your current symptoms and treatments, and the unpredictability of MS, avoiding these topics in the early days of a relationship is a set-up for stress and conflict down the road. It's impossible to build a strong relationship on a foundation of half-truths. Instead, it's better to get it all out in the open so that you can begin to work together to address this and other challenges in your lives.

Communicating Your Needs

Even though you may feel like it some days, your MS isn't written all over your face. Particularly if you're dealing with any of the disease's less visible symptoms, such as fatigue, weakness, bladder problems, or cognitive changes, other people may not have a clue what's going on with you or what you may need—or not need—from them. We've already said this, but it bears repeating: *No one can read your mind.* It's up to you to let people know when, and if, you need something from them and how they can be of most help. And by the way, don't assume you can read their minds either: The fact that people don't jump to offer assistance doesn't mean that they don't care. Two-way communication is the key.

Giving clear messages

You may have mixed feelings about getting assistance from others. On the one hand, you want to do all the things you used to do, just the way you used to do them. On the other hand, some days are better than others and some tasks are harder than they used to be. When it's a good day, you want to do everything yourself and you want others to know that you can. When it's a bad day, though, you wish someone

361

You can't have your cake and eat it too

Sandra's husband, Jim, was in a no-win situation. He wanted to be helpful to his wife but could never seem to figure out how and when to help. Sandra had always been a fiercely independent person who liked to do things in her own way and in her own time. When she was diagnosed with MS, Sandra made a point of saying that she wanted to remain as independent as possible. So, to respect her wishes, Jim tried to hold back and wait to be asked before he helped. But he quickly figured out that Sandra was pretty ticked off at him for not helping out more. When he finally asked what the problem was, she told him, "If you really love me, you would know when I was feeling crummy and needed your help." Poor Jim. The truth is that even people who love you a lot won't necessarily know how you feel unless you tell them. In fact, the people who love you the most may be so concerned about hurting your feelings or doing the wrong thing that they find it hard to do anything at all. Too much guesswork is an emotional minefield. So, the solution is to have a "heart-to-heart" talk about how you're going to let the other person know what you need and when — whether it's assistance of some kind, a pat on the back on a really good day, or just a hug.

would step up to the plate and help. The problem, of course, is that people aren't likely to know what kind of day you're having unless you tell them. See the sidebar "You can't have your cake and eat it too" for a case in point.

The best strategy for communicating your needs is to ask for help when you need it and to thank people and politely decline when you don't. However, when you do need help, always be sure to let people know exactly what kind of assistance would be most useful to you.

Staking out your independence

Everyone gives help in a slightly different way: Some people do it by telling you what to do; others by offering to do things for you (or simply doing them without asking); and some by asking whether you want help with anything. The last group is the easiest to deal with because they're relying on you to tell them if and when you need their assistance. The first two groups are more challenging because they assume that they already know what you need.

Your best strategy when dealing with those people who think that they know best is to thank them for their care and concern and promise them that you'll let them know when you need assistance. The important message to get across to them is that doing things for yourself—even if it takes a bit longer than it used to—is a source of pride and satisfaction that you don't want to give up.

If you're experiencing problems with walking or balance, you may find that some people—particularly those who love you the most—begin to hover protectively. If you find people looking like they're ready to catch you at any mo-

Seriously, I'm not drunk!

Jack resisted using a mobility aid for quite some time. Even though he had to rely on walls or furniture to help him maintain his balance, Jack was convinced that walking with a cane would make him look disabled. One day as he was making his way unsteadily down the street, a passerby called out to him, "Why don't you do your drinking at home?" That was all Jack needed to decide it was time for a cane. Not only would the cane provide stability, it would also send a clear message that his problem had nothing to do with alcohol consumption.

363

ment (or standing as far away as possible so they won't get crushed), that's a pretty good sign that you appear unsteady and at risk.

Even though the decision to use a mobility aid is distressing for many people (we talk about this in Chapter 7), using one is an effective way of letting the people around you know that you're doing everything that you can to get around safely and independently. It sends a clear message: "I have some difficulty with walking, balance, or fatigue, and I'm dealing with it." The important benefit here is that people will feel more relaxed and comfortable around you, instead of worrying all the time about what help you might need.

P.S. The doctor can't read your mind either

You're a key player in your MS care. Neither the neurologic exam nor an MRI can tell the doctor everything that's going on in your body. This means that even the most experienced of MS specialist physicians can't do the job alone—your input is essential.

Because the information you provide during your office visits enables your doctor to formulate treatment recommendations, this is no time to put on a show! Believe it or not, some patients cancel their appointments because they aren't feeling well (illogical, but true); some withhold information about their symptoms because they don't want to be a "bad" patient (even though this isn't school and no one is being graded); some put on a happy face because they don't want to be thought of as complainers (this isn't a popularity contest). We've even known patients who have told the doctor that everything was fine because they didn't want the doctor to "feel bad."

The point is, your healthcare providers need information that only you can provide. This information includes the following:

364

- Symptoms you're experiencing

- Physical or emotional changes you've noticed since your last visit

- Problems or side effects you're having with your medications

- Difficulties you're having with everyday activities—at home and work

Unfortunately, your time with the doctor or nurse may be limited. So, the best strategy for using that time well is to come prepared to talk about any problems you're having. If you're only concerned about one issue at the moment, give it all you've got: Make sure to describe what's been happening and how it's affecting your daily life. If you have a whole litany of problems, try to prioritize them in your own mind before telling the doctor. Chances are that everything can't be addressed at once, so you and the doctor need to tackle the most important things first.

Some of the most common problems people have are the most difficult to talk about. But, doctors and nurses don't blush easily, and those who are experienced in MS care know all about the bladder and bowel symptoms, sexual issues, and problems with thinking and memory (we call those the big three) that plague many people with MS. For heaven's sake, don't hold back. And if your doctor never asks about these kinds of problems, or doesn't seem comfortable when you bring them up, it's definitely time to start looking for another doctor!

Making MS a Part of the Family

*H*ere's a visual for you: Imagine that a stranger shows up on your doorstep one day. This stranger, who's all loaded down with suitcases and duffel bags, comes into your house, spreads his belongings throughout each room, and refuses to go home. You're the first one to meet this stranger, but in no time you're making introductions to the rest of the family. Over time, each person in the family needs to develop some kind of relationship with this new member of your household.

As you may have already noticed, multiple sclerosis (MS) plays the stranger role well. It can easily take over your

366

house and overwhelm your family. But, we come to the rescue with this chapter. We talk about how families can find room in the house for the MS stranger without giving it more space than it actually needs. The process starts with a recognition of each person's reactions and feelings and continues with good old-fashioned communication. Even though communication isn't the easiest challenge, with it comes teamwork and the ability to deal with the messy stranger's habits and quirks.

Addressing Your Family Members' Feelings about Your Diagnosis

People who have been diagnosed with MS can have all sorts of reactions and feelings over the course of the disease (see Chapter 3 for a complete discussion). But, you have to remember that all of these same feelings are shared by family members too. For example, here are just a few of the emotions that your family may experience:

- **Grief:** This normal expression of loss is common. Just like the person with MS, family members have developed a picture of their family and the life they share together. When MS changes one member's abilities to share in activities or carry out his or her everyday responsibilities, there's a sense of loss. Family members may think "Our family is different, and things will never be the same." or "Who are we now that MS has changed our family?"

- **Anxiety:** This is a normal reaction among family members when someone they love has been diagnosed with MS. Children and adults share some common concerns: They worry about what will happen to this person—right now and over the long haul. They also worry about how this illness will affect their own lives.

More specifically, the partner may wonder what will happen to the couple's plans and dreams, as well as to their partnership. The partner may also worry that all the responsibility will fall into his or her hands. The children may worry that their parent won't be there to take care of them, that they may catch the disease, or that they somehow caused the disease (see Chapter 17 for more information about how to help children with their concerns). And finally, aging parents may worry about who will take care of their adult child after they're gone and, more immediately, who will be able to help them as they're aging themselves (flip to the section "When Your Child Has MS" later in this chapter for more on this topic).

➤ **Anger:** Partners and children as well as aging parents may feel anger over this unexpected change in their lives.

"This isn't what I signed up for!" is a very real feeling for some partners. "It's not fair that my dad can't play ball with me!" is one variation on a pretty common theme for kids who have a parent with MS. And older parents who need to provide care for their disabled adult child may very well wonder what happened to that peaceful, well-deserved retirement they'd been anticipating for so long. Many times, angry family members look for someone to blame and somehow end up blaming each other or themselves.

➤ **Guilt:** This common feeling happens when a person feels responsible for a family member's MS. Parents and children are particularly prone to taking the

368

blame and feeling guilty. They may think "What did I do to cause this?"

Guilt is also a pretty common reaction to angry feelings that don't seem nice. For example, a partner may feel guilty for resenting an illness that the other person didn't ask for and can't control.

The tricky thing about families is that no two people are likely to experience or express these feelings at the same time or in exactly the same way. The result can be a bumpy ride on an emotional roller coaster. So, put on your seat-belts and get ready to acknowledge that each of you has a lot of feelings about this stranger called MS, and that it's going to take some time and practice to get comfortable with those feelings.

Communicating Effectively with Adult Family Members

Now that you've been diagnosed with MS, family life may feel a little different—and you and your family may find it difficult to talk to each other about it. So, just at the point when you need to communicate with one another about what's going on and what you're going to do about it, talking feels really difficult. The rest of this chapter focuses on the strategies adults need to talk comfortably with one another. We provide suggestions for talking with kids about MS in Chapter 17.

Recognizing communication barriers

It's common for people to have trouble talking to each other about stressful or frightening things. Here are some reasons why a family living with MS may find it difficult to discuss what's going on:

No two people have exactly the same coping style. One person clams up while another person talks. Or maybe one person wants to forget about the problem for as long as possible while the other wants to become an expert on the subject. Given that MS keeps changing over time, it's not too surprising that people's coping styles are likely to conflict on a routine basis.

The tendency, of course, is for everyone in the family to think his or her own coping strategies are the best. The fact is, however, that family members need to recognize and respect these individual differences before any kind of comfortable conversation can take place. And, everyone needs to be careful not to misinterpret the differences. For example, the fact that your partner doesn't want to read books about MS or go to support groups doesn't mean he or she doesn't care or isn't as sad or anxious as you are.

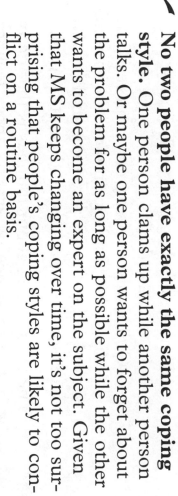

People have a lot of misconceptions about MS. Each person's ideas about the disease are based on someone with MS that they have met or read about. Because everyone's MS is different, the result is a hodgepodge of information. In addition, many people still confuse MS with muscular dystrophy or other disabling diseases.

Family members often worry about upsetting each other. In other words, family members feel so protective of one another that none of the tough stuff ever gets talked about.

For example, a partner may think to himself "She's so worried about her MS right now. I can't possibly talk to her about how moody she has been or about my concerns over our finances." Or, he may think

370

"She's trying so hard to have a positive attitude about her MS, I don't see how I can talk to her about planning for the future." And, the person with MS may be thinking to herself "My husband has already taken on so many extra chores around here, I can't possibly tell him I don't think I should be driving right now."

➤ **Some subjects are just uncomfortable.** Sex, bladder and bowel, and cognitive problems immediately come to mind. Under the very best of circumstances, many couples have trouble talking about sex. So, if MS begins to interfere with sexual activities, talking about it may be too difficult—particularly if the couple didn't talk about sex when it was great! The same can be true for bladder and bowel symptoms. Not too many people feel comfortable talking about bladder accidents or bowel problems—adults just aren't supposed to have to worry about those things. The common theme here, of course, is embarrassment. These are touchy issues that people find difficult to discuss—even with someone they love.

➤ **The subject of money can generate a lot of heat in any family—with or without a chronic disease to complicate things.** More couples argue about their finances than just about anything else. Given how costly MS can be (take a look at the section "Coping with the direct and indirect costs" later in this chapter for details), it isn't too surprising that couples sometimes disagree on how the family's resources should be divvied up.

371

Communication is essential—it's the foundation for just about everything else that families have to do in order to live comfortably with MS. Without effective communication, people can't support one another or problem-solve successfully.

Getting the ball rolling toward more open communication

Communication is a complex process, so don't expect to be a pro right off the bat—most people aren't. To get started, the following sections give you some tips for communicating with your adult family members.

Acknowledge your different communication styles

The starting point for good communication is recognizing that each of you may have a different way of going about it. For example, you strong, silent types may need to think about approaching things more openly—at least as far as MS is concerned. And you chatty types may need to remember that not everyone else is as fired up to talk about everything in such great detail as you are. Your goal should be to find common ground, beginning with the recognition that you can't begin to figure out how you're going to incorporate MS into your lives without talking about it.

Study up on MS

To enhance your communication, you need to make it a point to get better acquainted with your illness. This doesn't mean that you have to become the world's expert on MS, but you do need to know enough to make wise choices and sound decisions. Many of these choices and decisions are going to affect the whole family, so it's important to be able to talk about them and share opinions openly. Knowing your stuff and communicating it is the best way we know of to avoid confusion, resentment, and "I told you so" conversations down the line. Because people tend to like their information in different formats, here's a menu to consider:

↙ **Reading materials:** Printed stuff is great because you can take it with you and indulge at your convenience. Books that are appropriate for all ages are available at just about any bookstore or library (see the recommended readings in Appendix B). Also, the National MS Society has a library of brochures on virtually every aspect of MS. These brochures are available online (www.nationalmssociety.org/brochures) or by calling (800) FIGHT-MS (800-344-4867).

↙ **National MS Society Web Spotlights:** The Spotlight series is designed for folks who want to zero in on a particular topic without having to hunt around. You can access spotlights on a variety of topics at www.nationalmssociety.org/spotlight. Each spotlight will point you toward all the information on the site that relates to that topic.

↙ **Online programs:** These types of programs are attractive because you can access them 24-7 and you don't have to be sociable about it. Online programs can be the perfect venue for those of you who aren't comfortable disclosing your MS or seeing others who have it. The National MS Society offers programs on a wide variety of topics (www.nationalmssociety.org/webcasts). Many of the manufacturers of the MS medications offer programs as well.

↙ **Live programs:** These programs are just the ticket for people who like the personal touch. You can see the speaker and ask your questions first-hand, meet others with MS and exchange war stories and tips, and get to know a whole new group of people. Even though you may be reluctant to meet folks whose MS is worse or better or different than yours, remember this: Many people find that getting to know others who are living and dealing with different types of symptoms can actually be reassuring.

- **Support groups:** If you're one of those people who feels more comfortable, less anxious, and less alone when getting information in a group setting, support groups may be perfect for you. Call the National MS Society (800-FIGHT-MS) or the Multiple Sclerosis Association of America (800-532-7667) for information about local support groups.

  For those who like the group feeling but don't enjoy or can't get to a group meeting, chat rooms and bulletin boards also offer this kind of supportive environment. Check out the National MS Society's MS World chat room at www.nationalmssociety .org/chat and the forums offered by the MS Foundation at www.msfocus.org/services/svc_forums.html. Keep in mind, however, that the information you get will vary with its source—not everything you hear at a support group or online chat will be relevant to you or accurate. So be sure to check with your doctor or the National MS Society to verify any information that feels iffy to you.

When accessing any information, pay attention to the source so you can be on the lookout for subtle—or not so subtle—biases in the information. Whereas the National MS Society and other nonprofit groups are committed to providing unbiased information, the pharmaceutical companies are always wearing two hats when they develop consumer information: They're providing education about MS while trying to sell you their product.

Given all the avenues for accessing information, there's no reason why you and your partner or other family members need to pursue the same ones. The challenge is for each of you to find out your favorite way to gather information, and then figure out how to talk about it.

Make the time to talk

Given how busy everyday life is, it's easy to keep putting MS conversations on the back burner, particularly when you're a little uncomfortable about them in the first place.

A note about communicating long distance

For those of you who have parents or siblings that live far away, you need to think about what information to share and when. Families who are spread out tend to have different rules about sharing health information. Some families talk about absolutely everything (aches and pains, doctor visits, medical tests, diagnoses, treatments, and so on) — it's the shared expectation and everyone does it. Other families are more private, and they don't share any information until there's a treatment plan in place or a funeral (and maybe not even then).

Think about what the rules are in your family and whether they may need to be tweaked a tad. We advocate openness about health issues, but it's really up to you. Keep in mind, however, that after your loved ones know about your MS, they'll have reactions, questions, and concerns. And, the fact that your loved ones can't see you readily will usually heighten their anxiety. So, be prepared to educate, answer questions, and give periodic updates. Parents, in particular, tend to hover. They are, after all, still parents.

So, you may need to set aside some special time for this. It's important that you have some time when you won't be interrupted by kids or phone calls and that you have plenty of time to share everything that's on your minds (sort of like sex!). You may even think about scheduling regular times—a Sunday afternoon walk or a dinner out—to make sure that these conversations get the attention they need.

Avoid competition

Because everyone in the family is affected when MS joins the family, family members sometimes have a tendency to get into a contest about who has it worse—the person with the diagnosis or those whose lives have been changed by a disease they don't even have. This happens most when people don't have a comfortable way to talk about their feelings. The feelings stay bottled up and everyone feels unsupported. And when people start feeling unsupported they begin to say things like this:

➤ "You have no idea how I feel. MS is changing my whole life, I feel lousy, and you just keep going on about your business as though nothing were wrong."

➤ "You have no idea how I feel. I'm doing all the work around here—on top of my full-time job. I don't have any time for myself any more, and you're always too tired to do anything fun."

➤ "Just 'cause Mom's got MS, I'm stuck with more chores than any other kid I know."

Families do best when they can lay the blame on the MS rather than on each other. This reduces unhelpful competition and labels the problem for what it is—a challenge that everyone in the family needs to meet. Some families we know have even given the MS a name—like Fred or Mari-

376

etta—to help them remember that their shared goal is figuring out how to live with the MS.

Get a jump-start if you need it

Sometimes getting started is the most difficult part of communicating. Families that don't have a lot of practice with this kind of communication may need to practice a bit to get the hang of it. Educational meetings and support groups can be good places to practice.

For those of you who like to get your practice more privately, family therapists can be a great resource to help you start the conversation. Call the National MS Society at (800) FIGHT-MS for the names of therapists in your community who have experience with chronic illness and disability issues.

Keeping the Family Rhythm Going so Your MS Doesn't Steal the Show

All families have a rhythm of their own. You may not hear the music playing in the background, but over time, each family establishes patterns, procedures, and schedules for everyday living. This rhythm is part of what provides the feelings of safety and security that people look for from family life. Unfortunately, MS can disrupt your family's rhythm just the way that having weekend visitors temporarily changes the way you do things. But, because this visitor isn't going home, your challenge is to figure out how to fit MS into your lives with the least amount of disruption possible.

MS can be greedy. From time to time it can tap all the family's resources—money, energy, and time being the most obvious. This is why it's important to give MS some space in your life without giving it more than it needs.

Every member of the family is at a different place in his or her life, and each needs a share in the family's resources. If MS saps too much of any of these resources, the result is a disabled family—rather than a family with one person who has a disability.

Coping with the direct and indirect costs

The direct and indirect costs of MS in this country come to almost $60,000 per person per year (for an annual cost of $24 billion!). About half of this is related specifically to healthcare (medications, doctor visits, hospitalizations, and so on). The rest is accounted for by lost wages, unpaid caregiving activities, and other items. Fortunately, most people with MS have good health insurance coverage (flip to Chapter 19 for a detailed discussion of insurance issues). Nevertheless, the out-of-pocket expenses can be high.

Because the expenses for MS are high, we urge families to consult a financial planner early on. Even though it's never possible to predict how your MS will progress, or what expenses will be involved, it's a safe bet that you'll come across expenses that you never counted on having. A planner can help you anticipate possible expenses and identify strategies to meet these expenses should they arise (see Chapter 20 for some financial planning strategies).

One of the reasons that financial planning is so important is that MS isn't the only hungry mouth waiting to be fed. Summer camp, orthodontia, vacations, college expenses, and retirement are always on the sidelines waiting for their fair share of the pot. Unfortunately, these typical life expenses don't disappear just because MS comes along. The goal is to ensure that MS doesn't take more of the pie than necessary.

Managing energy and time

One of the big complaints about MS is that it takes a lot of time and effort. For the person with MS, the drain on time and effort is more obvious—it may take longer, with a greater amount of effort than before, to get the same things done. Simply getting around can sometimes be exhausting. In fact, basic activities may take so much of the person's energy that little is left over for extras, particularly if he or she is experiencing MS-related fatigue (check out Chapter 7 for info on this and other symptoms).

But, family members may feel their energy being drained as well. They may be pitching in to help with various activities, or they may be taking on more responsibilities than they had before. Everyone may find that MS calls on them to be more flexible, more creative, and more solution-focused—all of which can sometimes feel extremely tiring. In fact, another complaint from families is that "nothing is spontaneous any more"—they feel that everything takes more planning, more prep time, and more work.

Here are some strategies for making sure that your family's energy resources are used wisely:

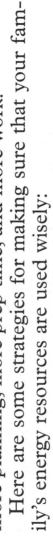

✔ **Focus on what's most important.** The key lies in figuring out where you—individually and collectively—want to focus your time and energy resources. Then, you should let those priorities guide your choices and plans. (Check out the section "Establishing family priorities" later in this chapter for details.)

✔ **Make sure that your home is arranged to maximize accessibility, safety, comfort, and ease of operation.** Doing so will enable the person with MS to navigate safely and independently while saving all of you a lot of time and energy. An occupa-

379

tional therapist can advise you on this kind of environmental design (see Chapter 4). And after you've arranged the house the way you want it, try to remember that keeping things in their proper places means less searching and organizing.

➤ **Make every effort to plan strategically.** Whether it's errands, a family outing, a household project, or a holiday gathering, take the time to think things through completely. Doing so will save all of you a lot of time and energy in the long run. (Flip to Chapter 12 for some tips on how plan your activities strategically.)

➤ **Share the workload.** Many families have traditionally divided the labor around the house into boy jobs and girl jobs—"You clean the gutters and I clean the floors" or "You deal with the kids and I deal with the lawn." However you have divided things in the past, you may need to begin thinking about tasks in a different way. You need to figure who can do which tasks with the best outcome and the least effort—even if a boy ends up doing a "girl task" and vice versa.

➤ **Use mobility aids.** Mobility aids can benefit the whole family. This is sometimes a hard sell, but the point is that the right piece of equipment—a cane or motorized scooter for example—can make it possible for family members to enjoy activities *and* each other's company. When mom uses a motorized scooter to go to the zoo, for example, the entire family can participate, everyone can move at a comfortable pace, and no one has to worry about her falling or getting exhausted.

380

Establishing family priorities

One of the things we hear a lot from families is "MS really helped us get our priorities straight." For these families, the MS made them stop and think about what things in life were most important to them, and what they needed to do to make those things happen. Obviously, the priorities are going to be different for each family, but the process is the same.

For example, one family may decide that quality family time is a top priority. Given that dad has a lot of MS fatigue, they need to figure out how to take that into account when planning shared activities. Maybe they decide that dinner will be 30 minutes later every day to give dad a chance for a power nap when he gets home from work. Or, maybe they decide that the kids can take over mowing the lawn so dad can use that time to rest up for the afternoon soccer game (and dad agrees to take his scooter to the field so he doesn't get too tired to cheer the team).

The examples are endless, but the point is that the family needs to identify a priority and then figure out how to make it happen. Other priorities may include making family trips accessible (see Chapter 23), increasing monthly savings, or having more company at the house so mom can stay connected with all her friends. The goal is to ensure that everyone's needs are balanced.

Problem-solving: Many heads are better than one

Living with MS takes creativity and flexibility. Each new challenge that comes along demands a response; otherwise MS threatens to run the show. Your best strategy for meeting MS challenges head-on is for you and your family to put your heads together to come up with a plan. This strategy provides more brain power to deal with the problem, and it also helps make sure that everyone buys into the solution.

If, for example, mom is having problems with balance, she and her family can think about ways to deal with it—perhaps by rearranging the furniture to make the house more convenient for her, helping her pick out a snazzy new scooter, or considering a move to a one-story house. Or, if the co-pay on her medications has increased, the family can work together to figure out where those extra dollars are going to come from each month. One of the advantages of this kind of shared approach to problem-solving is that everyone feels some ownership of the process.

Building and Maintaining Healthy Partner Relationships

MS can challenge even the best of partnerships. There isn't a young couple in the world—unless they grew up in families in which someone had a chronic illness or disability—that has a clue what "in sickness and in health" really means. The challenge is no doubt easier for those of you who already have a history together. You've had an opportunity to get to know another, build a partnership of whatever sort works best for you, and get comfortable with your individual tastes, strengths, and foibles. The same strengths and resources you have brought to bear in other difficult situations will help you with MS as well.

Those of you who are younger may have a tougher time simply because you may not know each other as well and may have less of a foundation together. Basically, you're getting to know each other at the same time as you're getting to know MS. Fortunately, no one needs to go it alone. Many resources and strategies are available to help couples

382

manage the stresses and strains that a chronic illness like MS can cause.

Making time for each other

As everyone knows, family life is busy under even the best of circumstances. Jobs, kids, and chores can be so time- and energy-consuming that many couples describe themselves as "ships passing in the night." And even the passing-in-the-night part isn't all that much fun because both members of the couple are so tired. We advocate quality time together for any couple, but it's particularly important after MS joins the family. Relationships need time and space to grow and thrive—it may sound hokey but it's true. For instance, the communication and shared problem-solving we talk about in this chapter can't happen unless you make time for them—and you won't make time unless you decide that communicating and joint problem-solving are high on the priority list.

We're big fans of "date night." Many couples find that if they don't actually schedule this kind of time together, it never seems to happen. Not every date needs to involve soul-searching discussions (although these are important every now and then). The important thing is that you're taking time to spend together, without all the distractions that grab your attention at home.

 Because fatigue can be such a major issue in MS, it's important to plan your time together when fatigue is at a minimum. Some couples grab a few minutes early in the morning, when energy is generally highest, to enjoy a chat or a cuddle before the family's day begins. Evening dates may be a problem because of the fatigue factor, so some couples stake out one weekend afternoon a month for themselves. It doesn't matter how you make it happen, it only matters that you do.

Keeping the intimacy alive

When the word "intimacy" is used these days, everyone tends to assume it's all about sex. But, there's definitely more to it than that. In fact, we purposely talk about sexual issues in another chapter to convey that intimacy is much more than just your sexual relationship (you can high-tail it to Chapter 8 right now if you're looking for the juicy stuff.). Intimacy involves all of the things that keep your partnership healthy and satisfying, including:

- ✔ **Communication:** The couples who communicate most successfully are those who can listen as well as talk, and who can recognize their points of agreement while acknowledging their differences. Too often couples clam up when they don't see eye to eye or when things start to get tense. Because MS is likely to throw a lot of new challenges your way, it's important to be able to talk about your issues and priorities—even if the conversations get a bit dicey at times.

- ✔ **Trust:** Partners need to be able trust that it's safe to express themselves without fear of rejection or ridicule. In other words, they need to know that the relationship is a safe place for revealing their feelings, needs, and concerns. They also need to feel confidence in the resilience of the relationship. If every bump in the road is a possible reason for one of you to jump ship, neither of you will ever feel safe, let alone intimate.

- ✔ **Mutual concern:** Every intimate partnership is a two-way street. Even when one partner has been diagnosed with a chronic illness, the other partner's well-being should be of equal concern. Try to make

384

sure that both of you are getting equal billing.

✔ **Respect:** Intimacy can't happen without mutual respect. Particularly if roles and responsibilities change as a result of MS, it's important that the person with MS continues to feel like a respected partner.

✔ **Sex:** The sexual relationship is an important way for couples to express and experience their intimacy. Because MS can sometimes alter sexual feelings and responses (and therefore interfere with sexual activities), it's critically important that couples get whatever help they need to deal with any changes that occur.

Unfortunately, MS seems to have its own don't ask, don't tell policy—doctors don't often ask and patients don't often tell—so sexual difficulties don't get proper attention. Don't let your doctor off the hook. If you're experiencing changes in your sexual relationship, speak up. Your doctor can help you figure out what is and isn't related to MS and can refer you to a counselor or sex therapist for help.

Maintaining a balanced partnership

Over time, every partnership develops its own set of ground rules. These ground rules are often unplanned and unspoken, but they're real just the same. According to these rules, each partner has areas of responsibility, such as breadwinner, chief cook and bottle washer, primary parent, gardener, grocery shopper, bill payer, and so on. The division of labor, however it evolves, ensures that the work gets done and that each person feels cared for. Sometimes something will come along to disrupt the pattern temporarily, but it generally rights itself pretty quickly. For example, families go through this when someone gets a cold or the flu. For a few days, everyone chips in to help the family member who's not feeling well. Then, as soon as the person feels better, everyone goes back to the usual routine.

When MS comes along, partnerships can get thrown out of whack. If one partner begins having difficulty managing his or her end of things, the ground rules gradually start to shift. The shift may last for weeks or months—until the current exacerbation is over—or forever. Here's the risk in this situation: The partner whose disability is getting in the way gradually begins relinquishing responsibilities. The other partner steps in to pick up the slack and pretty soon, the person with MS isn't contributing his or her share. And nobody feels good about it. The person with MS feels guilty and his or her partner begins to feel tired, overburdened, and perhaps resentful.

From the get-go, it's a good idea to assume that partnerships thrive best when they're balanced. For example, if the partner with MS begins to have difficulty with an activity, keep the partnership balanced by doing a swap of chores. It doesn't matter what the swap is as long as both of you still feel valued. Unfortunately, one of the biggest obstacles to this kind of swap tends to be people's sensitivity about gender roles. In these situations, you may hear things like "But *she's* supposed to do the cooking, the housework, and the carpooling." or "*He* always cut the grass, shoveled the snow, repaired stuff, and paid the bills." Our advice? Get over it! The strength of your partnership will depend on your ability to be flexible when and if you need to be (not on whether you're doing the "right" chores).

What to do when one partner can't participate in joint activities

Imagine what happens when a couple that has always played tennis or golf together, or hiked or skied together,

386

suddenly finds that these joint activities aren't possible any more because of MS. As you can probably guess, this change can be particularly challenging for those couples whose social lives have been built around these activities. Generally, the scenario plays out in one of the following ways: Both partners stop the activity (and one feels sad and guilty while the other feels sad and resentful) or one partner stops the activity (and one feels sad and angry and the other feels guilty). We don't think either of these options is a particularly good way to go. So, here are some alternative strategies:

✔ **Don't assume that you know what your partner is feeling about this.** Get the subject out in the open and figure out what's going to work best for your relationship.

✔ **Brainstorm about options that may work for both of you.** For example, here are some suggestions:

- Substitute another activity that you both enjoy as much as the one that you're now unable to do.
- One partner continues the activity while the other comes along to enjoy the social part.
- One partner continues the activity while the other finds an enjoyable alternative.
- One partner engages in the activity on a less frequent basis and you do something together the rest of the time.

✔ **Whatever option you choose, make sure that your together-time doesn't get lost.** Sharing time feeds and fuels your relationship, so do what you need to do to preserve some opportunities to enjoy time together (see the section "Making time for each other" earlier in the chapter for more details).

➤ **Maintain your social connections.** If, for example, your social life has revolved around the tennis club, you need to figure out how to maintain connections with friends even if you aren't playing as much tennis as you used to. This can be a real challenge, particularly if your "friends" turn out to be more interested in your tennis game than you. Obviously people like that aren't really your "friends," so you'll have to look around for ways to broaden your horizons with other people, such as friends from work, friends from your church or synagogue, or friends from neighborhood organizations.

Turning a caregiving relationship into a care partnership

Maintaining a healthy partnership can become especially difficult if MS progresses significantly (check out Chapter 13 for more on managing advanced MS). The more disabled a person with MS becomes, the more involved the partner is likely to be in his or her care. Caregiving activities can run the gamut from occasional assistance with daily activities like taking medications, buttoning buttons, and preparing meals to full-time, hands-on care with dressing, bathing, using the bathroom, and eating.

When one person is always on the caregiving end and the other is always on the care-receiving end, the relationship is no longer balanced. The give-and-take foundation for the partnership has been lost. But, it really doesn't need to be. Except in the case of severe cognitive impairment, which fortunately is relatively rare in MS (you can read more about this in Chapter 9), every person can contribute significantly to a partnership, even if he or she has to do it differently.

388

Here are some tips for creating a care partnership:

✔ **Make sure that each of you feels like a contributing member of the partnership.** Figure out together what the person with MS can do to support the activities of the household. Be creative and remember that assistive technology can make many things possible (see Chapter 7 for details).

✔ **Ensure that both of you are being givers and receivers.** Healthy partners need to let their MS partners know what they need; even if the partner with MS can't do much in the way of physical activities, he or she can give a lot in the way caring, support, humor, advice, and so on.

✔ **To the extent possible, keep caregiving activities separate from your couple time.** For example, hire outside caregiving help if you need it and can afford it. Make dates for together-time that doesn't involve caregiving activities. Or, come up with some activities that you can share and enjoy, such as watching movies, reading aloud, and going out to dinner.

When Your Child Has MS

As challenging as it can sometimes be to have MS, parents say that it's even more difficult when your child has it. No one ever wants anything bad to happen to their kids. When a child is diagnosed with MS—either as a youngster or as an adult—parents tend to feel overwhelmed with a lot of feelings, including anxiety, guilt, and anger. In this section, we talk about the issues confronting parents when their child has MS.

Helping your adult child with MS

Because MS is primarily a disease of young adults, a lot of middle-aged or elderly parents are left wondering what to do to help their kids who have been diagnosed. Clearly, the old "keep 'em home from school and give 'em lots of fluids until the fever goes away" doesn't really work. Yet the same feelings that made you want to care for and protect your kids from harm when they were little are still there even though your kid is now 30, 40, or even 50. The result is that you may tend to fall back on old parenting techniques that don't apply any more. Here are some tips on how you can still parent when your child is a full-fledged adult:

✔ **Have a heart-to-heart with your adult child, with the goal being to figure out how you're going to support each other in this situation.** Parent-child relationships are a form of care partnership, so you and your child need to figure out what each of you can do to take care of the other.

For example, your child needs to recognize that you're concerned and feel just as protective and parental as you always did. You, in turn, have to recognize that your child is now a grown-up who needs to deal with this life change in his or her own way.

✔ **Negotiate what you can expect from one another.** Your adult child may just want emotional support, or he or she may welcome advice, financial assistance, hands-on help, or a hundred other things. So, you need to be prepared to talk about what you can and can't provide. On the other hand, your child may want to sort things out alone for awhile. This is a reasonable request, but as concerned parents, you also have every right to request periodic updates.

390

✔ **In the event that your adult child becomes too disabled to manage on his or her own, discuss care options.** As we emphasize in Chapter 20, discussions about long-term care and related topics are most effective when they happen along the way. Even though most people don't ever require this level of care, discussing the options ahead of time gives family members the opportunity to sort our their feelings and needs so that difficult choices don't have to be made during a crisis. (You can find more info on the care options in Chapter 13.)

One option may be for your child to come back and live with you, but it's important to talk about all the options in order to make sure that everyone's needs are being met. If the solution doesn't work for you *and* your adult child, then it's not working.

✔ **If your child moves back into your home for health or financial reasons, renegotiate the parent-child "contract."** Otherwise, each of you will fall back on whatever rules were in place the last time you lived together (which was probably in your child's teenage years). Any child who has lived independently will want to continue to have a certain amount of privacy and freedom to come and go. You, on the other hand, may begin to worry about your child's welfare and safety just as you did in the old days—particularly if he or she now has mobility, visual, or cognitive problems that may affect driving or other activities.

An honest conversation will go a long way toward helping you sort out a plan that works for everyone. In general, we recommend that you and your child maintain as much independence as possible, while keeping each other informed of schedules and

391

whereabouts and coming together when you want to spend time together as a family.

- **Because this is a care partnership, everyone needs to be on both the giving and receiving end.** If your adult child finds it necessary to return to your home, he or she may feel guilty about imposing in this way, and may be concerned about not being able to provide you with the assistance that you may need as you get older. But, there are many ways for all of you to take care of each other. Work it out so that everyone is a contributor to the household.

- **If the situation gets too tense or emotional as you try to figure out a plan that works for all of you, consider talking with a family counselor.** This isn't an easy change for anyone, and an objective third party can often help the conversation along.

Young children and teens get MS too

This section is for those of you who have a young child or teen with MS. We want you to know up front that you aren't alone and that a lot of resources are available to help you and your child. So, before you do anything else, you may want to check out "Young Persons with MS: A Network for Families with a Child or Teen with MS," which is a support program developed collaboratively by the National MS Society and the MS Society of Canada.

You can get more information about the Network by calling (866) KIDS-W-MS (866-543-7967) or by going online (www.nationalmssociety.org/pednetwork).

Understanding childhood MS

Of the 400,000 people in the United States with MS, approximately 8,000 to 10,000 of them are children or adolescents. Initial symptoms have been seen as early as 13 months old, with a diagnosis as young as 2 years old. The majority, however, are diagnosed in their teens. An additional 10,000 to 15,000 youngsters have experienced at least one symptom suggestive of MS. Some—but certainly not all—of these will go on to develop MS. Although, in most cases they won't actually be diagnosed until they're adults.

The advent of *magnetic resonance imaging* (MRI) technology, combined with a growing awareness of pediatric MS among adult and pediatric neurologists and pediatricians, has made it possible to identify children with MS earlier than ever before. Even though the information about these kids is accumulating gradually, we want to fill you in on what's known so far:

✔ **As is true with adults, no one knows why one child gets MS and another doesn't.** In general, it's thought that a person with a certain genetic predisposition comes into contact with some kind of environmental trigger prior to adolescence that causes the disease to occur (you can read more about the genetic factor in Chapter 1). Doctors still don't know what the trigger is or what causes the disease to become active so early in some children. However, we guarantee you that neither you nor your child did anything to make it happen.

✔ **You can't predict how your child's MS will progress.** However doctors do know that most people with MS remain able to walk, even though they may need a cane or other assistive device to help them.

✔ **Right now, the diagnostic criteria for MS in children are the same as in adults.** As more in-

393

formation is gathered about these kids, however, the criteria may ultimately be revised somewhat for this younger group. You can read more about the diagnostic criteria in adults in Chapter 2.

Here's the challenge when it comes to diagnosing younger folks: When a child or teen goes to the doctor with a single episode of neurologic symptoms that are characteristic of *demyelination* (damage to the myelin coating and nerve fibers in the central nervous system), the doctor needs to decide if this is a one-time event in the child's life, or the first event in what will eventually turn out to be MS. To complicate matters, it isn't unusual for children to experience single neurologic events known as *acute disseminated encephalomyelitis* (ADEM). Although some neurologic symptoms and signs of ADEM are similar to those of MS—such as vision problems or difficulties with balance, sensation, or strength—others are quite different.

➤ **Like treatment in adults, the treatment of MS in children involves managing acute attacks, modifying the disease course, and managing the symptoms.** Unfortunately, though, many of the medical treatments described in this book have been studied extensively in adults but have not been studied in children under 18. And although several medications have been approved by the U.S. Food and Drug Administration (FDA) for use in adults with MS (see Chapter 6), none has been specifically approved for use in pediatric MS. This means that your child's physician has to rely on his or her clinical judgment—and that of experts in the field—when making decisions about what to prescribe.

➤ **Cognitive symptoms are an important issue for**

any person with MS, but they're of particular concern in kids because of their potential impact on school performance. Because cognitive changes (including problems with attention, memory, information processing, and problem-solving) can occur early in the disease—even as a first symptom—it's important to educate yourself about them so you can be on the lookout. (See Chapter 9 for a description of the cognitive changes in adults.) If you (or the teacher) notice any changes in your child's performance, consider a cognitive evaluation. The goal is to identify any changes early on so that the school can provide whatever assistance your child needs to learn comfortably and function at his or her best.

The Network for Families can give you additional information about the rights of children in public school districts, private schools, and post-secondary schools. Contact the Network by calling (866) KIDS-W-MS.

Parenting when your child has MS

Parenting is difficult enough without throwing MS into the mix. So, we included this section to give you some tips to handle it all. The following suggestions should address some of your most immediate concerns:

✔ **Talk openly with your child about his or her diagnosis.** It's far better to give your child accurate information about what's going on than to let his or her imagination fill in the blanks. The information you give also provides the vocabulary he or she needs to ask questions. Open and honest communication with kids also promotes feelings of safety and trust. In other words, when you feel comfortable talking about the difficult stuff, your child will feel confident that he or she is in good hands.

- **Be prepared for the reaction.** How a child reacts to an MS diagnosis will depend a lot on his or her age. In general, however, it's important to remember that most kids tend to take their cues from their parents. If you're anxious or upset, for instance, your child will be too. So, the truth (provided at an age-appropriate level) is important, but so is reassurance that he or she will be okay.

- **Involve your child in the treatment planning process from the get-go.** The treatment of MS is ongoing, so when kids are included in the decisions, they feel safer, more knowledgeable about what's happening, and more in control. Because all of the current treatments involve injections, it's important for youngsters to feel like part of the treatment team when decisions are made. For example, because the symptoms of MS tend to relapse, particularly in the early years, your child will be getting injections even when he or she is feeling absolutely fine. Without plenty of discussion, a child may not understand why he or she must continually be poked and prodded. After all, who ever heard of getting a shot when you're feeling fine?

- **Help your child deal with his or her doctors.** Kids with MS are going to have ongoing relationships with a variety of health professionals. They'll undergo a lot of medical tests, neurologic examinations, and evaluations of various kinds. You can help your child feel more comfortable and less afraid in the doctor's office if you stay calm yourself. We also

396

suggest trying to find out ahead of time what's likely to happen during the visit so you can give your kid a heads-up. Also, consider helping your youngster engage in age-appropriate conversations with the doctors, nurses, and other specialists—the more comfortable your child can become with each member of the treatment team, the safer and more relaxed he or she will feel in the long run.

Teenagers may gradually feel the need to handle some of the doctor visits on their own. If your child has been able to develop a trusting relationship with the doctor, he or she may prefer to be examined and talk to the doctor without you there. Even though this may be incredibly difficult for you, it's important to respect your teenager's need for privacy. We suggest a three-way agreement among you, your teen, and the doctor that acknowledges your child's wish for privacy and independence. But, make it clear that important medical decisions will be made by all of you together.

✔ **Don't be overprotective.** Because MS is so unpredictable, your child may feel really crummy one day and perfectly fine other days. Even though your first instinct may be to try and protect him or her from overexertion in an effort to keep the MS from doing its thing, your best bet is to let your kid be a kid whenever he or she feels up to it. Children's bodies will generally give them pretty good clues about what they can and can't do. If you have concerns about this, a three-way conversation with the doctor can help you and your child sort this out.

Introducing the first network of regional pediatric MS Centers of Excellence

In 2005, the National MS Society awarded $13.5 million for six regional Centers of Excellence to treat and study childhood MS. These centers offer optimal medical and psychosocial support to children under 18 and their families (with funds available to families in need of transportation, lodging, and medical care). The centers are located in geographically diverse areas in order to serve as many children and families living with MS as possible. They're staffed by teams of pediatric and adult MS experts who lead the field in MS diagnosis and treatment. The centers include the following:

➤ Center for Pediatric-Onset Demyelinating Disease at the Children's Hospital of Alabama (in connection with the University of Alabama at Birmingham)

➤ Pediatric MS Center at Jacobs Neurological Institute (in connection with State University of New York at Buffalo)

➤ Mayo Clinic in Rochester, Minnesota

➤ National Pediatric MS Center at Stony Brook University Hospital in Long Island, New York

➤ Partners Pediatric MS Center at Massachusetts General Hospital for Children in Boston

➤ San Francisco Regional Pediatric MS Center at University of California

398

Chapter 16

And Baby Makes Three, Four, or More: Planning a Family around Your MS

In This Chapter

▲ Understanding that parenthood is possible even if you have MS

▲ Knowing what issues to consider when it comes to parenthood

▲ Making your family-planning decisions easier with some strategies

*M*any people are in their 20s and 30s when they're diagnosed with multiple sclerosis (MS)—which is smack in the middle of the time when most folks are building their careers and starting their families. So, "Can I have children?" or "Will having a baby make my MS worse?" are among the first questions young women are likely to ask their doctors upon diagnosis. Similarly, men want to know if MS is going to affect their ability to father a child. And, both women and men worry whether MS will affect their ability to be good parents and whether their children are going to develop MS.

To help you make the best family-planning decisions for you and your family, in this chapter we answer all of your questions. We show you the impact of MS on fertility, pregnancy, childbirth, and breastfeeding, and then we show you the impact of pregnancy and childbirth on MS. We also discuss your medication options in the weeks preceding, during, and following pregnancy, and we provide suggestions on how best to think through your family-planning decisions, given how unpredictable MS can be.

MS and Babies: Here's the Good News!

The good news for couples is that women and men with MS can be effective, involved parents of healthy, happy children (check out Chapter 17 for info about the pleasures and pitfalls of parenting). Even though the message prior to about 1950 was that women with MS shouldn't even consider having kids, the research since then has confirmed repeatedly that MS and motherhood can go together just fine. Men with MS haven't received as much attention in this area, but no research suggests that MS interferes with a man's ability to father a healthy child or to be a good parent. To give you some solid reassurance, we include the following sections, which show you exactly what doctors today know about the connection between having babies and having MS.

Fertility isn't affected by MS

We're sure that you're thrilled to know that MS doesn't affect the production of eggs or sperm (or their ability to form healthy embryos). But, unless you're ready to hear the pitter-patter of little feet, the fact that your fertility factories are functioning means that you and your partner need to make the same decisions about birth control as everyone else. And, it's also important to know that some of the medications used to treat MS or its symptoms—including corticosteroids, anticonvulsants, and antibiotics—can reduce

400

the effectiveness of oral contraceptives. So, couples are advised to use additional protection if the woman is taking any of these medications.

Even though sperm production isn't affected by MS, problems with erectile function or ejaculation can interfere with conception. So, guys who are experiencing difficulty getting or maintaining an erection, or ejaculating, may want to consult a urologist about treatment for the problem. (Check out Chapter 8 for more information about changes in sexual function.)

Pregnancy hormones reduce disease activity

To understand how pregnancy hormones reduce MS activity, first consider what these hormones actually do: They suppress a woman's immune system so that her body doesn't reject the developing fetus as a foreigner. This, in turn, helps out your MS because as the hormone levels rise over the nine months of pregnancy, your likelihood of having a *relapse* (exacerbation) decreases—particularly during your third trimester when the hormone levels are highest. Lots of women with MS say they feel so good when they're pregnant that they wish they could stay pregnant forever.

As the pregnancy hormones return to normal levels during the three to six months following delivery (or the termination of the pregnancy by spontaneous or elective abortion), a woman's risk of relapse rises significantly before it levels off to her pre-pregnancy rate. So, as a group, women have about a 10 percent risk of having a relapse while pregnant, and a 29 percent risk of having a relapse soon after the pregnancy ends. However, the best way to predict your own risk of having a relapse following delivery is to look at your rate of relapses during the year before you got pregnant. The more active your MS was prior to your pregnancy, the more

401

likely you are to experience a relapse in the months after your baby is born. See the "Minding your medications" section later for tips on how you may be able to reduce your risk of relapse after pregnancy.

Pregnancies don't increase a woman's long-term disability level

Women with MS who have had one or more pregnancies don't become any more disabled over the long run than women with MS who have no pregnancies. In fact, some research even suggests that women with MS who have been pregnant fare slightly better than women who have not, although the reasons for this aren't clear. This means that even though your risk of having a relapse increases immediately following pregnancy, the risk is a short-term one, without any implications for your eventual disability level.

Childbirth isn't a piece of cake for anyone but women with MS do just fine

Despite popular belief, moms with MS deliver their babies just like other women do (you know, with lots of yelling, grunting, and gnashing of teeth). And just like women without MS, you have anesthesia options to make childbirth a little easier. If you want or need anesthesia, all types are considered safe for you to use—the choice is up to you and your physician.

A recent, large-scale study of all pregnancies in Norway suggests that the number of forceps deliveries and deliveries by Caesarian section is somewhat higher in women with MS than in the general population. The most likely explanation is that women with MS may become more fatigued during labor than other women. Or, they may have other symptoms such as sensory changes that make it difficult to

402

feel the contractions, or *spasticity* (stiffness) or weakness that may make pushing more difficult. If you're having significant problems with fatigue, weakness, or spasticity, be sure to discuss them with your obstetrician *before* you head to the hospital to deliver.

Even though evidence shows that moms with MS do well during pregnancy and delivery, some obstetricians and anesthesiologists in various parts of the country may be reluctant to take you on as a patient because they mistakenly consider pregnancy and delivery in a woman with MS to be "high risk." So, be sure to discuss your pregnancy and delivery with your obstetrician from the get-go, and make an appointment to meet with the anesthesiologist ahead of time. These conversations can help ensure that your big day is as comfortable and stress-free as it can possibly be. (Check out www.nationalmssociety.org/pregnancyinfo for information about pregnancy and delivery that you can share with your doctors.)

Parents with MS have healthy babies

As we've mentioned before, doctors used to think that pregnancy and MS didn't go together. They believed that pregnancy and delivery could make a mom's MS worse or that she could miscarry or have an unhealthy child. However, recent research has shown that women with MS can have healthy, full-term babies with no increased risk of miscarriages or fetal abnormalities.

Children who have a parent with MS do have a somewhat higher risk of developing MS than children in the general population, but the risk remains relatively low at approximately 3 to 5 percent. (Take a look at Chapter 1 for more information about the genetics of MS.) Unfortunately, no test or genetic study currently exists that can determine your child's risk of developing MS.

Breastfeeding is definitely an option

Women with MS who wish to breastfeed are definitely encouraged to do so—it won't increase your risk of an MS relapse and it's great for the baby. The only reason your doctor may discourage nursing is if he or she feels it's important for you to restart your disease-modifying medication right away to reduce your risk of relapses (see the section "Considering Key Issues when Making Family-Planning Decisions" later in the chapter for more on your medication options). Another consideration is that you may be very tired after your baby is born (the combination of MS fatigue and new-mom fatigue can be a real doozy), so you need to make sure that you have sufficient energy to nurse and that you have adequate help around if you need it.

If you're breastfeeding, your baby will nurse every two to four hours for the first several weeks. These frequent feedings will help you build up your milk supply, but they're also pretty tiring. So ask the happy dad or another support person to bring you the baby for the night feedings so you can conserve your energy. After the supply is well-established, you can pump milk during the day for nighttime bottle feedings, which dad or another helper can cheerfully provide at 2 a.m. Or, if necessary, you can use formula for those feedings.

Considering Key Issues when Making Family-Planning Decisions

Starting a family or adding to it is a big decision for any couple, and there are even more issues to consider when one of the parents has MS. All prospective moms and dads face some uncertainties in their future, but those with MS face even more because of the unpredictability of the disease.

Minding your medications

The goal during pregnancy is always to be taking as few medications as possible in order to avoid problems for your growing baby. Before trying to become pregnant, be sure to discuss all the medications you're taking (prescription and over-the-counter) with your physician so that changes or substitutions can be made prior to conception if needed.

The disease-modifying medications and pregnancy planning

We emphasize in Chapter 6 that early and ongoing treatment with one of the disease-modifying therapies—the interferon medications, Copaxone (glatiramer acetate), or Tysabri (natalizumab)—is important to controlling your disease. But, here's the hitch: None of these medications are approved for use during pregnancy or breastfeeding.

For safety reasons, the effects of the disease-modifying medications can't actually be studied during pregnancy, but the data collected from women who accidentally became pregnant while on an interferon medication suggest that the meds may cause a slight increase in the risk of miscarriage or fetal malformation. The data from Copaxone users so far show no increased risks but most neurologists and obstetricians still recommend that women stop the medication prior to becoming pregnant. At this time, there are no pregnancy data for Tysabri, but it isn't considered safe for use by pregnant women.

Until more information becomes available, we strongly recommend that you stop your disease-modifying therapy at least one month prior to trying to conceive (after consulting with your doctor, of course). And you should consult with your doctor right away if you become pregnant unexpectedly while on medication. If you haven't yet started a disease-modifying medication and are considering becoming pregnant within the coming year, you may want to wait until your baby is born to begin treatment in order to avoid having to start and stop.

But, you don't need to panic about being without your meds because pregnancy hormones actually provide some protection against MS disease activity (see the section "Pregnancy hormones reduce disease activity" earlier in the chapter for details). In fact, pregnancy hormones essentially reduce relapses by about the same amount as the disease-modifying therapies.

Unfortunately, none of the pharmaceutical companies have paid any attention to medication issues for men. No data have been collected regarding babies who were conceived while a father was taking one of the disease-modifying medications. Most physicians aren't concerned about the impact of the father's medications on the baby—but, if you prospective fathers want to be super-careful, you can talk to your physician about interrupting your medication schedule while you and your partner are trying to conceive.

Your options during and after pregnancy

It's great that pregnancy hormones provide some protection against MS disease activity during pregnancy, but what do you do while you're trying to get pregnant or if you choose to breastfeed? During these months you're obviously not receiving any protection against disease activity, so as you make your family-planning decisions, you need to be thinking about how long you want to be off your medication.

For example, if your MS has been particularly active in the year prior to your pregnancy and it remains active dur-

406

ing your pregnancy, you may want to consider getting back on medication as soon as you deliver, which means that you'll have to bottle feed your baby rather than nurse. Some neurologists are also prescribing intravenous immunoglobulin (IVIg) right after delivery to reduce the risk of relapses. However, if your MS has been pretty stable, you can probably postpone medication until you decide to stop nursing.

The effects of immunosuppressants on fertility

The immunosuppressant medications used to treat some progressive forms of MS can affect egg and sperm production and can harm a developing fetus (flip to Chapter 6 for more details on the immunosuppressant meds). So, you women out there should take a pregnancy test prior to starting any of these medications (and prior to subsequent doses of those medications that are taken every several months). Also, because of the potential of these drugs to cause sterility, men should consider banking sperm and women should consider harvesting their eggs for future use.

Remembering that babies don't stay babies very long

When women talk to us about their baby-making plans, they wonder how they'll feel after the baby is born or whether they'll be able to take care of the baby properly. These are all great questions, but it's also important to remember that babies grow up pretty fast. In other words, you need to consider how you and your partner will manage your growing child. So, as you talk through your feelings and thoughts about baby-making, try to imagine your new baby turning into an active toddler and your active toddler turning into a busy preteen and then—gulp—a teen. (Check out Chapter 17 for info on parenting with MS.)

Facing the uncertainties: The future doesn't come with guarantees

Everyone is faced with lots of uncertainties in life. However the unpredictability of MS—from day to day and over the long haul—makes big life decisions (like whether to start a family) even more complicated. Your best bet is to try and think through—individually and as a couple—what you would do if things got tough. Figure out how you would cope, what strategies you would use, and what resources you have available to you. Thinking through the future possibilities—rosy and not so rosy—helps you make more informed decisions. And whatever you decide, you'll know that your choices have taken into account the complexities of living with MS. (Refer to Part V for more details on planning for a future with MS.)

When you're making your family-planning decisions, keep in mind that all the good news we give you in this chapter (see the section "MS and Babies: Here's the Good News!" earlier in this chapter) is based on group statistics. The odds are in your favor—but they aren't guaranteed. In other words, if you're one of the women who has a severe, disabling relapse following delivery, it won't matter to you that the vast majority of women do fine.

Strategies for Smart Decision-Making

Family-planning decisions are never easy, especially when MS is present. So, in this section we provide you with some strategies that will help you as you're trying to decide whether you should have a baby.

Consult your MS doctor

No doctor has a crystal ball, but the level of disease activity you have experienced so far and the kinds of symptoms you have may give your neurologist some idea of how your MS is likely to behave over the long haul. Of course, you certainly have no guarantees, but talking about what *may* happen with your MS can highlight the important issues for you to consider.

For example, your doctor may suggest that you give yourself a year or two to stabilize on your disease-modifying medication before stopping it to become pregnant. Or, he or she may encourage you to begin your family sooner rather than later because you're doing well right now and the future is less certain.

Evaluate your financial situation

Even though financial considerations are important for any couple that's making family-planning decisions, the potential impact of MS on employment makes this a particularly important topic to discuss with your partner. You can implement strategies to keep your place in the workforce (see Chapter 18), but the bottom line is that you may not be able to work as long you had anticipated. The fact that you may not work as long as you would have hoped is important for a couple of reasons:

- Your family income may not be as great as you would like it to be down the road, particularly given the fact that two-income families are pretty much the norm these days.

- The partner without MS may need to take on a bigger share of the wage-earning responsibilities. For example, a mom who planned to stay home with school-age kids may find that she needs to work full-time because her partner with MS can't.

REMEMBER

Money worries are no fun, so make sure that you and your partner sit down and discuss your financial situation. If you need some expert advice, call the National MS Society at (800) FIGHT-MS (800-344-4867) for a free consultation through its Financial Education Partners program.

Take a good look at your teamwork

Parenting under the best of circumstances takes a lot of flexibility, patience, creativity, and endurance. With MS in the picture, it can require even more. So, given how unpredictable MS can be, one of the most important things to consider in your family-planning discussion is your teamwork.

For instance, ask yourself the following questions: Can you roll with the punches? How rigid are your roles and responsibilities in the household? Can you picture yourself as a stay-at-home dad or a working mom? How's your sense of humor? Can you talk about tough stuff when you need to? The answers to questions like these give you a sense of how well-oiled your teamwork is—and better teamwork sure makes for easier parenting.

Check out your support network

Some couples live surrounded by family, friends, and neighbors while others are pretty much out there on their own. There's no reason to run and join a commune, but it's worthwhile to think about the resources that you have available in the event that you need some assistance now and then. For example, you can find support people in all sorts of places: in your family, in your community, at work,

410

at your church or synagogue, and through your local National MS Society chapter.

Have a heart-to-heart with your partner

Decisions about if and when to have kids can be pretty emotional. People generally have strong feelings about this issue one way or another. And to top it all off, communicating about heavy stuff can sometimes be difficult. You don't want to upset your partner or give someone you love more to worry about than he or she is already dealing with. But, the fact is, holding back feelings or concerns—particularly about hot topics like family-planning decisions, family finances, and relationship issues—can come back to bite you later on (see Chapter 15 for more about family communication issues).

If you're scared to death about the future, about your partner's ability to take care of kids now that he or she has MS, or about your own ability to pick up the slack if you have to, now's the time to get those feelings out in the open. Chances are, you both have some worries, and now's the time to share them. The notion that "two heads are better than one" has some merit because together you can think through the stuff that's worrying you and figure out how you can deal with it.

If you need help having this kind of discussion, your healthcare provider or the National MS society (800-FIGHT-MS) can refer you to a counselor who can help mediate.

Talk to other parents living with MS

No matter what your concerns are, sometimes it's reassuring to talk to others who are in your same boat. For example, you can read everything there is to know about parenting (and Chapter 17 would be a great start), but there's

411

nothing better than a real-life chat. Picking the brains of moms and dads with MS who live the day-to-day joys and challenges of parenthood is by far your best way to get information about pregnancy, delivery, chasing energetic toddlers, or anything else that's on your mind. If you don't know anyone in your community who has MS, the National MS Society (800-FIGHT-MS) can help you get in touch with other couples to talk to. Or you can check out the Society's chat room at www.nationalmssociety.org/chat.

Remember that your plans can change

Many people arrive at adulthood with some preconceived ideas and dreams about parenthood. They know whether they want to have kids and they know exactly how many they want. And sometimes they have a detailed vision of what parenthood will be like. If, for any reason, you decide to change your parenting plans—to not have kids, to have fewer than you originally planned, or to adopt rather than having your own, it's important to remember that this change of heart can feel kind of like a loss. Even if you're comfortable with the decision, you're confident that it's the right one for you, and you're happy with the outcome, you may find that some grieving goes along with it. If you're feeling the need to grieve, go for it! Grieving is part of coping with a disease that sometimes upsets the apple cart (see Chapter 3 for more on healthy grieving).

Whatever you decide about having children, the choices are yours and only yours—not your doctor's, not your parents', and not your friends'. You may get a lot of opinions about what you should or shouldn't do, but the only right decision is the one that you and your partner make together.

412

Parenting: It Wasn't Easy *Before* You Had MS!

As a parent or prospective parent with multiple sclerosis (MS), you're probably worried about what effect your illness or disability will have on your children. You may wonder if you'll be able to give them what they need or whether they will have to take care of you. So, here are some things we've learned from our own research and clinical experience and from others who have studied this issue:

🗸 Kids who have a parent with MS generally do well emotionally, socially, and academically.

🗸 Many children develop a strong sense of responsibil-

ity and take pride in learning how to do things independently.

- Children learn a lot from watching a parent meet
  life's challenges—and it makes them proud.

- When children grow up with someone who has a
  disability, they tend to develop a greater sensitivity to
  the needs of others.

- Living with family challenges can bring family members closer to one another.

In other words, don't assume that having a parent with
MS has to be a downer for your children. On the other
hand, it's important to acknowledge your children's feelings and worries about MS because sweeping them under
the carpet doesn't really work in the long run. Your job as a
parent is to find the balance. And in the rest of this chapter, we help you do just that.

Keeping the Communication Lines Open

You may be wondering whether it's a good idea to tell
your kids about mom or dad's MS. You may worry that
the information will scare them or give them too much to
worry about. You may be afraid that they will see you differently or feel embarrassed. Or, you may simply not
know how to begin. So, in this section, we give you some
pointers that may make your decision a little bit easier. We
explain why we think it's so important for you to be up
front with your kids. We talk about how to respond to their
major worries and how to explain whatever symptoms you
may be having.

414

Telling the kids about your MS makes good sense

As you may have already figured out, MS doesn't just affect one person in the family—it impacts everyone—so each family member needs to develop some kind of relationship with the illness. And open discussion is the best foundation we can think of for building comfortable relationships.

You know your children better than anyone else does. So, ultimately, you're the one who needs to decide what's best for them and for the family. It's our experience, though, that there are some good reasons for introducing MS to kids early on. The following sections explain a few.

Kids have a sixth sense about what's going on anyway

Contrary to popular belief, kids of all ages are pretty quick to pick up on what's happening around them. If you're tense, worried, or upset, chances are that your children—no matter how young they are—are clued into it right away. Even if they don't quite know why you're upset, they sense your mood and interpret it as best they can. This means that without information from you, their imaginations will take over, and the problems they imagine are likely to be even more frightening than whatever the reality happens to be.

Big news items should come from you

Your kids need to hear about the important stuff directly from you for the following reasons:

- ✔ Someone else may not have the most accurate information or the best way of presenting it to your kids.

- ✔ Children don't like being the last to know about something important.

415

- When parents find it too difficult to talk about something, kids quickly conclude that it must be something really terrible or shameful.

- Hearing the information from you helps them feel secure and confident that you're on top of things.

The longer you put off talking about your MS, the more likely it becomes that your children will end up hearing about it from someone else—most likely a well-meaning friend or relative who accidentally spills the beans.

Hearing the information from you is a green light for asking questions

When a big, gray elephant is hanging out in the living room and no one's talking about it, it's easy for children to conclude that the subject is off-limits. But, when you talk about what's going on, your kids get the message that it's okay to ask their questions and tell you what's on their minds. And, you've given them the vocabulary they need to put their questions into words.

Accurate information about the disease relieves kids' guilt

Children have a tendency to see themselves as the center of the universe. Younger kids, in particular, are likely to assume that anything going on around them is somehow related to them. So, when you aren't feeling well or you're upset or tense, they're likely to assume that they're the cause of the problem. However, giving them accurate information about MS will reassure them that they haven't done anything to make you sick. Check out the sidebar "Tapping resources for kids" for some age-appropriate materials that you can share with your children.

416

Women are at increased risk for an MS relapse three to six months following childbirth (see Chapter 16 for more details). This means that for quite a few of you out there, your MS appeared right after the birth of a child. Kids can easily misinterpret this kind of family folklore as a statement of blame, and they can begin to feel guilty. A good discussion about the possible causes of MS can help lay these feelings to rest.

In the same way, statements like "You're really stressing me out; cut it out or you're going to make my MS worse" lay a heavy load on kids. So, try not to use your MS as a behavior-controlling tool.

Your openness about MS provides a good model of family sharing and problem-solving

If you have MS, believe it or not, you may have a bit of a blessing in disguise—you now have the opportunity to model for your kids how people help one another deal with life's challenges. Children who see that it's okay to talk openly within the family about problems that arise are much more likely to come to you when they hit snags along the way.

Sharing info with your children when secrecy is important

Sometimes your kids' needs conflict with your own. For example, say that you and your wife want to talk to the children about your MS, but you haven't told anyone at work yet because of concerns about job security (see Chapter 18 about MS and employment). You're worried that after the kids know, the information will gradually spread around the neighborhood and get to your boss's ears. What do you do?

417

From the mouth of babes

Here's what some kids have to say about having a parent with MS:

Joshua (age 12): "My life has been changed forever. My mom was diagnosed with MS in 2000. We have been fighting this disease for about five years. One morning my mom woke up and had double vision. She didn't know what was wrong. She went to the doctor to have some tests, and the tests showed that she had MS. My mom now has to stay cool so we sold our hot tub. She also switched from a full-time job to a part-time job. She can't do a lot of physical activity, so we bought a bicycle she can ride with one of us so she can still enjoy our family bike rides. With these changes, our family is still as strong as ever. MS has made our family much closer than we were before. We are thankful for everything — even MS."

Sarah (age 14): "My mom has MS. I have three brothers, so I'm the only girl. I always try to help my mom, because with MS, she gets weak in all sorts of places. Even though she's weak and hurts, she still does things for us. (It's like she has a million arms, because she loves us more than anything!) She takes us to the movies, our friend's birthday parties, out to lunch. Even though my mom has MS, she still is the best mom in the world!"

Amy Jo (age 12): "My mom has multiple sclerosis. It all started one morning when her hands were tingling. She just thought they were asleep, but soon her whole body was numb. When we got the news, we cried for hours. My mom was afraid to tell us, but says she found the strength because she was able to tell us two of the most important things: We could not catch this from her and she would not die from MS. She explained to us that although she didn't know everything about the disease, we could ask her anything, and if she didn't know the answer we would figure it out together. My mom has a very positive attitude. We have all learned a lot about the power of having a positive attitude."

418

This situation definitely has no easy answers. Ultimately, you need to make your decision based on what you know about your kids and about your work environment. Just remember that by the time they're 6 or 7 years old, most youngsters understand privacy and secrets pretty well. They can appreciate the idea that some things only get talked about at home. Any child who has had bed-wetting issues, for example, knows exactly how important it is to keep some stuff private.

Finding ways to broach the big issues

After you decide to talk to your kids about MS, you may be wondering what to say and how to say it. Here are a few basic things to keep in mind:

✔ **Children have individual needs and learning styles.** One wants all the details and another just likes the big picture. One wants to talk and ask questions while another wants to read a book or watch a video. Some kids will ask a lot of questions and show a lot of interest while others won't appear to have the slightest bit of interest or curiosity. Because one size definitely doesn't fit all, you have to tailor your conversations to each child's needs—preferably one-on-one.

✔ **One conversation won't do it.** Don't expect to be able to gather all your children in the living room, give a short explanation of MS, and be done with it. Talking to kids about MS is a lot like talking to them about sex—you start with the amount of information they need at the time, and gradually expand on it as they get older and their needs (and your worries) change.

419

➤ **Regardless of how old they are—preschoolers or teens—all kids share a few major worries.** Here are a few of those worries:

- **"Are you going to die?"** When they ask this question, you can tell younger children that "Once in a while, MS can make someone so sick that they die, but most people live to be old. But, you don't need to worry about that because we will always take care of you." Tell older children "People sometimes die of complications of their MS—like serious infection—but most people live very close to a normal lifespan."

- **"Am I going to catch it?"** Here's what to tell younger children: "You can't catch MS like a cold or the chicken pox—it isn't contagious." Tell your older children: "MS isn't contagious, but some people have genes that make them more likely to develop it than other people. The risk, however, is low."

- **"Did I make you get sick?"** Tell both younger and older children the following: "No, you didn't make me sick. There's nothing that you or anyone else did to make this happen."

Your children may not come right out and ask these questions, but they need the answers in whatever way you feel most comfortable giving them.

➤ **Let your kids know what you're doing to take care of yourself.** Nothing is more reassuring for your children than knowing that you have a good doctor who's working with you to treat your MS in the best possible way. Also, don't worry about keeping your treatments and medications a secret. When you share info about your treatments, your kids feel

420

more confident that you're in charge and that your illness is under control. In fact, if you take an injectable medication to manage your MS, your kids are will be very impressed with how brave you are.

Depending on your children's ages and level of interest (and your neurologist's bedside manner) you may want to schedule a time for the kids to come to the office with you so they can watch the neurologic exam and ask the doc some questions.

At one time or another, you may need to go into the hospital for treatment—perhaps during a relapse—or into an inpatient rehabilitation program. Children may be frightened about your hospital stay, particularly if grandma or some other friend or relative died during a hospital stay. Take the time to explain exactly why you're going to the hospital, what's going to happen while you're there, and when you expect to be home. Daily phone conversations and visits, if possible, can help reduce kids' worries.

Explaining those pesky invisible symptoms

Children have a difficult time understanding symptoms they can't see. For instance, they can see that you trip or lose your balance and need a cane or scooter to help you walk. And they can see (and probably think that it's funny) that you drop things a lot. But kids have a much harder time getting a handle on fatigue, cognitive, mood, or vision problems, or other symptoms that aren't as visible to them. For example:

✔ Children know that when they're tired, they can go to bed or take a nap and feel much better when they wake up. But, it's difficult for them to understand that sometimes you feel just as tired when you wake

421

up as you did when you went to sleep. Older kids, in particular, may think that you aren't interested in doing stuff, or that you aren't trying very hard (this is a situation when open communication is particularly helpful).

- Children know that many people wear glasses. So, they may find it difficult to understand why your vision problems can't be fixed with a new pair of glasses or contact lenses.

- Kids understand pain—something hurts until it's better, and then the pain goes away. Chronic pain, however, is likely to be much more difficult for them to comprehend.

- Problems with thinking and memory are particularly difficult for children to understand and easy for them to misinterpret. They may think that you aren't interested enough to pay attention to what they're saying, or that you're "getting dumb." You can help your kids understand the challenges you're experiencing by involving them in some of the strategies that you use to compensate for your cognitive problems.

You may want to give your kids the opportunity to "try on" some of your physical symptoms. Obviously, these "try-ons" don't give the full picture, but they offer kids a hint of what some MS symptoms can feel like. Here's how to do it:

- Let your kids wear some light ankle weights while they walk around for a little while. This will give them a sense of what it feels like when your legs and ankles feel tired and weak.

- Put an elastic bandage around their knees or elbows so they can feel what *spasticity* (stiffness) feels like.

- Place an elastic bandage around your kids' chests or tummies. This can give them a pretty good imitation of the uncomfortable sensory symptom that feels like an "MS hug."

- Smear a little petroleum jelly on a pair of sunglasses to demonstrate what blurry vision looks like.

- Stick a little square of cellophane tape in the center of each eyeglass to show what patchy vision can look like.

- Have your kids put on kitchen gloves, and then tell them to try and button a shirt, pick up pennies, or unwrap a piece of hard candy. This will help them see how sensory changes in your hands can make it difficult for you to do things.

- Tell you kids to spin in a circle until they're dizzy. When they're dizzy, tell them that is what vertigo can feel like for you.

 Mood changes are more difficult to demonstrate, but they're just as important to explain. Kids definitely know when you're down or cranky. And they're quick to assume that they're the cause—particularly if you take your moods out on them. So, it's a good idea to talk about your mood swings if you have them. And be sure to tell your kids that your moods aren't because of them.

Parenting around Your MS Symptoms

You probably have some set ideas about what parents ought to be able to do with and for their children. If you don't

423

Tapping resources for kids

The National MS Society offers a lot of good resources to help you explain MS to your children. Here are a few of them:

➤ *Timmy's Journey to Understanding MS* is a fun cartoon about Timmy and his dad that helps explain MS to younger children. Call (800) FIGHT-MS (800-344-4867) to request a copy (DVD or video).

➤ Keep *S'myelin* is a free newsletter for children who are 6 to 12 years old. Each issue has information about a specific MS symptom or issue, cartoons, games, and a pull-out section for parents that provides information and resources to help you talk to your kids about MS. You can subscribe by calling (800) FIGHT-MS. Or, you can find the interactive, online version of each issue at www.nationalmssociety.org/ks.

➤ Two brochures are available specifically for children:

➤ *Someone You Know Has MS: A Booklet for Families* (for kids 5 to 12 years old). You can access this brochure at www.nationalmssociety.org/familybook.

➤ *When a Parent Has MS: A Teenager's Guide*. To access this brochure, visit www.nationalmssociety.org/teen guide.

➤ "The Journey Club" is a chapter-sponsored education program for parents with MS and their children who are 5 to 12 years old. The sessions provide entertaining activities designed to help families discuss issues related to the family's journey with MS, including symptoms, emotional issues, and changes in family life.

➤ Chapter-sponsored children's camps give kids who have a parent with MS the opportunity to discover a lot about MS while enjoying recreational activities.

✔ Chapter-sponsored "Family Days" offer families the opportunity to socialize while learning about MS in lectures and workshops.

To find out about the programs your chapter has to offer, call (800) FIGHT-MS.

Parents are sometimes reluctant to make use of these resources with their children. They have all kinds of reasons, including busy schedules, a reluctance to make MS a focus of attention, and a worry that their children will be upset by what they read, see, or hear. Parents also say to us (and themselves), "Oh, we're doing fine — we don't need that yet." But, these resources are for everyone — even those families who are "doing fine." Don't wait for some kind of family crisis to get involved in these activities. It's much easier to help your kids understand your MS as you go along than to wait for a crisis that will be much more difficult to deal with.

---

have kids yet, you may be picturing the way your mom and dad did things with you. If you already have children, you're probably busy comparing what things were like before you got MS with how you're feeling now. Whatever your situation, you're probably worrying about how MS can or will get in the way of doing stuff with your kids. So, in this section, we talk about some ways to get around your symptoms and think more flexibly about being a parent with MS.

"I'm so tired that I'm in bed before they are!"

If you experience MS fatigue, you know that when you hit

that wall, there's no way around it—all of a sudden, you're simply out of gas (we talk about strategies for managing MS fatigue in Chapter 7). Unfortunately, MS fatigue is likely to peak just about the same time that the kids are coming home from school, dinner needs to be cooked, and the family is getting together for the evening. If you're coming home from a long day at work, you may not have much energy left for anyone or anything. Here are some ideas to help you make the most of your family time:

- **Make good use of power naps.** If you can carve out 30 minutes to rest before the kids get home, do it. Or, if you can come in from work and rest for a little while before joining the family, do it. Kids will understand your need for rest time as long as you explain the plan and promise to do something with them afterwards.

  If you don't need or want to sleep during your rest time, you can invite your kids to read with you, tell you about their day, or play a quiet game.

- **Set your priorities.** If quality time with your kids is high on your list, spend less time on the things that aren't as important. Figure out what you want to do with each child—help with homework, read a bed-time story, or watch a program—and plan around it. You don't need to spend a lot of time—you just need to make the time you have count.

- **Keep things simple.** Dinner doesn't need to be a banquet. Come up with some simple but nourishing menus, and do things the easiest way possible (for example, by using pre-cut salad ingredients or plan-ning menus that provide plenty of leftovers).

  Take a look at the book by Shelley Peterman Schwarz called *Multiple Sclerosis: 300 Tips for Making*

426

Life Easier (Demos Medical Publishing, 2006) for ideas on how to save your energy for the important stuff.

✔ **Ask for help.** It's okay to ask family members to pitch in and help—and to remind them how everyone will benefit in the long run. For instance, consider these examples: "Sara, if you help me with the dishes tonight, we'll have more time to spend on your science project." Or, "Honey, would you make the kids' lunches so I can sit and read with them for a while?" Just remember that teamwork makes the chores go faster and you may even have some fun while you're doing them.

Sometimes, MS fatigue has the last word. If you need to lie down, invite your kids to join you for a bedtime story or a nice chat and a cuddle.

"How can I be a good dad if I can't even play ball?"

In spite of what you may think, there are lots of ways to be a good parent. Take some time to think about what kids need most. Sure, every child is different, but they all need to be loved, and to feel safe, secure, and cared for. Even though you may think that playing catch, building tree-houses, or baking elaborate desserts is what being a dad or mom is all about, the reality is that it's about being there for your kids—no matter how you're able to do that.

We've known a lot of dads who couldn't run around and play catch, but who still coached the team or cheered loudly from the sidelines. And we've know a lot of moms who went on class trips, volunteered at school, or became Brownie or Cub Scout leaders even though they were using

More from the mouth of babes

Here's some more of what kids have to say about living with a parent or grandparent with MS:

Sean (age 8): "When I was 5 years old, my mom lost her eyesight in one eye. So, we went from one doctor to another and after many tests, they found out she had MS. I remember her being happy to finally know what was happening with her body. I can't say we are happy she has MS, but at least we can do things to make things easier for her. We go to her doctor's as a family sometimes. Her doctor is so cool. He always sits down with us to make sure we understand what is happening to her body. My favorite parts of the day are spent with my mom. She swims a lot and plays lots of games. The part about MS that is hard is watching her take a shot every day. But I don't like anything that hurts her. I know the most frustrating part of MS for her is that she is so tired and gets frustrated easily. I do more chores than most of my friends, but that's okay. That's what family is all about."

Sallie (age 9): "My mom has MS. Sometimes it's hard having a mom with MS but I know that she needs help. I love my mom a ton. Me and my brother think MS can be a bother but I love my mom for who she is and I hate MS for what it is."

Timothy (age 6): "My mom got MS. She said she wouldn't lose MS until they find a cure. It made me want to find a cure right away. I was very scared when my mom went to the hospital. I didn't know if she was going to die but my dad said she wasn't going to die from MS. She has trouble walking sometimes but she is still a good mom. I try to help her when I can. I don't know a lot about MS but I know it is [in] her central nervous system. But sometimes it makes her drop stuff or forget things. My mom said she could be in a wheelchair too but I told her that would be okay and that I would push her. I know some day they will find a cure and my mom will be better forever."

428

Kelles (age 11):

My Hero Grandma

I have a special hero,
her name is Grandzanne.
She teaches me lots of things,
most important that "I can!"
She's had lots of hard things in her life,
she's in a wheelchair, too.
But that has never stopped her,
from what she wants to do.
For years she was a teacher,
and now she writes a book.
She's always like to fight MS,
no matter how much control it took.
Grandzanne is my role model.
She's never down . . . instead,
she always looks on the bright side,
eager to see what's ahead!

a scooter or wheelchair. The point is that your kids want you to care about what they do and they want you to be involved—even if you have to do it differently than you ever imagined.

"How can I discipline 'em if I can't catch 'em?"

Moms and dads who can't get around as quickly or easily as they used to worry about how they'll be able to discipline their children. In other words, if they can't outrun their kids, how can they maintain any kind of control? Well, the fact is that most kids can outrun their parents eventually

429

anyway—with or without MS. So, discipline has to be about more than just moving fast enough to catch kids or give them a wallop on the bottom. When it isn't more than that, any smart kid will quickly realize that staying out of reach is the best strategy.

Discipline needs to be about clear, consistent expectations, firm limits, predictable consequences, and mutual respect—all of which are possible with or without MS. Obviously, the earlier the groundwork is laid, the easier it is. If discipline in your household has always depended on your ability to move faster, it will be tougher now to restructure things. So, think about having some family discussions about rules and expectations. Even young kids can participate in this kind of family powwow. Let them help in setting some of the rules and determining some of the consequences—you'll be surprised at how much more willing your children are to live by these rules when they've had some say in the situation.

Parental teamwork is key to effective discipline. In other words, it's important for parents to agree on the rules and be consistent in enforcing them. Here are a few suggestions to reinforce your teamwork:

- **Agree to support each other's decisions.** The quickest way to sabotage your disciplinary efforts is to let your kids play one of you off against the other. If Johnny gets a "no" about something from mom, and then gets a "yes" from dad, guess who Johnny's going to ask first the next time around?

  So, if you aren't sure whether the answer to Johnny should be yea or nay, talk it over with your partner first and then give Johnny the answer. If you aren't sure whether Johnny has already asked his other parent, find out before giving your answer.

430

✔ **Try to avoid the "Just wait until your father (or mother) gets home!" school of discipline.** First of all, this method diminishes your own parental role, and second, it sets the other parent up as the tough guy (or gal). If a kid's behavior demands some consequences, make those consequences clear right then and there.

✔ **Make sure that the MS doesn't diminish your parental role in anyone's eyes—starting with your own and your partner's.** If the consistent message to the kids is that you're in charge (no, this isn't a democracy), you'll find that your ability to set and enforce limits with your kids will be greatly enhanced.

Employing Effective Parenting Strategies

Parenting is never easy—it wasn't a piece of cake before MS came along and it won't be now. So, this section gives you some strategies to keep in mind.

Call a spade a spade: Let MS take the blame when it needs to

Sometimes MS is going to get in the way of things that you or your kids want to do. But, by being open about the disease and your symptoms, you make it easier for your kids to understand why plans sometimes need to be changed or activities need to be postponed. It's okay for them to be angry at the MS (just like it's okay for you to be angry at it). And, in the end, they'll feel a lot less guilty about expressing anger at the disease than at you.

431

To get the ball rolling, you can start by sharing your own anger at the disease—by saying, for example, "I get so mad at my MS when it keeps me from doing something I want to do with you. I was really looking forward to our bike ride today, but I'll give you a rain check on the bike ride and we can think of a fun substitute for today."

Polish up your creativity and flexibility

Whether you like it or not, MS is going to get in the way sometimes. Relapses or day-to-day symptoms have a way of interfering with the best-laid plans. The key for anyone, particularly for parents, is to have a backup plan. In fact, we recommend having a backup strategy for any major outing, trip, or activity. This may sound like negative thinking, but it's actually a way for families to hope for the best while planning for the worst. Kids (and adults) learn to roll with the punches more easily when they know that they can count on something really good in the near future.

It's important not to let MS steal the show. If your MS symptoms are affecting your ability to enjoy some favorite family activities, don't be shy about doing them in a different way than you normally do. Ask the rehab professionals for suggestions on how to adapt some of those activities to the demands of your MS (see Chapter 7 for more information about the role of the rehabilitation team in managing your MS). If, for example, fatigue or balance problems are making bike riding more difficult, think about investing in a tandem bike or a three-wheeler. Flexibility is the key—if you're willing to think about doing things differently, you can do almost anything.

Call on your support network

Grandparents, uncles, aunts, neighbors, and friends can be wonderful sources of support. Even though you may want

432

Other recommended parenting resources

For some more helpful tips on parenting and communicating more effectively with your kids, check out the following resources: Books

✔ *How to Talk So Kids Will Listen & Listen So Kids Will Talk* by Adele Faber and Elaine Mazlish (Collins Publishing, 1999).

✔ *Positive Discipline* by Jane Nelson (Ballantine Books, 2006).

Web sites

✔ Dolls with Disabilities (www.multiculturalkids.com): This Web site sells cute rag dolls that come in a variety of skin tones and hair colors and that can be outfitted with a variety of assistive devices, such as a wheelchair, a cane, forearm crutches, a walker, a hearing aid, and more.

✔ Family Food Zone (www.familyfoodzone.com): At this Web site, parents with MS who are looking to improve their diet can get recipes and tips for healthy family eating. Family Food Zone also provides a link to its fun, interactive kid's site that teaches kids about nutrition.

to do everything with your kids all of the time, the reality is that you may need to pick and choose your activities. So, instead of asking your kids to give up the activities that you can't participate in, think about getting some other folks involved to take your place. Children can get a lot of support and enjoyment from other adults in their life.

For example, if you're fortunate enough to have your kids' grandparents in the area, this week's soccer game may be a great opportunity for them to enjoy their grandchild. They go cheer at the game while you rest up, and then give you the play-by-play as soon as they get home. Or, if you can't be chauffeur this month, perhaps a neighbor could take over driving the kids for a while—and you do something for her after you're back on your feet.

Remember, MS isn't always to blame— other people's teenagers are a pain too

Parents with MS have a tendency to blame everything on their MS—if Susie's moping around the house, Jimmy's not doing well in school, Carol's having nightmares, or Sam's locked in his room all the time, it must be the MS. Even though MS may certainly be the problem, it generally isn't (take a look at the section "Handle little problems before they get bigger" later in the chapter to be sure).

Kids hit all kinds of bumps in the road that may have absolutely nothing to do with you or MS. By jumping to the wrong conclusion, you may miss other things going on with your children that need your attention. Or, you may beat yourself up with a lot of guilt when it's just standard teenage stuff. It's important to keep an open mind (as well as open eyes and ears) so you can figure out what's making your child upset. For example:

➤ Susie may be moping because she's angry at you for being different from other dads, *or* she may be ticked off that you wouldn't let her get that tattoo she's been wanting for months.

➤ Sam may be locked in his room because he's fed up with your MS, *or* he may be sad because he hasn't been able to get a date for the prom.

434

Handle little problems before they get bigger

When your kids are acting up or you've noticed differences in their behavior or mood, you may want to know how to tell if they're running into problems due to your MS or if something else is going on. Even though you don't want to jump to the conclusion that MS is the root of all evil, you also don't want to miss the times when it is.

Here are some typical scenarios and the best ways to handle them:

✔ **Your 5-year-old starts wetting his bed after two years with a "clean" record.** You're reading a bedtime story and he tells you that he's afraid something bad is going to happen to you. He saw all the medicine in the refrigerator and peeked at those needles in the box, and now maybe he thinks that you're going to die.

Explain to him that the medicines are good for you and that they're helping your MS. Also, consider going online with him to look at some issues of *Keep S'myelin* (see the sidebar "Tapping resources for kids" for details), so that he can understand more about how you take care of your MS.

✔ **Your 10-year-old suddenly stops bringing friends home.** When you have a heart-to-heart, you discover that his friends have been teasing him about your scooter and he's feeling embarrassed.

Consider calling his teacher and volunteering to come in and talk to the kids about MS and give them a chance to see the scooter up close.

✔ **Your 14-year-old suddenly becomes preoccupied with her health.** While you're riding in the car one day (this is the best place for conversations because everyone's a captive audience), your daughter asks what her chances are of getting MS.

To best deal with this question, call the National MS Society for some info about genetics. You can also ask her if she'd like to come to your next neurologist appointment to get some reassurance from a pro.

- **Your 17-year-old starts making noises about living at home for college.** When pressed, she tells you that she's worried about the costs of living on campus and thinks she should stay around to help.

  In this case, reassure her that the college money is set aside—and that it's important to you that she has this college experience. You can work out a deal that she will get a part-time job to help pay for her extras. And, be sure to reassure her that you'll keep her posted on how you're doing and let her know immediately if her help is needed.

Obviously, not all problems are this easily resolved, but these scenarios point out how youngsters' worries can show up in their everyday behavior. With a little prodding, though, you can usually get to the root of things and get your kids talking about what's on their minds.

Allow kids to be kids

Moms and dads with MS may need to look to others—their partners, children, extended family members, and friends—for help with their daily activities or their care (see Chapter 15 for details about care partnerships in MS). But sometimes, children are given more caregiving responsibilities than they can handle. Even though this doesn't happen often, in this section, we want to emphasize that kids need to be able to be kids—not miniature adults. So, we give you several tips on how to avoid overloading your kids.

Avoid assigning too many chores

Having chores around the house is not a problem for kids. Many kids who have a parent with MS end up doing a few more household chores than their peers, but it's generally not a big deal. Particularly if everyone in the household pitches in, and the chores are done on a rotating basis so that no one person always get stuck with the yucky ones, the kids don't seem to mind much. In fact, children and teens are often pretty proud of their contribution to the household and the skills they develop.

The problem begins when household chores interfere with schoolwork, social activities, sports, and so on—the activities that are important to a child's development and well-being. So, if your children don't have time to do their own stuff, you probably need to reassess and adjust the situation.

Be careful not to heap on too much responsibility

Developing a sense of responsibility is healthy for kids. However, being given responsibilities that are more than they can handle isn't. Kids get anxious when your expectations exceed their abilities, particularly when they believe that your safety and well-being depend on them.

For example, consider the story of Wendy, a 5-year-old who became upset when her mom started falling a lot. She felt that it was her job to take care of her mother, but didn't have the strength or the know-how to help. After awhile, Wendy was scared to be home alone with her mom. When the mom's neurologist heard about the problem, he referred Wendy's mom to a physical therapist (PT) to learn how to use a walker, and an occupational therapist (OT) to learn how to make their home safer and more accessible.

The OT also helped Wendy and her mom develop a plan to handle any future falls. Now, emergency numbers are posted by the phone, her mom is more stable on her feet, and Wendy isn't scared to be home alone with her any more.

So, while developing a sense of responsibility is a good thing, too much of a good thing isn't healthy for any child. If you need more help than your children are able to provide safely and confidently, talk over your options with your healthcare team and call the National MS Society (800-FIGHT-MS or 800-344-4867) for tips on finding help in your home.

Establish boundaries

Sometimes kids—particularly those of single parents—end up having to provide more personal care than is appropriate. For example, a mom or dad who needs help with dressing, bathing, or toileting may call on a son or daughter for help. Even though this kind of situation is sometimes unavoidable, young children and teens shouldn't be involved in a parent's intimate care because it's too uncomfortable for both the parent and the child. Every effort should be made to make other arrangements, either by enlisting the help of adult relatives or by hiring someone to provide the assistance.

Contact the National MS Society by calling (800) FIGHT-MS if you need assistance finding resources in your community to help with your care.

438

Part V

Creating Your Safety Nets

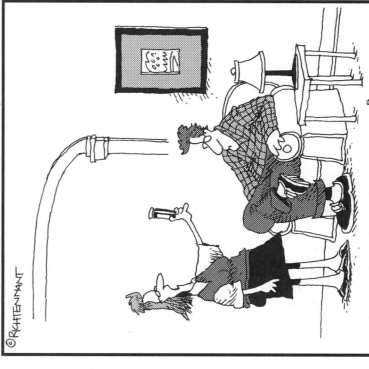

The 5th Wave · By Rich Tennant

"It says to avoid strenuous activities such as wing walking, bear wrestling, or trying to find out if this medication is covered by your insurance company."

In this part . . .

Planning ahead isn't usually high on most people's lists of fun things to do. But, when you've been diagnosed with a chronic, unpredictable disease, one of the best things you can do for yourself and your family members is to create some safety nets for the future. So, in this part, we go over the laws that are designed to help you remain in the workforce as long as you're interested and able. We also give you tips on getting the most from your health insurance, and we show you the importance of managing your finances right from the get-go.

Chapter 18

Keeping Your Place in the Workforce

In This Chapter

▲ Understanding why people with MS leave the workforce
▲ Recognizing important benefits of continued employment
▲ Stepping up to your employment challenges
▲ Exploring the ADA and how it works for you
▲ Exhausting your options before leaving the workforce

I t wasn't all that long ago when one of the first "prescriptions" for someone newly diagnosed with multiple sclerosis (MS) was to "quit your job and go home and rest." So, following the doctor's advice, lots of people trudged home, put their feet up, and then got really bored. Today things are different. Even though MS may affect your employment situation at some point along the way—depending on the types of symptoms you have and the kind of work you do—we now know that quitting work doesn't have to be part of your treatment plan.

This chapter, then, is about how you can keep working as long as you're able and eager to do so. We explain why people leave their jobs—the symptoms, the attitudes (their own and other people's), and the environmental obstacles that nudge them out of the workforce. And, we give you the information you need to make the choices that are right for you and your family.

Understanding the High Rate of Unemployment in MS

So, you want to know why people with MS leave work. Well, even though lots of different factors are to blame, an underlying theme is a lack of information about available options. Here are a few of the most common reasons why people end up leaving the workforce:

✔ **Their symptoms are making it difficult for them to function at work.**

More folks leave the workforce because of fatigue and cognitive issues than any other symptoms. Others may leave because they're experiencing embarrassing problems—with their bladder or bowel, for example. What isn't clear is how many of these individuals are unaware of the treatment strategies and on-the-job accommodations that may help them remain comfortably on the job (check out Chapters 7, 8, and 9 for detailed information about managing symptoms and the section "Knowing Your Rights under the ADA" later in this chapter for more details on job accommodations). They may quit before learning about the resources that are available to help them, only to discover that they feel much better in a few weeks or months but have no job to go back to.

✔ **Their well-meaning families, friends, and health professionals may be encouraging them**

to get away from all the stress. If this sounds like your situation, just remember that the relationship between stress and MS is murky at best, and unemployment (and therefore lack of money) isn't such a hot antidote to stress. Instead, take a look at Chapter 12 for some more practical (and less expensive!) stress management strategies.

✓ **They're just too uncomfortable about their diagnosis to disclose it to anyone else.** Because some amount of disclosure is required to request work accommodations, these folks never get to see how modifications in their work environment or schedule could help them do their job (flip to "Disclosing your MS in the workplace" later in this chapter for details).

✓ **Their symptoms are causing problems with driving and transportation.** Without information about possible car modifications, community carpooling programs, or community transportation options, they leave work because they think they can't get there. Check out Chapter 4 to see how occupational therapists (OTs) can get you on the move again, and call the National MS Society (800) FIGHT-MS (800-344-4867) to be referred to a qualified specialist in your area.

Counting the Reasons to Keep on Truckin'

Apart from the obvious—that working brings in a paycheck—you can find lots of other reasons why staying in the workforce may be in your best interest. For example, consider the following:

443

- **Adding to your financial security is a good thing.** The longer you remain in the workforce, the more you can put into savings and the higher your benefits are likely to be in the event that you do need to take disability retirement someday. In the long run, building financial security is likely to reduce your stress a lot more than leaving the workforce does.

- **Fringe benefits are valuable.** The fringe benefits provided by your job—such as health insurance—may be among your most valuable assets. So, you really want to think twice before giving those up (flip to Chapter 19 for more detailed information about insurance).

- **Your work is a key part of your identity.** People often define themselves, at least in part, by the kind of work they do. When you leave the workforce, you may be giving up a big chunk of your identity—not to mention an important source of self-esteem and self-confidence—without even realizing it.

- **Feeling productive is important.** Most folks like to feel as if they're contributing—to their families, to their communities, and to society as a whole. In fact, one of the biggest issues for people who become severely disabled, by MS or any other condition, is how to continue to feel valuable to the world around them. So leaving the workforce early because of MS can short-circuit those feelings of productivity.

- **Self-sufficiency feels good.** Feeling self-sufficient is a big part of feeling like a competent grown-up. Feeling dependent—and not in control of your own financial resources and choices—can be a real bummer. So, while the idea of being able to rely on disability benefits or other people can be comforting when you're in the throes of a relapse, you may find that it isn't so comfortable over the long haul.

✔ **Being a role model for others feels good, too.** When you find ways to meet challenges in the workplace (or anyplace else for that matter), you become a role model for others—your kids, other people with disabilities, and anyone else who's paying attention. And that's something to feel really good about.

Speed Bumps Ahead: Recognizing the Job-Related Challenges

Depending on your symptoms, the kind of work you do, and the environment in which you work, you're bound to run into challenges along the way. Some of these challenges may be related to your symptoms and others may have more to do with attitudes (yours and other people's) about your MS. Being on the alert for these challenges will make it a lot easier for you to meet them head-on.

When symptoms get in the way

For many kinds of jobs, some combination of good symptom management and reasonable job accommodations from your employer can keep you working for a long time. We know that approximately 40 percent of people with MS are still employed 20 years after their diagnosis. This means that lots of people are finding ways to work around their symptoms. (Check out Chapters 7, 8, and 9 for details on how to manage your specific symptoms.)

Sometimes, however, your particular line of work and your MS simply don't mix. If your job is a physical one, problems with weakness, balance, or coordination may make it impossible for you to be safe and productive. A construction worker, for example, may have relatively mild symptoms but may still be unable to do the job. If your work is all in your head, so to speak, then cognitive changes may interfere with your effectiveness as a lawyer or scientist (even though problems with walking may not). In other words, there are some job functions that are so dependent on particular abilities that even the slightest changes in those abilities interfere to a significant degree.

If and when you hit the fork in the road—where you've exhausted the possible on-the-job accommodations and you're unable to function in your current job because of your symptoms—you have two options:

➤ Make use of your talents in other types of employment

➤ Retire on disability and perhaps put your talents to work in some volunteer capacity

Even though making changes in your work life can be difficult and painful, keep in mind that a fork in the road can also provide unexpected opportunities to try something new, explore a hidden talent, or go in a new direction. Take a look at the National MS Society's publication, *A Place in the Workforce*, at www.nationalmssociety.org/workforce for some eye-opening info about what people with MS can do when they put their minds to it.

The members of your healthcare team are your key allies in your employment efforts. (Check out Chapter 4 for more information on these helpful professionals.) For example:

➤ The neurologist and nurse can help you implement optimal symptom management strategies.

446

✔ Physical and occupational therapists can recommend the tools, mobility aids, and environmental changes you need to be effective in your job.

✔ A *vocational rehabilitation counselor* can help you identify strategies to stay in your job or sort out your options if you think a change is in order.

When attitudes get in the way

Sometimes attitudes—your own or other people's—get in the way of your job even more than MS symptoms do. For example, many people mistakenly assume that anyone with a chronic illness or disability can't be a productive employee or a valuable member of the team. Fortunately, attitudes can be changed with a little patience, some good information, and effective communication.

Dealing with your own attitudes

It's a good idea to take a look at how you think about MS and disability in general because negative attitudes can trip you up as easily as weakness, stiffness, or any other physical MS symptom can. For example, maybe you've always thought that a person with MS couldn't or shouldn't work; that anyone who used a mobility aid wasn't very smart; that your job could only be done one way; or that no one at your workplace would ever understand your situation. In other words, your attitudes may interfere more with your creativity and productivity at work than your MS does.

If your knee-jerk response to managing your MS symptoms at work tends to be a negative one—"It'll never work" or "It's not worth the effort"—you may want to think about a little attitude tuneup. We talk a lot in this book about getting comfortable with the idea of doing things differently, because the more flexible and creative you can be, the more easily you'll be able to come up with strategies to work around whatever physical or cognitive challenges you have. After you have these workarounds sorted out for yourself, you'll be ready to confidently pitch your ideas to your boss and co-workers.

If you're more of a rose-colored-glasses type, you may have a tendency to plow ahead without thinking things through. Even though cockeyed optimism can be a wonderful thing, it's also helpful to be informed and cautious where employment is concerned so that the choices you make are in your own best interest. Slow down just enough to get your ducks in a row by

➤ **Giving some careful thought to how your MS may impact your productivity at work—now or down the road.** The situation generally works out a lot better if you can identify and address the problems you're having *before* you boss does it for you.

➤ **Getting familiar with the provisions of the Americans with Disabilities Act (ADA) so you know what protections the law provides—and doesn't provide.** Check out the section "Knowing Your Rights under the ADA" later in the chapter for details.

➤ **Thinking carefully through your disclosure decisions.** These decisions can have long-lasting consequences because once the information about your MS is out there, you can't take it back. (For more info, check out the section "Disclosing your MS in the workplace" later in the chapter.)

Dealing with other people's attitudes

After you've done your own attitude check, you're ready to deal with whatever other people may be thinking. Your

Get to know your employment resources

The legal and financial issues involved in your employment decisions are complex for even the savviest of folks. So, it's well worth your while to get acquainted with the resources that are out there to help you with questions, concerns, and legal issues related to your employment. Here are a few of those helpful resources:

✔ ABLEDATA: A free national database of assistive devices and rehabilitation equipment
8630 Fenton Street, Suite 930, Silver Spring, MD 20910; phone: (800) 227-0216; Web site: www.abledata.com

✔ U.S. Equal Employment Opportunity Commission (EEOC): A commission that enforces federal employment discrimination laws
1801 L Street NW, Washington, DC 20507; phone: (800) 669-4000; Web site: www.eeoc.gov

✔ ADA&IT Technical Assistance Centers: Regional centers providing information on the Americans with Disabilities Act and accessible information technology
Call or check out the Web site for the center in your area; phone: (800) 949-4232; Web site: www.adata.org

✔ Job Accommodation Network (JAN): A free consultation service designed to increase the employability of people with disabilities
West Virginia University, P.O. Box 6080, Morgantown, WV 26506-6080; phone: (800) 526-7234; Web site: www.jan .wvu.edu

✔ National Multiple Sclerosis Society: Offers consultation and educational programs about employment-related issues
Call or check out the Web site for the chapter in your area;

449

phone: (800) FIGHT-MS (800-344-4867); Web site: www
.nationalmssociety.org/employment

U.S. Department of Labor Office of Disability Employment
Policy: A federal office that develops and influences disability-related employment policy

200 Constitution Ave., NW, Washington DC 20210; phone:
(866) 633-7365; Web site: www.dol.gov/ODEP

boss, for example, may have known someone with MS who became severely disabled. He may assume that anyone with MS will have the same problems and will therefore be a big liability on the job. Or, he may worry that your MS will drive up the company's insurance rates. Your colleagues may assume that you won't be able to hold your own weight, which could mean extra work for them.

People tend to carry around a lot of misconceptions and prejudices, so your job will be to help folks understand more about your MS. Flip to Chapter 14 for some sugges- tions on how to present your MS face to the world. And if you decide you're ready to disclose your MS, you may want to give your boss and colleagues a copy of the National MS Society brochure, *Information for Employers* (www .nationalmssociety.org/employerinfo). The Society's gen- eral information brochures (www.nationalmssociety .org/generalinfo) are also great for giving people back- ground info about the disease.

You'll be giving the people in your workplace a helpful at- titude check when you work around your MS symptoms to remain a productive employee.

450

Knowing Your Rights under the ADA

The Americans with Disabilities Act (ADA), which was passed in 1990, prohibits discrimination on the basis of disability—in employment, public services, public accommodations, and telephone services. When it comes to employment, the ADA basically says that personnel decisions—hiring, promoting, and firing—must be made without regard to a person's disability status. This means that the provisions of the ADA, which we discuss in this section, are your best legal protection on the job. That being said, the ADA isn't a bulletproof vest, so you need to proceed with care.

Disclosing your MS in the workplace

When you're trying to decide who in your office should know about your MS, it's important to remember that disclosure in the workplace should generally be on a need-to-know basis. So ask yourself the following questions:

- Who needs to know?

- Why do they need to know?

- How much do they need to know?

- What's the best way to provide the information that they need?

Take the time to think through the answers to these questions carefully. Before disclosing your MS to anyone at work, you should research the issues and consult with the experts to ensure that you're making the right decision. The reasons for all this caution are pretty straightforward: After the information is public, you can't take it back; you can

451

never be sure that other people will have your best interests at heart, particularly if your interests conflict with theirs; and you want to keep as many options open for yourself as possible.

When it's best to disclose

After you've asked all of the appropriate questions, you're ready to survey the situation and decide whether you're ready to tell your boss or your office mates. Here are the best reasons for disclosing your MS at work:

➤ **You have visible symptoms.** After you begin having symptoms that others can see or that require you to use some kind of mobility aid, you may want to explain what's going on before they come to their own conclusions. Particularly if you aren't as steady on your feet as you used to be, you want to make sure that no one mistakes your imbalance for problems with drugs or alcohol.

➤ **Your productivity is down or you're missing a lot of work days.** If you become concerned that your productivity isn't what it used to be, it's a good idea to bring up the subject before your boss does. But, make sure you're ready to explain what the problems are—and what you're planning to do about them—before having the conversation. Any boss will feel better knowing that you have a plan for solving the problem.

➤ **You feel more comfortable with things out in the open.** Being open about things may simply be your style. Or you may feel that your work environment is such that total frankness is the best way to go. Use your best judgment, but keep in mind that even the most supportive employers can become less

452

supportive when they believe that their own interests are threatened.

Some people feel strongly that they need to be totally frank in a job interview. Even though this honesty may be admirable, it may not be smart. Remember that under the ADA, a prospective employer can't ask if you have a disability unless your need for an accommodation to do the job is visibly apparent. So, unless you need an accommodation for the interview process or for the job itself, you may want to keep mum.

There's no reason for you to include information about your MS on your resume! Even if you have a gap in your work history, don't include information about your MS diagnosis. Of course, if you're asked during a job interview about the gap, it's important not to lie. At that point, it will be up to you decide how much information you want to share. You can, for example, say that you were dealing with some health issues, or you can go into an explanation about your MS.

✔ **You want to request accommodations.** Maybe everything is still going fine on the job—you make it through the day, your productivity is good, and no one has a clue what's going on. But, you're wasted by the end of the day and convinced that you're going to crash if you don't make some changes. In this case, even though you have no obvious or visible reason to disclose, you're required to disclose that you have a disability if you want to request some on-the-job accommodations.

Planning your disclosure strategy

After you've decided to disclose your MS, it's important to

plan your strategy carefully. Follow these steps for a smooth disclosure:

1. **Figure out who's the best person at work to talk to.**

   You may need to talk to your boss, someone in the human resources department, or maybe your project manager. The answer will differ depending on your work setting. Your goal is to get the information to the people who need to know, not to be a source of office gossip.

2. **Plan your disclosure statement with someone who is knowledgeable about the provisions of the ADA.**

   A National MS Society staff person can provide guidance for the disclosure process. You can request assistance by calling (800) FIGHT-MS. You can also discuss disclosure issues with someone at the Job Accommodation Network (JAN) at (800) 526-7234. After you have your strategy all figured out, rehearse it several times with a couple of family members or friends.

3. **Make your disclosure, but stick with the minimum amount of information that will get you what you need.**

   If you're planning to ask for an accommodation, the law only requires that you provide some verification from your physician that you have a disability. Technically, you aren't even required at the outset to say that you have multiple sclerosis. In reality, though, most employers want more details.

   If your employer asks for more information, including your diagnosis, you may not have a whole lot of options. After you disclose your diagnosis, you need to be prepared to help the person understand what MS is and how it affects you. And you have to keep explaining if your situation changes over time. Be open to questions—this is an educational process.

In making your disclosure, you're letting your employer or prospective employer know that you have a condition that affects you at work and that with the appropriate accommodations you can excel at the job.

Understanding the terms used in the law

One of the key provisions of the ADA requires any employer with 15 or more employees to provide *reasonable accommodations* for qualified workers who have *disabilities* that make it possible for them to perform their *essential job functions.* (However, remember that not all employers are covered by this law. For example, the federal government isn't required to comply with the ADA employment provisions because it's prohibited from discriminating against employees with disabilities by the Rehabilitation Act of 1973.)

To help you make sense of these laws and terms, consider the following definitions:

- A *disability* is any impairment that substantially limits a major life activity (seeing, hearing, walking, working, reading, and so on).

- An *accommodation* is a modification that makes it possible for a person with a disability to apply or test for a job and perform the major functions of the job. Here are examples of accommodations that could be made for a person with MS:

  - Altering the job application or testing procedures

to accommodate a person's fatigue or mobility problems

- Providing special equipment, such as air conditioning for someone with heat sensitivity or adaptive computer software for someone with a vision problem

- Creating a flexible work schedule, such as allowing for telecommuting, part-time schedules, or rest periods during the day

- Modifying the office space or bathrooms to make room for a motorized scooter

- Providing a parking space close to the office entrance

✔ *A reasonable accommodation* is one that doesn't cause the employer *undue hardship.* In other words, the employer is expected to make every effort to meet the employee's needs unless the accommodation would be too expensive or disruptive for the business. In reality, most accommodations requested by people with MS aren't particularly costly.

✔ *Essential job functions* are the key activities in a particular job. They're the functions that require special expertise and that are specifically written into the job description.

Even though employers are required to make reasonable accommodations, they aren't required to lower the standards that exist for all employees, eliminate important job functions, or provide accommodations that would hurt the business in a significant way. If you're unable to perform the essential functions of the job, even with reasonable accommodations, an employer can terminate your employment.

456

Requesting reasonable accommodations

Under the ADA, the responsibility for requesting accommodations lies with you. So, you need to be the one to figure out exactly what you need, and you need to be the one to initiate the conversation. Don't wait until your supervisor starts complaining about your performance. We encourage you to keep an eye on your own performance, recognize when it's slipping, and figure out what changes could be made that would help bring your performance back up to snuff. Here are some tips to keep in mind when you're thinking of asking for workplace accommodations:

✔ Consult with your healthcare team. For instance, vocational rehabilitation counselors and occupational therapists are particularly good at identifying helpful accommodations.

✔ Request accommodations that will specifically enhance your performance, and be prepared to explain how your employer will benefit.

✔ Be open to counter-suggestions. Your employer may have ideas that could be just as useful as your own.

✔ Think creatively about ways in which assistive technology of various kinds may be helpful. Some great resources include the Job Accommodation Network (JAN), the ADA&IT Technical Assistance Center, ABLEDATA, your local vocational rehabilitation agency, and your occupational therapist (check out the sidebar "Get to know your employment resources" for more details on these resources).

Some of your fellow employees may resent any accommodations that are made for you—particularly if your symptoms are mostly invisible and they misinterpret the

457

changes as preferential treatment. If you think that people are getting a little hot under the collar, be ready to explain how the accommodations help you get the job done. After your co-workers understand the purpose of the accommodations, they'll get the picture that everyone benefits from the outcome, not just you.

 TIP

Calling in the EEOC

The *U.S. Equal Employment Opportunity Commission* (EEOC), which oversees enforcement of the employment title of the ADA, is a good resource to know about in case you and your employer can't come to an agreement about accommodations. Before calling in the big guns, however, it's a good idea to try to work things out with your employer if at all possible in order to avoid the legal hassles. For instance, if you don't get your first choice accommodation—because your employer thinks it would be too expensive or too difficult to provide—see if you can come up with a compromise solution. If, after your best efforts, no agreement is reached, you can file a complaint with the EEOC.

The EEOC can also assist you if

- ➤ You believe you've been terminated unfairly.

- ➤ Your work environment is hostile or discriminatory.

- ➤ The work environment has negatively changed since your disclosure.

- ➤ You believe you've been overlooked for job promotions or training because of your disability.

If you need to file a complaint with the EEOC, be sure that you're prepared with careful documentation (which you've stored on your computer at home rather than at the

458

office!). Take the time to research the system so that you know the ins and outs and can get the most help possible. For instance, it's important to know that EEOC claims have to be filed within a specific timeframe after the alleged incident.

To find the EEOC office nearest you, go to www .eeoc.gov/offices.html. To read more about how to file an EEOC claim, go to www.eeoc.gov/charge/overview_ charge_filing.html.

Thinking about Leaving Your Job

At one time or another (particularly after a really long, hard week, month, or year of feeling crummy or battling difficult symptoms), you may find yourself thinking about packing up and heading out of the office.

Deciding to leave your job is a complex decision that needs to be made carefully and in consultation with the experts, such as your physician, your vocational rehab counselor, your rehab team, and anyone else whose expertise you value. In this section, we provide you with some basic information to jump-start those important conversations, as well as some significant issues to keep in mind when making your decision.

Exhausting your short-term leave options

Before you make any long-term decisions, it's important to make sure that you've made full use of any available short-term leave options. For example:

✔ Find out if your company offers any kind of short-term disability policy that would allow you to leave work for a defined period of time.

✔ Check out the provisions of the *Family and Medical*

459

Leave Act (FMLA) at www.dol.gov/esa/whd/fmla. This act, which was passed in 1993, requires that any employer with 50 or more employees who live within a 75-mile radius of the work locations (and all public or government employers) to provide up to 12 weeks of unpaid leave *per year* for qualified individuals who are dealing with a personal or family medical situation. The 12 weeks can be taken at one stretch or in chunks, with no impact on your job or health benefits. To be eligible for FMLA, you need to

- Be working for an employer who's covered by this law
- Have worked with that employer for at least 12 months
- Have worked at least 1,250 hours in the past 12 months

Looking into long-term disability options

If, in spite of all necessary accommodations and short-term leave options, you're still unable to perform your essential job functions, it's time to look at the alternatives. Perhaps other positions in your company would be more suitable. Or maybe you could be retrained for work in some other field. If neither of these options seems feasible, you need to find out what disability options you have. We discuss the most common options in the following two subsections.

Long-term disability

Before making any final decisions, be sure to check out your company's long-term disability plan—particularly the definition of *disabled* that's being used by the plan (the definition tends to be very specific and very strict) and the benefit it provides. The benefit provided is usually a per-

460

centage of your last salary earned, so going to part-time employment before going out on this type of disability plan is generally not a good idea. Make sure that you understand how your company's policy works so that you can compare it with the benefits provided by Social Security. Most private long-term disability carriers require you to apply for Social Security Disability Insurance (SSDI) as well because they can subtract from their benefit whatever you receive from SSDI.

Social Security Disability Insurance

Social Security Disability Insurance (SSDI), which is a program run by the Social Security Administration (SSA), is based on your prior work history. For easy-to-understand information about SSDI, go to www.socialsecurity.gov or www.nationalmssociety.org/SSDI.

Here are the requirements you must fulfill in order to be eligible for SSDI:

 You must have worked for a sufficient number of years (some of them recently) and paid Social Security taxes.

 A physician must determine that you're too disabled to work at any job.

 You can't be working at the present time—or if you are, you must be earning less than the level of "substantial gainful employment," which is $860 per month or $1,450 per month for those who are blind. These amounts are periodically adjusted to reflect changes in the cost of living.

For a person with MS, the SSA recognizes four impairments: gait (walking), vision, cognitive problems, and fatigue (you can read more about these symptoms and their

461

management in Chapters 7 and 9). In order to qualify for SSDI, your neurologist must be able to document a significant deficit in at least one of these four areas. Most SSDI applications are initially denied, in part because physicians, including neurologists, have no training in how to fill them out, and the application is a generic one that doesn't lend itself well to the impairments caused by MS. Be sure to check out the National MS Society Web site at www.nationalmssociety.org/SSDI for a toolkit that helps you and your neurologist file effective SSDI applications. If your initial application is denied, don't despair—you can appeal the SSA's decision. If needed, the National MS Society (800-FIGHT-MS) can refer you to an attorney who can help you with the process.

If you qualify for SSDI and later decide that you want to try returning to work, the SSA offers various kinds of work incentives to help you gradually transition back into the workforce. You can read more about the SSA's work incentives at www.socialsecurity.gov/work.

Making the choices that are right for you

When all is said and done, you know yourself and your situation better than anyone else does. You're the only one who can decide what works best for you. If you're pouring every ounce of energy into your job—leaving little or no energy for yourself or your family—continuing to work may not be in anyone's best interest (yours or your family's). If, on the other hand, your work is a major source of personal gratification, take the time to look for gratifying alternatives before leaving the workforce. All in all, achieving balance in your life is important to your overall health and wellness.

In this situation, the "right" and "wrong" answers are never clearly marked. So, you need to think carefully about your options and go for the one that feels right for your situation. Fortunately, you don't have to do this alone. Your healthcare team and the National MS Society can help you find the information you need to make an informed decision.

Chapter 19

Getting a Grip on Insurance

*Y*ou've probably noticed that doctors, hospitals, prescription drugs, mobility equipment, and a lot of other things that you may need to stay healthy despite your multiple sclerosis (MS) cost a lot of money. But, luckily, the bitter pill of healthcare costs is a lot easier to swallow when health insurance picks up the tab—and the more your insurance covers, the better it tastes.

In this chapter, we explain some of the basics of health insurance, as well as disability, life, and long-term care insurance, so that you can take advantage of the coverage and benefits for which you're eligible. Our goal is to help you figure out how to get and keep the insurance that you need

464

so you can spend less money out of your own pocket and less time worrying about it.

Considering Your Health Insurance Options—It's All about Eligibility

Because the United States doesn't have universal health coverage, different people come by their insurance eligibility in different ways, as the following sections explain.

No matter how you get your health coverage, make sure that you know the basic facts about the eligibility rules for your health plan. Without that knowledge, you may make some faulty assumptions that could cost you a bundle.

For more detailed info about your insurance options, check out *Health Insurance Resource Manual: Options for People with a Chronic Illness or Disability*, 2nd edition, by Dorothy Northrop, Stephen Cooper, and Kimberly Calder (Demos Medical Publishing, 2007).

Employment-based insurance programs

Most people in the United States have health insurance because they're eligible for a *group health plan* from their employer or a family member's employer. Members of trade unions (and their dependents) are usually eligible for group coverage through the union.

If you're eligible for group health benefits from an employer or union, it's best to enroll as soon as possible. In most cases, you'll pay a small portion of the premium through a regular payroll deduction, and your employer will pay the balance. Federal law guarantees that no one can be singled out and denied group health benefits on the basis of his or her health status (check out "Protecting your coverage with HIPAA later in the chapter). Even if you don't enroll in the health plan until after your MS diagnosis, you're still eligible. But, anyone who delays enrollment for any reason is likely to be charged a higher premium when they do enroll.

Keep in mind that employers aren't required by law to offer health insurance plans to their employees or their family members, and they're free to make changes in their insurance packages at any time.

Public health insurance programs

Many people are covered by a government-funded, public health insurance program because they meet the established eligibility criteria. Public health insurance programs are designed to meet the needs of people working for the military or the government, or who don't have access to other coverage because of unemployment, age, income level, or disability. Public insurance includes the following programs:

➤ **Government employee benefits:** Federal government employees can enroll in the Federal Employee Health Benefits Program (FEHBP). State and municipal employees are offered comparable programs.

➤ **Medicare:** This government entitlement program is designed to provide health coverage for people outside the work force. To be eligible for Medicare, you must meet one of the following requirements:

- You must be at least 65 years old.
- You must have been deemed "disabled" by the Social Security Administration (SSA) for at least 24 months. (Check out Chapter 18 for more info about Social Security Disability.)

466

✔ **Medicaid:** This government entitlement program provides health insurance for low-income people. To be eligible, you must meet the specific criteria determined by your state government. (Check out 64.82.65.67/medicaid/states.html for information about each state's program.). Although the states vary considerably, eligibility is based on your income, your assets, and your marital and immigration status.

✔ **State Child Health Insurance Programs (S-CHIPs):** These public insurance programs provide coverage to children 18 and under in every state. Eligibility benefits are determined by each state, but families with incomes too high for Medicaid eligibility can often enroll their children in S-CHIP programs.

✔ **TRICARE:** This program provides health benefits for people in the Active, Reserve, and Guard forces of the uniformed services and their dependents.

✔ **VA benefits:** The Veterans Administration provides health benefits to people who were honorably discharged from active military service.

Self-employment options

People who are self-employed—and therefore not eligible for coverage from an employer's group health plan or a public program—need to go shopping for it themselves. And, we warn you now: Shopping for insurance isn't easy. If you're self-employed, you'll be shopping for *individual insurance.*

With this type of insurance, you not only have to pay the full cost of the coverage yourself (shop around because the costs can vary a lot), but the eligibility for it is typically

467

based on your health status. In other words, it's more difficult to qualify for individual insurance if you have a medical condition. Those people with a diagnosis of MS (or any other expensive health condition) are routinely (and legally!) denied coverage because insurance companies want to avoid the responsibility of insuring people who are known to pose a significant financial risk.

Options if you don't have health insurance

If you have MS (or any other serious health condition) don't start your search for insurance by calling insurance companies or brokers, or filling out lots of application forms for insurance. Instead, begin by finding out what you are eligible for in spite of your "high risk" condition. The good news is that most states have, or are moving toward, some mechanism to provide health insurance for people who aren't eligible for any of the programs we talk about earlier in this section, or who are "un-insurable" due to their high risk. Read up on your state's laws and programs on www.healthinsuranceinfo.net; the site also provides info on programs such as "high-risk pools" that may meet your needs.

Keep in mind that finding a plan for which you're eligible doesn't mean that it will fit your budget. But, we recommend that you get yourself insured if at all possible, even if your only option is a plan with a monthly premium of $1,000 or a $4,000 annual deductible. If you're physically able to work, your best option is to find a job with an employer who offers health benefits. As we discuss in the next section, you can't be denied enrollment in a group employer-sponsored health plan because you have MS.

Keeping a Tight Hold on Your Health Insurance

To get and keep health insurance in this country, you have to be eligible for it. Unfortunately, keeping the insurance you have can become difficult as your life situations change. But, Congress and many states have passed laws to protect your eligibility as you go through the most common life transitions, such as getting too old to be covered by your parents' insurance policy, getting divorced, getting laid off from your job, or retiring. We discuss the two biggies in the following sections: COBRA and HIPAA.

Continuing coverage with COBRA

COBRA (the Consolidated Omnibus Reconciliation Act) was passed into law by Congress in 1986. It protects your right to continued eligibility under your group health plan for a certain number of months after coverage would otherwise end—which is a particularly valuable protection for anyone with high or unpredictable medical costs like those associated with MS care.

COBRA is also important because lapses of sixty-three days or more in health insurance coverage make it difficult for a person to enroll in a new plan. With a few exceptions, COBRA guarantees this right of continued eligibility for all qualified beneficiaries (covered employees and their covered spouses and dependents) for a limited time period after employment ends, provided the former employee pays the former employer (or a designated third party) the full premium plus a 2 percent surcharge. After you pay this premium and surcharge, your employer no longer pays any part of the cost of your coverage.

Qualifying for COBRA

COBRA protection is triggered by several different kinds of events:

➤ For employees:

- Your employment is terminated voluntarily or involuntarily for any reason except gross misconduct.
- You change your work status to part-time and become ineligible for your employer's health plan.

➤ For spouses of covered employees (domestic partners aren't covered):

- Your husband or wife (the covered employee) is terminated voluntarily or involuntarily for any reason except gross misconduct.
- Your husband or wife changes his or her work status to part-time, resulting in ineligibility for the employer's health plan.
- Your husband or wife becomes entitled to Medicare.
- You get a divorce or legal separation.
- Your husband or wife dies.

➤ For dependent children:

- The qualifying events for dependent children are the same as for spouses (see the previous bullet)
- Child loses dependent status according to the plan rules (typically by passing the age limit).

Putting COBRA benefits into action

The law requires your employer to notify you about your

470

COBRA rights when you join the group health plan and then again when you're about to leave the plan because of one of the triggering events listed in the section "Qualifying for COBRA." As a qualified COBRA beneficiary, you have 60 days from the date of the COBRA offer to tell your employer whether you plan to elect or reject the continued coverage. COBRA coverage begins on the same day that the other coverage ends—without any gap in protection.

You can elect COBRA for yourself and any family member who's covered under the same plan. If your spouse is the covered employee, he or she can elect it for you if you're covered under the same plan.

Determining how long you receive COBRA benefits

The length of time that you receive COBRA benefits depends on what triggered your COBRA eligibility. For example:

✔ If your job is terminated or your work hours are reduced, the COBRA benefit period is 18 months.

✔ If the triggering event is loss of dependent status for an adult child, a divorce or legal separation from, or the death of, your insured spouse, the benefit period is extended to 36 months.

✔ If any qualified beneficiary (employee, spouse, dependent child) becomes disabled during the first sixty days of COBRA coverage, he or she may extend coverage for an additional 11 months.

To be eligible for this extension, you must give the insurance plan administrator a copy of the Social Security Administration's disability determination within 60 days of receiving it. But bear in mind that the premium can legally be increased by 50 percent

471

for months 19 through 29. For more info on Social Security Disability, flip to Chapter 18.

Some additional facts about COBRA

COBRA is a complex federal law with a lot of twists and turns. So, if you're stumped, check with your health plan administrator or with the U.S. Department of Labor (www.dol.gov) for more details. In the meantime, here is some additional info:

- ✔ Federal law requires every employer with 20 or more employees to offer COBRA benefits. However, many states go beyond this to require smaller employers and other federally exempted employers to offer COBRA-like benefits.

- ✔ By law, qualified beneficiaries (covered employees and their spouses and dependents) are guaranteed benefits identical to those received immediately before qualifying for COBRA.

- ✔ The cost of COBRA isn't standardized because group health insurance plans vary. Prepare for some sticker shock—but take comfort in the fact that the COBRA premiums are lower than those for an individual plan (because COBRA is an extension of group coverage).

- ✔ People who retire early on Social Security Disability are at risk of being uninsured during the 24 months they must wait before Medicare kicks in (check out the section "Public disability insurance: SSDI" later in the chapter). So, it's critically important for anyone leaving the workforce to use their right to COBRA benefits to cover that gap. These same people should also plan their finances accordingly (check out Chapter 20 for more on financial planning with MS).

✔ When you elect COBRA, you're agreeing to pay the premium for continued health benefits for yourself and, possibly, your dependents. Failure to pay in a timely manner can result in termination of coverage—and reinstatement is unlikely.

✔ Every piece of information that you receive in writing from your former employer or COBRA administrator is a legal document, so keep it for your personal protection.

Protecting your coverage with HIPAA

HIPAA (the Health Insurance Portability and Accountability Act), like COBRA, is another complex federal law designed to help protect people who have or who are seeking insurance. However, unlike COBRA, this law specifically provides protection to people with a history of health problems. Here's the gist of what HIPAA does:

✔ **It provides antidiscrimination protections.** HIPAA guarantees that you can't be denied enrollment in a group health plan (generally an employment-based plan) on the basis of your health status, and you can't be charged a higher premium because of a disease or disability.

✔ **It limits preexisting condition exclusions.** HIPAA limits the length of time (12 months for first-time enrollment in a health plan and 18 months if you enroll any time other than the official open-enrollment period) that a health plan can deny coverage for a *preexisting condition*. A preexisting condition is any health condition you had during the

473

six-month period before your new plan started—in other words, any health problem for which you saw a health professional or for which you were treated (including taking a prescribed medication).

HIPAA also gives you (and your covered dependents) credit for the amount of time you were insured by your previous plan (referred to as *prior coverage*) and applies that credit to the preexisting condition exclusion period of your new plan. This is called *creditable coverage*.

To help you prove your creditable coverage, HIPAA requires health plans to give anyone who leaves a plan a *certificate of coverage* indicating the amount of time he or she was covered. However, keep in mind that prior coverage is *not* creditable if you have a gap of 63 or more days without coverage.

HIPAA's protections apply to most health plans, including employment-related group policies, union and association plans, Medicare, Medicaid, high-risk pool insurance, and more. Exceptions include so-called "temporary" health policies, certain student plans, catastrophic or disease-specific policies, private disability policies, and dental or vision coverage.

When considering the purchase of *any* health insurance policy, be sure to ask if it would be considered creditable coverage under HIPAA. For more information about HIPAA, consult your employer, your health plan administrator, or your state department of insurance.

The following section provides a few examples to help you get your head around the logistics of COBRA and HIPAA.

Seeing COBRA and HIPAA work as a team

Making sense out of COBRA and HIPAA may be easier

with a few examples. Here are three that illustrate how these two complex laws can work together to help you:

➤ George was diagnosed with MS while working for the ABC Corp. and was insured by ABC's group health plan. After three years at ABC, he took a job with XYZ International and enrolled in their group health plan. George was uninsured for nine days between the end of his ABC coverage and the start of his XYZ coverage. For any new employee that has been uninsured for 63 or more days, XYZ's plan excludes coverage for preexisting conditions for the first 12 months of the employee's coverage. Because George was uninsured for only nine days, all of his care costs were covered as soon as his new plan went into effect.

➤ Annette, who has MS, was covered by her husband Greg's group health plan for the ten months he worked for DEF Corp. At ten months, he was laid off. They didn't elect COBRA because they couldn't afford the premiums. Within a month, Greg got a new job at HIJ Co. and immediately signed up for the health plan they offered him and his family. Unfortunately, Annette's MS qualified as a preexisting condition, and HIJ's plan had a 12-month preexisting condition exclusion period. But, HIPAA enabled Greg to apply the ten months of Annette's prior coverage from DEF to the 12-month exclusion period so that they only had to absorb the uncovered costs for anything specifically related to her MS for two months.

➤ Janet, a person with MS, lost her job and health benefits when her employer downsized. She didn't elect COBRA because of the expense. Janet found

475

another job three months later. Because more than 63 days had elapsed between the two jobs, Janet didn't get any credit for her prior coverage and she had no insurance for MS-related healthcare expenses for a full year. But, other, non-MS-related costs were covered.

If Annette or Janet had elected COBRA, they would have remained covered until their new group coverage took over. When you have an expensive health condition, it's worth your while to invest in COBRA in order to stay covered until you have a new policy, even if you have to borrow the money to do it.

Understanding the Ins and Outs of Your Health Insurance Plan

Given the soaring cost of healthcare in the United States, health insurance coverage may be a person's most valuable asset. And it's particularly valuable for anyone with MS because the costs related to managing this disease—including medications, hospital stays, and mobility equipment—can be high. This section is designed to help you ask the right questions about your current coverage or about any health plan that you're considering joining in order to make sure that it offers the greatest possible coverage for your MS needs.

To take best advantage of your health coverage, you need to make careful choices based on the cost and practical implications of the following factors:

- ✔ Who's covered under the policy—employee, spouse, dependents? (Those who are covered are considered *qualified individuals*.)

476

✔ Is this a managed care plan in which you can save money by going to in-network doctors, hospitals, and pharmacies? Is it worth it to you to see MS specialists who aren't in the network? Do you know exactly how the referral system works and how much more expensive it may be to use specialists that aren't in the network?

✔ Is there a waiting period before a qualified individual is covered? Is there a period of time during which your MS or other preexisting condition will not be covered? If yes, how long?

✔ How much is the annual deductible? Is it for each family member separately, or for the whole family in combination? Is there a separate deductible for prescription drugs, mental health benefits, or other services?

✔ How much of the cost of covered services (*co-insurance percentage*) do you have to pay after the deductible has been met? Is there a fixed dollar amount (*co-payment*) for services such as doctor visits?

✔ What are the renewal conditions? Under what circumstances can your health plan (or employer or union) increase your premium?

✔ Is there a *stop loss provision* that limits the amount of your out-of-pocket expenses? If yes, what's the maximum out-of-pocket amount you would have to pay for the deductible, co-insurance, and co-payments per year before the plan begins picking up the full tab?

✔ Is there a maximum amount that the health plan will pay while you're eligible for coverage (or in your lifetime)?

✔ What services, medical equipment, and supplies does the plan cover? You may want to check out things like physical therapy, occupational therapy, mobility aids, catheters, and so on.

✔ What's the prescription drug benefit? Are there tiers of drugs that require different co-insurance or co-pay amounts (as is happening increasingly with the approved disease-modifying medications)? Are all of your medications included in the formulary?

✔ Does the health plan have arrangements with a mail-order pharmacy or medical equipment supplier that could save you money?

✔ What isn't covered by the policy? For example, what are the limits on

- Your choice of hospital and the number of covered hospital days? Are other hospital expenses covered?

- The amount paid for doctor visits, including in-network and out-of-network doctors?

- The number of visits or the amount of annual coverage for mental health benefits?

Filing Successful Insurance Appeals

It turns out that it isn't enough to know how to get and keep your health insurance—you also need to know how to file an appeal if your insurance plan refuses to pay for something your doctor has prescribed for you—which can happen with a lot with the medications and services that are used to manage MS. Many people don't pursue their right to appeal because they don't think they can win. But the fact is, when done properly, over 50 percent of appeals are successful. So, in this section, we show you the steps to take.

Step 1: Check your coverage

Start by reexamining your health plan manual to make sure that what you thought would be covered actually is. If the service (such as physical or occupational therapy) or treatment (such as injectable medication) you need is specifically excluded by your policy, the chances of winning coverage for it on appeal are slim to none. If the policy doesn't specifically exclude it, however, it's definitely to your advantage to try the appeals process.

Step 2: Confirm why coverage was denied or was less than expected

Carefully review the *explanation of benefits form*—the insurance company's official response to your claim—to see why coverage was denied or is being reimbursed for less than the cost. These explanations often appear as codes, with explanatory notes at the bottom of the page or on the back. If the problem requires a simple fix, such as correcting a code number or supplying a bit of missing information, make the change and resubmit your claim to the same place you or your doctor sent it originally. If everything's in order on the claim, and they're still denying coverage, your next step is to appeal.

Step 3: File an appeal

To give yourself the best chance at success, study your plan's *appeal procedures* (sometimes found in the section on grievances and appeals in your plan manual). It's important to follow these procedures carefully—especially the deadlines. Here are some basic guidelines:

✔ **Write a clear and simple letter.** Give the facts

479

and a concise explanation of why you believe your claim should be paid. This letter should be no more than one page.

Be sure to include your insurance ID number, the specific claim number (if applicable), the name and contact information of your healthcare provider, and the date of service (if applicable).

- **Keep detailed records.** Health insurance policies and anything else that the insurance companies give you in writing are legal documents—so hang on to them.

  Also, keep detailed notes about all interactions with your insurer, including dates and names of company representatives you speak with on the phone. Save copies of claims and bills, appeal letters and any attachments, and other relevant communications.

- **Follow up.** If your appeal is denied, go to the next level of appeal—don't assume that this happens automatically. The second appeal will still be an *internal appeal*, but it will involve a reconsideration of your original claim among a higher level of professionals within your plan.

  If your second appeal is denied, you *may* be eligible for an *external review* of your claim by a panel of health professionals who have no affiliation to your health plan. Contact your state department of insurance to ask about any external appeal rights you may have in your state.

- **Discuss your appeal with your healthcare provider.** If the dispute is over the medical necessity of a treatment, your physician's input in the form of a letter that includes studies demonstrating the treatment's benefit will be invaluable. Make sure that your healthcare providers have a copy of your appeal letter on file. Be sure to let them know about the National MS Society's publication *Health Insurance Appeal Letters: A Toolkit for Clinicians* at www .nationalmssociety.org/appealletters.

Replacing Your Income with Disability Insurance

Whereas health insurance helps pay for your healthcare costs, *disability insurance* helps replace your income if you become too disabled to earn a living. You can purchase disability insurance on your own. Or, some employers offer disability insurance (through a commercial insurance company) to their employees as a benefit. In addition to this type of commercial insurance, the Federal government provides public disability insurance through programs administered by the Social Security Administration (SSA). These programs are financed via the taxes paid by workers and employers.

Commercial and public disability plans define "disability" differently (the following sections explain the differences). Both, however, put the burden of proving your disability on you and your doctor.

Commercial disability insurance

Commercial disability insurance (as distinguished from public disability insurance) is available through some employers or may be purchased privately to protect you in the event that you become unable to continue in your current job because of a disability. Because every commercial disability policy is a contract, the definition of "disability" can vary a lot depending on the terms of that contract. So, don't make any assumptions about your coverage. Take the time to familiarize yourself with your policy's definitions and conditions early on—well before you ever consider filing a claim.

After you've been diagnosed with MS (or a variety of other conditions, including common problems such as lower back pain), it can be difficult (if not impossible) to qualify for commercial disability insurance. Employers can't deny it, but the insurance companies may not be willing to take you on. If you decide to try and buy it on your own, it may help to work through an insurance broker or to speak with someone in the underwriting department (rather than the sales department) of an insurance company because the underwriting folks are less likely than the sales folks to turn you down outright. If you've already been diagnosed, the chances of approval will probably depend on how well you're doing when you apply.

Never lie about your medical condition or history on an application for insurance! Don't volunteer anything you aren't asked for, but don't commit fraud by providing inaccurate information—doing so will seriously jeopardize your ability to buy any type of insurance ever again.

Even if you have commercial disability insurance, you can still apply for benefits from SSA (see the following section "Public disability insurance: SSDI"). In fact, commercial insurers are eager to transition disabled policyholders into Social Security Disability Insurance (SSDI) and are likely to require you to file the application.

Public disability insurance: SSDI

The main public disability insurance you need to be aware of is *Social Security Disability Insurance* (SSDI). SSDI pays benefits to you and certain members of your family if you're *insured*, meaning that you worked and paid Social Security taxes for a sufficient period of time.

The eligibility criteria for SSDI are clearly defined in the law, and this program is strictly for those who are unable to be gainfully employed because of a physical or mental impairment that lasts at least 12 months. An *impairment* isn't simply a diagnosis of a disease or condition; it's a measure of how impaired one is as a result of that disease or condition. Check out the SSA Web site at www.ssa.gov for lots of helpful information about the eligibility criteria and the application process.

If you're considering applying for SSDI benefits, review the eligible MS-related impairments (vision, walking, and cognitive problems, and fatigue) carefully and honestly with your doctor to make sure that you're in agreement about which may apply to you. To help with this discussion, take a look at the SSDI toolkit on the National MS Society Web site at www.nationalmssociety.org/socialsecurity.asp. The components of the kit will help you understand the application process and the criteria used by the SSA. The kit also provides you and your doctor with the information and template letters you need to file an effective application.

The SSA will notify you in writing when you've been deemed disabled, and it will provide the exact start date of the disability. Beginning with that start date, you'll have a waiting period of five months until the payment of benefits begins. Make sure you factor this waiting time into your personal financial plans.

Twenty-four months after your SSDI benefits begin (29 months after the onset of disability) you'll automatically qualify for Medicare. Contact Medicare at www .medicare.gov or at (800) MEDICARE (800-633-4227) if you don't receive information regarding the program before your 29th month of disability. The move to Medicare coverage (from your group insurance plan or from COBRA) is another critically important transition period for your personal financial planning because you'll need to make important decisions about your coverage, including your prescription drug plan. (Check out the section "Continuing coverage with COBRA" earlier in the chapter for more info.)

People with disabilities who gain eligibility for Medicare when they're under 65 must make all the same choices about their Medicare benefits as those who retire into the program. So, if this is you, go to www.medicare.gov and click on "Compare Medicare Prescription Drug Plans" to get started. And don't hesitate to contact the National MS Society by calling (800) FIGHT-MS (800-344-4867) if you need to consult with someone about your options.

Finally, it's good to know that Social Security Administration offers incentives to people who think they may want to try returning to the workforce. You can return to work on a trial basis (referred to as a *trial work period*) without jeopardizing your eligibility for benefits. Check out more information about SSA's work incentives at www.ssa.gov/work.

A Brief Word about Life and Long-Term Care Insurance

Life insurance, which is designed to help support your family in the case of your death, is sold exclusively through the commercial marketplace. The commercial marketplace includes many financial institutions and commercial insurers. Even though many employers offer life insurance as an elective benefit to their employees, they aren't required to. A diagnosis of MS generally doesn't disqualify a person from obtaining life insurance, but it may jack up your premiums a bit or result in some limitations to your coverage.

Many people use their life insurance as a tool for planning their personal and family finances. It's a good idea to talk this over with an experienced financial planner to figure out how to put your insurance policies to work for you. Call the National MS Society (800-FIGHT-MS) to obtain free financial education and advice services through the Society's partnership with the Society of Financial Service Professionals. (Check out Chapter 20 for more details on planning for a life with MS.)

Long-term care insurance, which helps pay for home healthcare and nursing home care, generally isn't available for anyone who has already been diagnosed with MS. However, your family members may want to look into this type of coverage for themselves—either through their employer or with a private insurance company.

485

Chapter 20

Planning for a Future with MS

*E*ven though you may not think of yourself as a big-time gambler, chances are you've bet on quite a few things in your life. You may bet that good things will happen—by buying a lottery ticket, for example. Or, you may bet that bad things will happen—by buying car insurance, life insurance, or liability insurance. And all this betting is normal for just about anyone. But, when you throw in multiple sclerosis (MS), you now have one more wild card to contend with. Whether you're into betting or not, the fact is that life with MS is a bit of a crapshoot. The only surefire bet for anyone living with MS is that the future is unpredictable.

So, in this chapter, we talk about ways to look that unpredictability in the eye and figure out how to plan for it—fi-

486

nancially and otherwise. We also explain how to assess your current situation so that you can anticipate the kinds of challenges or changes that could arise in the future. With this groundwork laid, you can begin to construct a safety net for yourself and your family.

Preparing for the Worst While Hoping for the Best

Encouraging folks to plan for the worst is a hard sell. Who, after all, wants to spend time thinking about all the yucky things that can happen in life? Some people even think that it's bad luck—they believe that planning for those things may make them happen. Other people don't want to "waste" the good times worrying about possible bad times. And people with MS often say that they don't want to give any more time, energy, or thought to MS than they absolutely have to. They say "We'll deal with that problem (disease progression, disability, job change, and so on) if and when we need to."

In this section, we're going to try and sell you on the idea that careful planning is one of the best gifts that you can give yourself and your family. If you gear up to deal with whatever challenges MS can bring, and then find down the road that your MS has actually remained pretty stable and manageable, you haven't lost anything except some planning time. But, if you lay down some plans and the disease progresses enough to interfere with your life in a significant way, you'll already have some safety nets in place to meet the challenges head on.

Facing those scary "what-ifs?"

When you heard the words, "You have MS" from your doctor, you may have had some scary thoughts: "What if I end up in a wheelchair?" "What if I can't work?" or "What if my vision doesn't clear up?" It turns out that most people have one or two what-ifs that scare them more than anything else, and with human nature being what it is, those are exactly the things they don't want to spend time thinking about.

The best way to deal with the stuff that scares you the most is to take the time to think about what you would do if those scary things actually happened. Formulating a strategy—by consulting with the experts, identifying helpful resources, and developing a contingency plan—helps you feel prepared. And when you feel prepared, you can worry less about the future and enjoy the present more.

So if, for example, you're worried that your MS symptoms will interfere with your ability to stay employed, now is the time to meet with a vocational counselor or occupational therapist to figure out what kinds of accommodations in the workplace may help you stay on the job or what other kinds of work you may be able to do. It's also the perfect time to meet with a financial planner to talk about what you can begin doing now to protect your financial security down the road.

Taking charge of your future

In spite of the unpredictability of MS, you can do a lot to feel prepared. Because MS is so variable from one person to the next, and people's life circumstances are so different, no one-size-fits-all solutions exist. But, the process involved in developing a safety net is basically the same for everyone. When you're ready to take charge of your future, follow these steps:

1. **Take the time to learn about the ways MS can change over time.**

488

Additional resources about planning your future

Planning for an uncertain future isn't easy for anyone. So, here are some additional books to help you think through your personal situation, formulate the right questions, and identify the best resources:

✔ *Adapting: Financial Planning for a Life with Multiple Sclerosis* by the National Endowment for Financial Education (2004). You can order this book from the National MS Society by calling (800) FIGHT-MS (800-344-4867) or by going to the National MS Society Web site (www.nationalmssociety.org/adaptingbook).

✔ *Multiple Sclerosis: The Questions You Have; The Answers You Need*, 3rd edition, edited by Rosalind Kalb (Demos Medical Publishing, 2004).

✔ *Multiple Sclerosis: A Guide for Families*, 3rd edition, edited by Rosalind Kalb (Demos Medical Publishing, 2006).

For example, even though MS is an unpredictable disease, it's helpful for your planning purposes to know that the majority of people who are diagnosed with relapsing-remitting MS transition to a more progressive course within twenty-five years. (Check out Chapter 1 for more details on the course of MS.)

2. **Let yourself think ahead (even if it's scary).** Even though a head-in-the-sand approach may feel more comfortable, it won't serve you well in the long run. But, thinking ahead about ways that MS may affect your lifestyle can help keep you one step ahead if and when you experience major changes.

3. **Ask the right questions of the right people.**
   You don't have to figure everything out alone. Legal, vocational, and financial experts can help you get your thoughts in order. Share your concerns about employment and your financial future—whatever they may be—and let these folks guide you.

4. **Develop the plan that feels right for you.**
   Even with input from all the experts, you're the only one who can decide exactly what's right for you. So, gather all the information you can, and then take whatever steps you need to in order to feel prepared—whether that means increasing your savings, requesting accommodations in the workplace, or training for a different kind of career.

5. **Take steps now to begin putting the plan into action.**
   At this stage, you bravely forge ahead, bringing your plan to life. Acting on your plan will help you feel stronger and more prepared no matter what MS brings your way.

6. **Go on with your life.**
   We want smart planning to be part of your life, but we certainly don't want it to be the most important part. Don't get so wrapped up in planning for your future that you forget to live your life and enjoy the present.

490

Navigating the Planning Process: It's as Easy as One, Two, Three

Financial planning is all about figuring out how to pay the piper—now and in the years to come. It's designed to ensure that you have adequate resources to meet your present needs as well as any needs you anticipate down the road.

So, successful planning depends on your anticipation of as many of your future needs as possible.

The planning process starts with the following three basic questions—and your answers to these questions form the basis for your plan:

➧ Where are you now?

➧ What might the future bring?

➧ What can you do now to be ready?

These questions may seem daunting, especially when your MS is acting particularly unpredictable. So, in the following sections, we go over each of these questions in detail.

Where are you now?

It's inventory time—but don't worry, it's not as difficult as it sounds. The key areas to focus on include your health, finances, insurance coverage, employment situation, and family life. Taking this kind of inventory allows you to step back and take a look at the big picture of your life, with an eye to how these five important areas may interact in the years ahead and how you may tweak the picture to meet your future needs.

Taking a look at your health

Your health is about more than just your MS. So, when you review your current situation, remember to take into account your overall health and fitness as well as what's going on with your MS. For example, ask yourself if you're up-to-date with the health screening exams for people your age. Also, keeping in mind that like everyone else, people with MS are likely to die of heart disease, cancer, and stroke, ask

491

yourself about your risk factors: Do you have a family history of any of these health problems? Are you overweight? Do you smoke? Do you exercise regularly and eat a balanced diet? (Take a look at Chapter 11 for more info about wellness strategies.)

When it comes to surveying your MS, ask yourself whether your disease course is active or stable (your doctor can help you answer this one if you aren't sure), and whether you're following the doctor's recommendations for slowing disease progression and managing your symptoms. Even though it isn't the most fun thing to do, take the time to think about how your symptoms are affecting your everyday activities. For example, are things feeling pretty manageable at the moment, or not? If the answer is no, be sure to talk that over with your doctor to see what other strategies may be helpful.

Checking out your finances

As you can imagine, when you have an unpredictable disease like MS, taking a long, hard look at your financial health is important. Even though you don't want to think about it now, your medical bills may end up rising later due to disease progression (or you may need to hire extra help), and so you want to be prepared financially for whatever happens.

When you're checking out your finances, be sure to include the plus column and the minus column. You can do this in a variety of ways—by writing lists of your sources of income and expenses, by keeping a daily journal of monies coming in and monies going out, or by filling out a loan application (by the time you fill in all those blanks, you'll know your situation pretty well!). Just keep in mind that it always feels better to start with the plus column. Here are the specifics you should consider:

492

- **Sources of income:** These incoming sources can include income, assets, all forms of financial support (including child support and alimony), VA benefits, interest and dividends, food stamps, public assistance, rental income, life insurance policies, employee benefits, and anything else you can think of.

- **Expenses:** These outgoing sources can include housing, food, transportation, utilities, clothing, loans, mortgages, car payments, interest on credit balances, employer deductions, alimony, property taxes, insurances, medical care, prescriptions, rehab, personal assistance, and anything else that drains the coffers.

You may consider getting a credit report from one of the three credit reporting agencies—Equifax, Experian, or TransUnion—to see where you stand. You're entitled to one free report per year from each of these agencies. Check out www.annualcreditreport.com, which is the central Web site that the three companies created so that the public can easily request free reports.

Reviewing your insurance coverage

Having good health insurance coverage is important for the average person, but for someone who has a long-term disease, it's even more important because things can get costly. So, for the purposes of financial planning, the important thing is to figure out the costs associated with the coverage you have. For example:

- Review your health insurance plan to see exactly what it does and doesn't cover, keeping in mind that non-covered expenses end up coming out of your pocket.

- Calculate what you're paying now for premiums, co-pays, co-insurance, deductibles, prescription coverage, and any other associated expenses. When you figure this number into your health-related expenses, keep in mind that costs can vary significantly from year to year.

- If your employer offers more than one health plan, take the time to compare them, keeping in mind that the plan with the lowest premium is likely to give you higher out-of-pocket expenses down the road. And if you chose your current plan before your MS diagnosis, check to see if it's still the most appropriate one for you in terms of what it covers, the doctors you see, and the medications you take.

- If your insurance comes through your employer (or your partner's employer), check to see if it's a *fully insured* or *self-insured plan*—the difference can have some financial implications.

   With a self-insured plan, your employer acts as the insurance company and doesn't have to follow any state regulations—which means that you have to go to court to fight any unfavorable decisions. A fully insured program, which the employer purchases from an insurance company, provides greater consumer protection because it's regulated by the state. With this kind of plan, you can request an independent review by the state if you have an unsuccessful appeal concerning your coverage. About 60 percent of people with employer-based coverage have self-insured plans.

- Check out whether you have any *disability insurance* through your employer. It turns out that most people think they have it but they actually don't. Remember

494

that after you've been diagnosed with MS, chances are you won't be able to purchase a new policy.

If you're fortunate enough to have disability coverage, read the find print to find out how it defines disability, how much it pays and for how long, and how long you have to wait for it to kick in after you've filed for it. And check to see if you're allowed to do any kind of work when you're receiving benefits.

Getting a handle on insurance coverage now—before you run into any kind of crisis, is a critical piece of your financial safety net. Check out Chapter 19 for detailed information about insurance coverage—how to get it and how to keep it.

Scoping out your employment situation

Employment equals income for most people—so it's definitely in your best interest to take a hard look at your current work situation. The key to good planning is to ask yourself some difficult, but important, questions:

✔ **Is your job stable?** Are there mergers or layoffs in the offing? Is a new boss coming in who's likely to clear the ranks? Is the company in good financial shape? Have your recent performance reviews been positive?

✔ **What's happening with your MS?** Is your MS behaving lately? Is it pretty stable? Are your symptoms pretty much under control? Do you feel pretty good?

✔ **How's your job performance?** Are you performing up to snuff? Are you able to handle the essential functions of your job? Do the symptoms you have interfere with the kind of work you do? Do you need some accommodations to help you function at your best—and if so, have you already asked for them?

This is no time to be a cockeyed optimist (optimist, yes; cockeyed optimist, no). Providing honest answers to these questions will help you do whatever you need to do to stay productively employed for as long as you want and are able to do so. Being honest with yourself will also help you plan effectively if a change in your work situation is looming. (Check out Chapter 18 for all the ins and outs of working with MS.)

What might the future bring?

By this point in the planning process you should have assessed your current situation (see the section "Where are you now?" earlier in the chapter). Now it's time to bring out the crystal ball. You can't predict the future, but you can try to anticipate some of the changes or challenges that may crop up down the road. And anticipating these changes can help you stay in control of your life.

Life changes

With or without MS, life is full of changes—some more expected than others. Marriage, starting a family, moving to take a new job, caring for elderly parents, getting a divorce, and going back to school for an advanced degree are just a handful of those changes you can expect. As you develop your financial plan, it's important to take these kinds of changes into account and think about how your MS fits into the picture. For example, are there any changes you would like to make sooner rather than later—such as returning to school or having a child—because of concerns about your MS progressing? Or does your partner need to alter his or her career plans based on the possibility that you may not be able to remain in the workforce as long as you planned?

Changes in your MS

We talk a lot in this book about how unpredictable MS can be. Nevertheless, an important part of good planning is letting yourself think about the changes that *might* happen.

For instance, your symptoms may continue to be more annoying than disabling—requiring only minor tweaks in the way you do things. Or, you may find that you need a mobility aid, additional medications, or some help from the rehab team to keep yourself functioning at your best (take a look at Chapter 7 for more information about rehabilitation strategies to manage your MS). Sometimes, though, MS symptoms can have a greater impact that calls for some heavy-duty help—perhaps some personal assistance with your care, modifications to your home or car, a motorized scooter or wheelchair, or whatever else it takes for you to stay active and comfortable.

All of these modifications have financial implications that are important to keep in mind as you try to create a financial safety net for yourself and your family. A motorized scooter, for example, can be quite expensive, so you may want to check how much of the cost would be covered by your insurance. Also, your insurance plan may cover some of the MS medications and not others, or cover physical therapy services but not those provided by an occupational therapist. You may consider building a medical savings account for yourself to help pay for some of the extras that your insurance doesn't cover.

Employment changes

Changes in your employment situation may be planned or unplanned, positive or negative—but they all need to be taken into account when you plan for the future. If you or a family member retire from the workforce or cut down on your hours, your income inevitably goes down. On the other hand, a promotion for you or your partner can add a big chunk to the plus column.

Also, if your MS progresses to the point that you're unable to work—even with the job accommodations we talk about in Chapter 18—your disability retirement income is likely to be lower than your current salary. Private disability insurance generally only covers a portion of your current income. Social Security Disability Insurance payments are also significantly lower than your current salary. Anticipating the possibility of this kind of change in your finances can help you plan for it more effectively.

Financial changes

Your financial situation can change in either direction for many reasons. Windfalls happen and so do unexpected problems. For example, your incoming funds could get a hefty boost from Aunt Bertha's will or from the piece of property your parents left to you and your sibs. Or, you may pay off the car loan, send in your last mortgage check, or finally get that last kid through college. Any of these would significantly up your disposable income. Of course, losing child support or alimony or buying a new car or house could significantly zap your disposable income.

Unanticipated expenses are obviously the real challenge. The best strategy, then, is to assume that you'll have some of these unexpected expenses, and then you can try to build in enough give in your budget to absorb them. Here are some expenses you can plan for (even if they never actually happen):

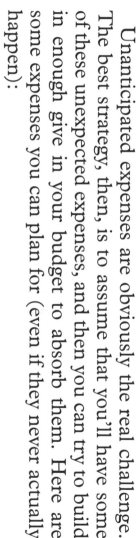

➤ **Home modifications to stay as active as you want to be:** These modifications, such as widening doorways for wheelchair access or building a ramp,

498

can be costly, but they're worth their weight in gold. Remember, however, that many state vocational rehabilitation services will cover the cost of home modifications that make it possible for you to remain in the workforce, so be sure to call the National MS Society (800-FIGHT-MS or 800-344-4867) for the names and numbers of people to contact in your state.

✔ **Medical treatments or wellness interventions that aren't covered by your insurance plan:** As you can imagine, these out-of-pocket expenses can also pack a wallop. Your insurance company, for example, may deny coverage for your physical therapy visits or the massages that are so helpful for your *spasticity* (stiffness). Or, you may want to join a gym or exercise class to help reduce your fatigue or build your endurance. Even though these costs are related to your MS, they, too, would likely come from your own pocket.

Changes in your insurance coverage

Insurance is a moving target these days—the industry is changing so rapidly that it's often difficult to keep up. Companies can change the benefits they offer, increase their co-pays or co-insurance amounts, and fiddle with their *formularies* (the list of drugs they cover). And your employer can raise your portion of the premium from year to year. Even worse, some employers are now pulling back from providing insurance coverage altogether, or they're providing such bare-bones coverage that you're pretty much on your own. (Check out Chapter 19 for more information about how to maximize and protect your health insurance coverage.) We encourage you to read your insurance plan carefully, as well as any updates provided by your

499

employer or the insurance company, in order to avoid too many unpleasant surprises.

CALL A PRO

Changes in your family

In addition to trying to anticipate changes within your immediate family—such as having children and saving for their college education—it's important to think about whether your extended family is available to help you in the future. In the old days, people could pretty much count on assistance from family members if the need arose because family members usually lived close together and more women stayed home to raise their children. Today, families are more spread out, with many couples relying on two incomes just to get by. And their own life changes—new babies, retirement, illness, returning to the workforce—may make it impossible for relatives to assist you with your own life changes. This means that any help you may need down the road may have to be hired from the community, which obviously would be an added expense (whether you planned for it or not).

What can you do now to be ready?

After you've surveyed your current situation and you've looked into the future to see what changes may happen, it's time to begin the actual planning process by talking to the right people and gathering all the information you need. Like other complex issues related to your life with MS, you don't have to do this alone.

Talking to the right people

The most important piece of advice we can give you regarding the actual planning process is to get your guidance from the experts. Even though you can—and should—get input from your friends and family, your best help will

500

come from the professionals who have a working knowledge of the rights and protections that are available to folks with chronic illnesses or disabilities.

The folks you may need to get in touch with include the following:

✔ **Financial planners:** These professionals help people set financial goals and then figure out how to meet them. The goals may include investments, tax planning, asset protection, retirement planning, and estate planning. It's never too early to have a chat with one of these folks. You can go to the Web site of the Certified Financial Planner Board of Standards (www.cfp.net) to see a listing of certified financial planners in your area or to determine if your accountant is a certified financial planner. Or, you can call the National MS Society (800-FIGHT-MS) to find out more about the free financial education and advice offered through Financial Education Partners, a collaborative program with the Society of Financial Service Professionals.

✔ **Accountants:** Your accountant knows how to help you get the best return for your money. He or she may be able to inform you if you're overlooking certain tax deductions that you could be taking because of your disability. Or, he or she may be able to show you ways to use the equity in your house to generate some needed funds. If you have no disability insurance, the accountant may also be able to advise ways to invest some money now that would provide the same kind of benefits later on.

✔ **Elder law attorneys:** These attorneys specialize in legal issues affecting the elderly and people with disabilities. They're particularly skilled in public benefits, such as Medicaid and Medicare (see Chapter 19), but they also can help with wills, trusts, long-term care planning, and estate planning. Find an attorney in your area who's certified by the Board of Certification of the National Elder Law Foundation (NELF), by going to www.nelf.org/findcela.asp.

➤ **Social Security attorneys:** These professionals specialize in helping people obtain Social Security Disability Insurance (for those who have worked and paid Social Security taxes) and Supplemental Security Income (for those with little or no income) if and when they need it. The primary resource for these specialists is the National Organization of Social Security Claimant Representatives (NOSSCR). You can contact the NOSSCR referral service at 800-431-2804 during East Coast business hours.

➤ **Care managers:** These experts navigate the health and social service systems, and they know the eligibility requirements for available services. They're the perfect matchmakers—they help you get the care and services you need. Care managers are typically social workers or nurses (hint: they usually have the initials CMC or CCM after their name). The National MS Society can refer you to a professional care manager in your area. To contact the Society, call (800) FIGHT-MS.

➤ **Credit counselors:** A credit counselor can help you if you have accumulated significant debt and need assistance regaining sound financial footing. The National Foundation for Credit Counseling is a non-profit organization with member agencies around the country. You can talk with a credit counselor in your area by calling (800) 388-2227.

502

In addition to tapping the right professionals, it's important to keep the communication lines open with your family members. Some (or all of you) may shy away from discussions about the future, but, in the end, the best way to relieve everyone's anxieties is to get them out in the open. Talking over what you would do if the MS progressed to the point that more day-to-day help was required is a good place to start. If getting this kind of conversation going proves to be a challenge, think about sitting down with a family counselor to jump-start the process. (Flip to Chapter 15 for more details on making MS a part of the family.)

Maximizing your employment options

Now's the time to make sure that you have all of your ducks in a row at work. Check out Chapter 18 for recommendations on how to maximize your productivity on the job and maintain your place in the workforce as long as you're willing and able to. If you haven't already taken the time to review your job situation (your current performance, the impact of any MS symptoms you're having, the kinds of accommodations that may help you function more comfortably and effectively, and the short-term disability and leave options that are available at your job), don't put it off. Too many people wait until their job is in jeopardy before trying to take steps to protect it—and by that time, it's often too late.

Becoming familiar with the appropriate laws and regulations

To plan effectively, you need to be aware of the laws and regulations that exist to protect you. We talk about them in more detail in the chapters on employment (Chapter 18) and insurance (Chapter 19), but here they are in one tidy list:

➤ **The Americans with Disabilities Act (ADA):**
This act provides rights and protections that help
people with disabilities stay employed and involved
in the community.

➤ **COBRA:** These health benefit provisions from the
Consolidated Omnibus Budget Reconciliation Act of
1985 help people maintain health insurance when
they leave their jobs and lose their job-related health
benefits.

➤ **HIPPA (Health Insurance Portability and Accountability Act):** This act prohibits employers
who provide health coverage from discriminating
against an employee because of a *preexisting condition* (a health problem he or she had before the current coverage began).

➤ **The Olmstead Decision:** This legislation, which
was approved by the Supreme Court, makes it a re-
quirement for states to provide home- and
community-based services to help people with disabilities remain in their homes and their communities.

Now is as good a time as any to check out these important laws and regulations to see how they may benefit you
in the future, if the need arises. It's always better to become
familiar with them before you hit a bump in the road than
when you're smack in the middle of a crisis.

Part VI

The Part of Tens

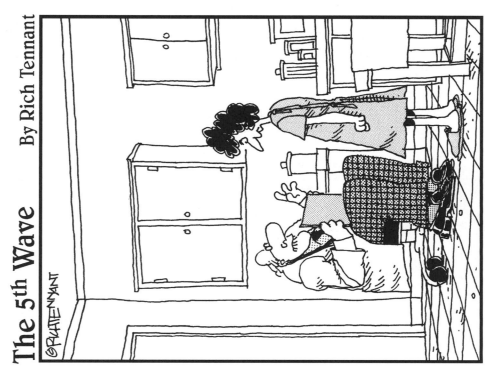

The 5th Wave   By Rich Tennant

"I was just surprised you put the word 'marriage' next to the question asking if you suffered from a chronic condition."

In this part . . .

In this part, we give you some little gems—they're small, but they're worth a fortune! You can find ten must-do's for living with multiple sclerosis (MS), ten myths that you want to toss out as quickly as possible, and ten suggestions for how to globe-trot with comfort and confidence despite your MS.

Chapter 21

Ten Must-Do's for Living with MS

*N*o one asks to be diagnosed with multiple sclerosis (MS) and no one's happy when it happens. But long gone are the days when a person could do nothing but "go home and learn to live with it." No matter what you've heard elsewhere, you can live a full and satisfying life with MS, and this chapter gives you the top ten strategies for doing just that.

Educate Yourself about MS

Information can help put you in the driver's seat. Armed with accurate info about MS, you'll feel more in control and more prepared to be an active partner in your care. Because doctors still haven't found a cure for MS, managing it involves a lot of choices (check out Part II for details on managing your MS). And informed choices are better choices.

MS information is available from lots of sources—of which some are better than others—so pick carefully! The best information sources are your healthcare team (flip to Chapter 4 to find out how to create your team), the National MS Society and other MS organizations, and government Web sites (take a look Appendix B for additional resources). And don't forget this book—it's chock-full of information. Just check out the table of contents or the index to find the topic you're interested in. The pharmaceutical companies that manufacture the MS medications also provide excellent information, but it's important to be able to distinguish the marketing messages from the educational messages. Because the Internet is a mixed bag of good and bad info, be sure to check stuff out with your healthcare team.

Work with Your Neurologist

MS is a long-term disease that requires an ongoing partnership with your neurologist. So, it's well worth the effort to find a doctor you trust, respect, and can talk to. See your neurologist at least once a year and come prepared with plenty of information: Your input—how you feel and the symptoms you've been having—is essential to effective treatment planning (Chapter 5 gives you tips on creating a mastery plan). For a list of ways to make the most of your partnership with your MS doctor, check out the Cheat Sheet at the beginning of the book.

Start Treatment Early

If you've been diagnosed with a relapsing form of MS—or your doctor believes that you're heading in that direction—

you may be a perfect candidate for one of the approved disease-modifying therapies (see Chapter 6). Irreversible nerve damage can occur early in the disease course, so getting on treatment early is the best way to head off some of that damage. If you aren't a candidate for one of these therapies, you still have many options to feel better and manage your symptoms (see Part II for management tips).

Make MS a Part of the Family

When one person in a family gets MS, the whole family lives with it. So, education for family members—including kids—is important. And learning how to communicate comfortably and openly about the disease and how it affects all of you will make it a lot easier to plan, problem-solve, and support one another (flip to Chapter 15 for more on these family matters).

 Voluntary health organizations like the National MS Society (www.nationalmssociety.org) and the Multiple Sclerosis Association of America (www.msaa.com) have educational materials and programs for every member of the family. The Multiple Sclerosis International Federation even has information about MS in six languages (www.msif.org). And if you need help starting the family powwow, call the National MS Society at (800) FIGHT-MS (800-344-4867) for a referral to a family counselor to get the ball rolling.

Develop Your Support Network

In spite of how alone you may have felt when you first heard your diagnosis, you don't have to deal with it on your own. It's never too early to start building your support system—beginning with your healthcare team and close family and friends, and gradually branching out into your community. You'll be amazed at all the resources that are available to help you. Call the National MS Society at (800) FIGHT-MS for the names of MS specialists and the Multiple Sclerosis Association of America at (800) 532-7667 for info about their support programs and services. As you reach out to others, be ready to let them know how they can help—most people are more than willing to pitch in when they know what you need.

Plan for the Future

MS is an unpredictable disease—and this unpredictability is what tends to scare folks the most. The best way to deal with uncertainty is to plan for it—financially, vocationally, and any other way you can think of. As it turns out, planning for the *best* doesn't prepare you for much of anything because the best hardly ever happens in life. Planning for the *worst*, however, helps you feel more prepared and less vulnerable no matter what comes along. Check out Part V for three helpful chapters regarding how to prepare for the future.

Planning doesn't have to be a downer. Wise planning can help you pursue your goals with confidence and optimism—without having to focus too much attention on your MS.

Feel Healthy and Well

Despite popular belief, you can actually be healthy with MS. And the healthier you are, the better you're going to feel no matter how your MS is behaving. So, don't let MS hog all your attention.

Because having MS doesn't protect you from other medical problems (see Chapter 11), it's important to protect your health with a balanced diet, regular exercise, and pe-

510

riodic medical and dental checkups (your neurologist won't be worrying about your heart, lungs, or gums, or reminding you to get a Pap smear or a mammogram). You also need to find healthy ways to manage the unavoidable stresses of daily life (see Chapter 12). If you find it difficult to do all these healthy things for yourself, don't panic. Whatever you eat, drink, or do, you're not going to make your MS get worse. And keeping active isn't going to make your MS worse either—your body will let you know if you need to take a rest or cool down—so enjoy yourself.

Create Your Tool Chest

The key to keeping MS from getting in your way is to figure out strategies to work around it. When problems with fatigue, vision, mobility, or any other MS symptom interfere with your daily activities, your choice is to either give up the activities or find some tools, mobility aids, or other gizmos to help you get the job done (see Chapter 7 to check out some helpful devices).

Using tools doesn't mean you're giving in to MS. Instead, it means you're figuring out how to take charge of it. The more creative and flexible you're willing to be in the way you do things, the more things you'll be able to do.

Monitor Your Mood

Depression is one of the most common and treatable symptoms of MS (check out Chapter 9). In fact, you have at least a 50 percent chance of developing a significant depression at some point along the way—and it can happen early or late in the disease, regardless of what your physical symptoms may be. Depression isn't about being a wimp or a chicken. Depression is a part of this disease just like any other symptom, which means it deserves to be treated.

Facing the challenges of MS is difficult enough without being depressed, so talk to your doctor if you experience a significant change in your mood. Counseling or antidepressant medication have both been shown to be effective in treating depressive symptoms.

Keep Your Sense of Humor Well-Oiled

MS certainly isn't a laughing matter, but finding things to laugh about, and people to laugh about them with are key to making peace with this disease. For some, laughing about bladder or bowel symptoms, problems with thinking and memory, or wheelchairs can be difficult. But support groups and Internet chat rooms are hotbeds of humor. Get a group of MS folks together and you'll quickly see that humor is part of the game plan for living with this disease.

Being able to laugh about something has a way of taking the sting out of it, which is the first step toward making the problem feel more manageable.

Chapter 22

Ten MS Myths Debunked

In This Chapter

▲ Ignoring the top ten MS myths
▲ Understanding that each person's MS is unique

• •

Chances are that if you've heard about multiple sclerosis (MS) before, you haven't heard much that was good. In fact, you may have heard only about wheelchairs, nursing homes, or even death—not a pretty picture. You tend to hear more about the bad stuff because the good stuff isn't as visible. When people with MS are busy living their lives, other folks may not even know that they have MS. So, just in case you've got some mistaken ideas about what MS is and isn't and what it does and doesn't do, this chapter will clear up some of the myths.

MS Is Fatal

Maybe you've heard about someone who died from MS. The fact is that most people with MS die from cancer,

Everyone Eventually Needs a Wheelchair

Even though they may need to use a mobility device, such as a cane or motorized scooter, to help with balance or fatigue, the fact is that two-thirds of people with MS remain able to walk. Think of it this way:

✔ Approximately one-third of people with MS have a relatively *mild* disease course with manageable symptoms and little or no disability.

✔ Approximately one-third of people have a *moderate* disease course with more bothersome symptoms and a greater disability as time goes on.

✔ Approximately one-third of people experience a severe course that's significantly more disabling.

So, while most people with MS *don't* need a wheelchair on a full-time basis, doctors currently have no way to predict which path a person's MS will take.

514

heart disease, and stroke—just like everyone else. Statistically speaking, the MS life span is very close to normal. But, of course, there are some situations that can shorten a person's life, including a very rare and rapidly progressive form of MS that leads to an early death. Sometimes severe complications of MS, such as serious infections that don't respond to treatment, can eventually be fatal, too. And severe depression that isn't treated can sometimes end in suicide. So, be sure to let your doctor know about any big changes in your mood (see Chapter 9).

Because There's No Cure, There's Nothing You Can Do about Your MS

True enough—there is no cure for MS yet. But, the good news is that over the last 15 years, more progress has been made in the treatment of MS than in all the time since the disease was described in 1868 by Jean-Martin Charcot. MS treatment is now a package deal—complete with medications to manage your relapses and the disease course (check out Chapter 6), rehabilitation strategies to keep you safe, active, and complication-free (check out Chapter 7), and emotional support to help you sort it all out (check out Chapter 9).

People with MS Can't Handle Stress

After diagnosis, one of the first things you may hear from well-meaning family members and friends, from some health professionals, and from info on the Internet is that stress isn't good for you. Even though it's clear that too much stress isn't particularly good for anyone, the fact is that the relationship between stress and MS just isn't all that clear. Whatever the final conclusion turns out to be, the bottom line is that life is stressful, so trying to rid your life of stress can become a *stressful* and ultimately fruitless effort.

Before you rush to try and eliminate all the stresses from your life—particularly a major activity such as employment (which also provides income and a sense of accomplishment) take time to think through your decision. Being unemployed isn't exactly a stress-free bed of roses. We'd rather see you figure out how to manage the stresses in your life more comfortably (see Chapter 12) than to give up those things that give your life meaning, purpose, and sat-

515

isfaction (flip to Chapter 18 for info about MS and employ-ment).

People with MS Shouldn't Have Children

Fortunately, this myth is on the way out. Since about 1950, the research has shown that men and women with MS can have healthy babies and happy kids: MS doesn't affect pregnancy, childbirth, or breastfeeding. And these events, in turn, have no long-term effect on a woman's level of disability. In fact, the hormones of pregnancy offer some protection against MS relapses. Even though children who have a parent with MS have a somewhat higher risk of developing MS than other children, the risk remains fairly low. (Check out Chapters 16 and 17 for some in-depth info about parenting with MS.)

"Natural" Treatments Are Safer

Don't be seduced by advertising for "natural" treatments. Even though prescription medications are strictly regulated in this country, dietary supplements aren't. For example, the manufacturer of a prescription medication can't make any claims about its product that haven't been proven in rigorous clinical trials, but the manufacturer of a supplement can make any claims it wants—calling the supplement "safe," "healthy," "effective," or anything else to catch your eye and pocketbook. And, the fact that something comes from nature doesn't make it safe, non-toxic, or free of side effects. (Check out Chapter 10 for more on supplements and other alternative treatments.)

No One Can Understand How You Feel

It's certainly true that no one else is standing in your shoes. Given that everyone's MS is different, your experience is definitely your own. But, there are lots of folks in the MS circle (in support groups, online, at the National MS Society and other MS organizations, and on your healthcare team) who get it. They understand the feelings of loss, anger, and anxiety that you live with, as well as the challenges and frustrations that crop up every day. And they understand the sense of accomplishment you feel when you overcome them. The more you're willing to share, the more understanding you'll find in others. Check out www .faceofms.org to hear people's stories and share your own if you choose.

Having a Relapse Means Your Medication Isn't Working

The available medications can't cure MS or stop the disease in its tracks. This means you're likely to have some relapses (hopefully fewer) and experience some disease progression (hopefully less) even though you're faithfully taking your medication.

Remember, having a relapse or some disease progression doesn't mean that the medication isn't working or that you need to switch medications. You and your doctor can decide together when and if it's time to try something else.

Scientists Aren't Making Any Progress

Actually, progress has never been faster! In the 1970s, scientists found new and better ways to explore the workings of the immune system. In the early 1980s, magnetic reso-

517

nance imaging (MRI) technology gave doctors the first "picture" of the damage done by MS to the brain and spinal cord. This amazing technology provides a bird's-eye view of the underlying disease process and a sensitive way to evaluate new treatments. Researchers are collaborating on a hunt for MS genes. And the research into how damaged tissue in the central nervous system may be repaired has moved into high gear. For a glimpse of the exciting world of MS research, check out the work of The Myelin Project (www.myelin.org), the Accelerated Cure Project (www.acceleratedcure.org), and the Nancy Davis Center Without Walls (www.erasems.org) as well as the National MS Society's overview of progress in MS research at www.nationalmssociety.org/researchprogress.

If You Can't Walk, Your Life Is Over

For those who fear being unable to walk more than anything else in life, nothing we say is likely to reassure you. But we've known countless men and women who have stayed mobile, productive, adventurous, and involved while sitting down. They work, play, travel, make love, make babies, and make a life. If you want to be convinced, we urge you to meet some of those folks for yourself—in support groups, at educational meetings, or in your community—and get to know them. They may even tell you that it's easier to smell the roses when you're a little bit closer to the ground.

518

Chapter 23

Ten Tips for Trouble-Free Travel

*T*he world is your oyster. People with multiple sclerosis (MS) travel all over the world—on business, on vacation, and so on. They sightsee, trek, snorkel, and go white-water rafting, and you can too. In this chapter, we suggest ways to go where you want to go and do what you want to do when you get there.

The key to your travel enjoyment is a readiness to be creative and flexible. The more willing you are to adapt your activities to the demands of your MS, the more places you'll be able to go and the more fun that you'll have.

Tap the Right Resources

Even though you may feel like an intrepid explorer the first time you venture out on a long trip with your MS, remember that many, many others have gone before you—so be sure to tap into their expertise. Here are some resources to check out:

- Take a look at *The Access-Able Travel Source* (www .access-able.com) for detailed information about traveling with a disability.

- Visit the National MS Society's travel page (www. nationalmssociety.org/travel) for additional resources and travel ideas.

- Check out the books *There Is Room at the Inn: Inns and B&Bs for Wheelers and Slow Walkers*, and *Barrier-Free Travel: A Nuts and Bolts Guide for Wheelers and Slow Walkers*, both by Candy Harrington (Demos Medical Publishing).

Calm Your Medical Concerns

Have a frank talk with your neurologist about any concerns you have regarding your trip. Although very little of what happens with MS is a medical emergency, you'll feel more relaxed if you've talked about what to do and whom to call if you have a relapse far from home. (See Chapter 6 for info about MS relapses.)

Keep in mind that heat and overexertion can cause your symptoms to act up temporarily, so take time to cool down and rest up before jumping to the conclusion that you're having a true relapse. Infections can also kick your symptoms into high gear, so if you're prone to urinary tract infections, ask your doctor for a supply of medication to take with you just in case.

You'll also feel reassured by having the name and phone number of a local medical facility in your destination city or cities. Take a minute to join the International Association for Medical Assistance to Travelers (www.iamat.org). This nonprofit organization lists English-speaking doctors all over the world.

Save Energy for the Fun Stuff

In addition to budgeting your money for a trip, it's important to budget your energy. Figure out how much you can comfortably do each day, leaving time for rest breaks along the way. Don't plan such a jam-packed trip that you get exhausted just thinking about it. And most importantly, don't stand when you can sit or walk when you can ride. By making the best use of mobility aids, you can conserve the energy you need to have fun (check out the Cheat Sheet at the beginning of the book for more tips on saving your energy).

Check Ahead for Accessibility

Everyone defines *accessibility* differently. Your definition will depend on your personal needs—do you need an elevator, air conditioning in your hotel room, or a grab bar in the shower? Travel agents that specialize in accessible travel know how to check whether a certain place or activity is accessible, but they can't do the detective work without knowing what your needs are. So, take the time to think through exactly what you're likely to need at every step along the way. Of course, nothing is fail-safe, so prepare yourself for some occasional creative problem-solving.

Rent Accessible Vehicles

In this day and age, you can rent just about anything anywhere. A knowledgeable travel agent can help you find accessible equipment in cities all over the world. For example, you may want to rent an RV (it's great to have a bathroom handy for long car trips!), a car with hand controls, a wheelchair-accessible van, or a motorized scooter for gadding about. Just be sure to give your agent plenty of notice and details about your specific needs.

Keep Your Cool

Getting overheated is one of the quickest ways to sap your energy and cause your symptoms to act up. So try to schedule your trip for the coolest, least humid seasons, and plan your activities during the early and later parts of the day. Wear layers of lightweight, light-colored clothing and a head covering, and invest in a commercial cooling vest or bandanna that you can wear when it's really hot. Make the most of air conditioning and sip cold water throughout the day.

Navigate Air Travel with Confidence

Air travel has become a lot more complicated for everyone, but you can do several things to make it easier and more comfortable for yourself including the following:

➤ Call the airline a few days ahead of time to let them know of any special needs you may have.

➤ Pick your seat carefully by figuring how much legroom you need and how close to the bathroom you want to be.

➤ If you have access to a computer, print out your boarding pass ahead of time (most airlines make them available up to 24 hours prior to departure) to reduce waiting time at the airport and to guarantee your seat.

- ✔ Get to the airport early to allow for long security lines and to avoid having to rush. And use curbside check-in to save your energy.

- ✔ Pack smart so the things you need to access easily are right on top, and pack lightly so you aren't lugging around more luggage than you need.

- ✔ If you check any mobility equipment, such as a motorized scooter, tag all parts with your name and telephone number, and consider bringing the manuals in case your equipment needs to be disassembled (and therefore reassembled).

Safely Pack Your Prescriptions

Be sure to pack all of your medications in your carry-on bag, along with a complete list of all your prescription and non-prescription drugs.

If you take an injectable medication, carry the vials and syringes in their original package, complete with the prescription label so that the security guards won't confiscate it. A letter from your doctor isn't good enough—you really do need the prescription label. If any of your medications need to be refrigerated, make sure you have adequate packaging to protect them until you arrive at your destination (and check ahead to make sure there's a refrigerator where you're going). And don't forget to bring along a safe used-needles container.

Get Vaccinated

Traveling outside of the United States often involves a vaccination of one kind or another. Vaccinations for the flu, hepatitis B, tetanus, measles, and rubella are safe for you unless you're currently having a major relapse (in which case you should wait four to six weeks after the onset of the relapse to have the vaccination) or you're taking a medication that suppresses your immune system, such as Novantrone (mitoxantrone), Imuran (azathioprine), Cytoxan (cyclophosphamide), or methotrexate. If you're currently on one of these immunosuppressants, you need to avoid the live, attenuated vaccines, such as varicella or the vaccine for measles, mumps, and rubella, because you're at greater risk of developing the disease.

The consensus among MS experts is that you shouldn't be denied access to health-preserving and potentially life-saving vaccines because of your MS. Follow the Centers for Disease Control (CDC) guidelines for each vaccine (www.cdc.gov/travel/vaccinat.htm).

Look for Adventure

The most important thing to remember is that you can have fun just like everyone else. Spend a little time scouting on the Internet for accessible options—safaris to Africa, European tours, sky-diving, deep-sea diving, ski trips to Vail—whatever suits your fancy. Don't assume that you can't do something until you've taken the time to research it carefully. You'd be surprised at all the things that people with MS are up to.

Part VII

Appendixes

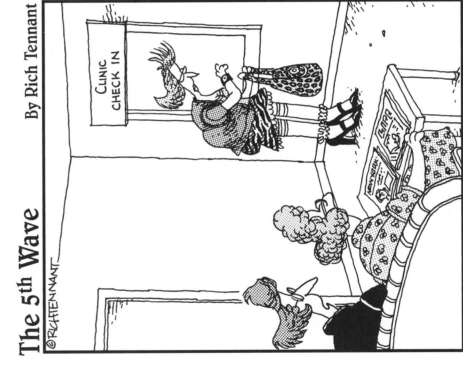

The 5th Wave   By Rich Tennant

CLINIC CHECK IN

"I can't believe her MS is affecting her body any worse than her sense of style is."

In this part . . .

The three appendixes in this part are the frosting on the cake. We start with a glossary so you can check out all those words you hear in your doctor's office or stumble over in multiple sclerosis (MS) publications. Then we give you a list of medications that are commonly used in MS—either to manage the disease or treat the symptoms. And we end with a menu of helpful resources—including books that focus on particular topics in this book, Web sites, and agencies and organizations. You'll no doubt find these resources useful along the way.

Appendix A

Glossary

adrenocorticotropic hormone (ACTH): A hormone that's extracted from the pituitary glands of animals or made synthetically. ACTH stimulates the adrenal glands to release glucocorticoid hormones, which help reduce inflammation. ACTH may be used to treat acute relapses.

advance (medical) directive: A directive to medical personnel and family members that preserves a person's right to accept or reject a course of medical treatment even after the person becomes mentally or physically incapacitated to the point of being unable to communicate those wishes. Advance directives can be in the form of a living will or a healthcare proxy.

ankle-foot orthosis (AFO): An ankle-foot orthosis is a brace, usually plastic, that's worn on the lower leg and foot to support the ankle and correct foot drop. The AFO promotes correct heel-toe walking. See *foot drop*.

antibody: A protein produced by certain cells of the immune system. The protein is produced in response to bacteria, viruses, and other types of foreign antigens.

antigen: Any substance that triggers the immune system to produce an antibody; generally refers to infectious or toxic substances such as viruses or bacteria.

aspiration: Inhalation of food particles or fluids into the lungs.

aspiration pneumonia: Inflammation of the lungs due to aspiration.

assistive devices: Any tools (canes, walkers, shower chairs) that are designed, fabricated, or adapted to assist a person in performing a particular task.

assistive technology: A term used to describe all of the tools, products, and devices, from the simplest to the most complex, that can make a particular function easier (or simply possible) to perform.

ataxia: The incoordination and unsteadiness that result from the brain's failure to regulate the body's posture and the strength and direction of limb movements. Ataxia is most often caused by disease activity in the cerebellum.

attack: See *relapse.*

autoimmune disease: A process in which the body's immune system causes illness by mistakenly attacking healthy cells, organs, or tissues in the body that are essential for good health. Multiple sclerosis is believed to be an autoimmune disease.

axon: The extension of a nerve cell (neuron) that conducts electrical impulses to other nerve cells or muscles.

axonal damage: Injury to the axon in the nervous system, generally as a consequence of trauma or disease. This damage may involve temporary, reversible effects or permanent severing of the axon.

B-cell: A type of lymphocyte (white blood cell), manufactured in the bone marrow, which makes antibodies.

Babinski reflex: A neurologic sign in MS in which stroking the outside sole of the foot with a pointed object causes an upward movement of the big toe rather than the normal bunching and downward movement of the toes. This abnormal response indicates damage to the motor pathways in the brain and spinal cord. See *sign.*

black hole: A dark area on a T1-weighted MRI scan that indicates destruction of myelin and nerve fibers. Black holes occur in areas where repeated inflammation has occurred.

blinding: An attempt to eliminate bias in the interpretation of clinical trial outcomes by having at least one party involved in the clinical trial be unaware of which patients are receiving the experimental treatment and which are receiving the control substance. See *double-blind clinical study* and *single-blind clinical study*.

blood-brain barrier: A cell layer around the blood vessels in the brain and spinal cord that prevents large molecules, immune or white blood cells, and potentially damaging substances and disease-causing organisms from passing out of the blood stream into the central nervous system.

brainstem: The part of the central nervous system extending from the base of the brain to the spinal cord that contains the nerve centers of the head as well as the centers for respiration and heart control.

catheter: A hollow, flexible tube made of plastic or rubber, which can be inserted through the urinary opening into the bladder to drain excess urine that can't be excreted normally. See *indwelling catheter*.

central nervous system: The part of the nervous system that includes the brain, optic nerves, and spinal cord.

cerebellum: A part of the brain situated above the brainstem that controls balance and coordination of movement.

cerebrospinal fluid (CSF): A watery, colorless, clear fluid that bathes and protects the brain and spinal cord. The composition of this fluid can be altered by a variety of diseases, such as MS. See *lumbar puncture*.

chronic progressive: An old-fashioned catch-all term for progressive forms of MS. See *primary-progressive MS*, *secondary-progressive MS*, and *progressive-relapsing MS*.

clinically isolated syndrome (CIS): A first neurologic episode that lasts at least 24 hours and produces MS-like signs or symptoms caused by either a single demyelinating lesion (referred to as monofocal) or more than one lesion (referred to as multifocal) in the central nervous system. A person with CIS may or may not

529

go on to develop MS.

clinical trial: Rigorously controlled studies designed to provide extensive data that allow for a statistically valid evaluation of the safety and efficacy of a particular treatment. See *double-blind clinical study*, *single-blind clinical study*, and *placebo*.

cognition: High-level functions carried out by the human brain, including comprehension and use of speech, visual perception and construction, calculation ability, attention (information processing), memory, and executive functions, such as planning, problem-solving, and self-monitoring.

cognitive impairment: Changes in cognitive function caused by trauma or disease process.

cognitive rehabilitation: Techniques designed to improve the functioning of individuals whose cognition is impaired because of physical trauma or disease. Rehabilitation strategies are designed to improve the impaired function via repetitive drills or practice, or to compensate for impaired functions that aren't likely to improve.

controlled study: A clinical trial that compares the outcome of a group of randomly-assigned patients receiving the experimental treatment to the outcome of a group of randomly-assigned patients receiving a standard treatment or inactive placebo.

corticosteroid: Any of the natural or synthetic hormones associated with the adrenal cortex (which influences or controls many body processes). See *glucocorticoid hormones*, *immunosuppression*, and *relapse*.

cortisone: A glucocorticoid steroid hormone, produced synthetically or by the adrenal glands, that has anti-inflammatory and immunesystem-suppressing properties. Prednisone and prednisolone belong to this group of substances.

demyelination: A loss of myelin. In MS, this occurs in the white matter of the central nervous system. See *myelin*.

deoxyribonucleic acid (DNA): The chemical basis for genes. See *gene*.

detrusor muscle: A muscle of the urinary bladder that contracts

530

and causes the bladder to empty.

diplopia: Double vision or the simultaneous awareness of two images of the same object that results from a failure of the eyes to work in a coordinated fashion. Covering one eye will "erase" one of the images.

disability: As defined by the World Health Organization, a disability (resulting from an impairment) is a restriction or lack of ability to perform an activity within the range considered normal for a human being.

double-blind clinical study: A study in which none of the participants, including experimental subjects, examining doctors, attending nurses, or any other research staff, know who's taking the test drug and who's taking a control or placebo agent.

dysarthria: Poorly articulated or garbled speech resulting from the dysfunction of the muscles controlling speech. The dysfunction is usually caused by damage to the central nervous system or a peripheral motor nerve.

dysesthesia: Distorted or unpleasant sensations experienced by a person when the skin is touched. The sensations are typically caused by abnormalities in the sensory pathways in the brain and spinal cord.

dysmetria: A disturbance of coordination, caused by lesions in the cerebellum.

dysphagia: Difficulty in swallowing. It's a neurologic or neuromuscular symptom that may result in aspiration, slow swallowing, or both.

dysphonia: Disorders of voice quality (including poor pitch control, hoarseness, breathiness, and hypernasality) caused by spasticity, weakness, and incoordination of muscles in the mouth and throat.

erectile dysfunction: The inability to attain or retain a rigid penile erection.

etiology: The study of all factors that may be involved in the development of a disease, including the patient's susceptibility, the nature of the disease-causing agent, and the way in which the per-

531

son's body is invaded by the agent.

evoked potentials (EPs): Recordings of the nervous system's electrical response to the stimulation of specific sensory pathways (for example, visual, auditory, or general sensory). EPs can demonstrate lesions along the pathways whether or not the lesions are producing symptoms.

exacerbation: See *relapse*.

Expanded Disability Status Scale (EDSS): A part of the Minimal Record of Disability that summarizes the neurologic examination and provides a measure of overall disability (also called a "Kurtze score" after the neurologist who developed it). The EDSS is a 20-point scale, ranging from 0 (normal examination) to 10 (death due to MS) by half-points. See **Minimal Record of Disability**.

experimental allergic encephalomyelitis (EAE): An autoimmune disease resembling MS that has been induced in some genetically susceptible research animals.

failure to empty (bladder): A type of neurogenic bladder dysfunction in MS resulting from demyelination in the voiding reflex center of the spinal cord. With this dysfunction, the bladder tends to overfill and become flaccid, resulting in symptoms of urinary urgency, hesitancy, dribbling, and incontinence.

failure to store (bladder): A type of neurogenic bladder dysfunction in MS resulting from demyelination of the pathways between the spinal cord and brain. Typically seen in small, spastic bladders, storage failure can cause symptoms of urinary urgency, frequency, incontinence, and nocturia.

finger-to-nose test: A test of dysmetria and intention tremor, in which the person is asked to touch the tip of the nose with the tip of the index finger (with the eyes closed).

Food and Drug Administration (FDA): The U.S. federal agency that's responsible for enforcing governmental regulations pertaining to the manufacture and sale of food, drugs, and cosmetics.

foot drop: A condition of weakness in the muscles of the foot and ankle, caused by poor nerve conduction, which interferes with a

532

person's ability to flex the ankle and walk with a normal heel-toe pattern. The toes touch the ground before the heel, causing the person to trip or lose balance.

gadolinium: A chemical compound that can be administered to a person during magnetic resonance imaging to identify inflamed areas where immune-system cells have passed from the blood, through the blood-brain barrier, and into the central nervous system.

gadolinium-enhancing lesion: A lesion appearing on magnetic resonance imagery, following injection of gadolinium, that reveals a breakdown in the blood-brain barrier.

gene: A basic unit of heredity containing coded instructions for manufacturing a protein. Genes are subunits of chromosomes, which are strands of deoxyribonucleic acid (DNA) contained within most cells.

glucocorticoid hormones: Steroid hormones that are produced by the adrenal glands in response to stimulation by adrenocorticotropic hormone (ACTH) from the pituitary. These hormones, which can also be manufactured synthetically, are used to treat MS relapses.

healthcare proxy: See *advance (medical) directive*.

heel-knee-shin test: A test of coordination in which the person is asked, with eyes closed, to place one heel on the opposite knee and slide it up and down the shin.

immune-mediated disease: A disease in which components of the immune system are responsible for the disease either directly (as occurs in autoimmunity) or indirectly (for example, when damage to the body occurs secondary to an immune assault on a foreign antigen, such as a bacteria or virus).

immune system: A complex network of glands, tissues, circulating cells, and processes that protect the body by identifying abnormal or foreign substances and neutralizing them.

immunology: The science that concerns the body's mechanisms for protecting itself from abnormal or foreign substances.

immunomodulation: In MS, a form of treatment that alters certain actions of the body's immune functions, including those directed against the body's own tissues.

immunosuppression: In MS, a form of treatment that shuts down the body's natural immune responses, including those directed against the body's own tissues.

impairment: As defined by the World Health Organization, any loss or abnormality of psychological, physiological, or anatomical structure or function (due to injury or disease). It represents a deviation from the person's usual biomedical state.

incidence: The number of new cases of a disease in a specified population over a defined period of time.

incontinence: The inability to control passage of urine or bowel movements.

indwelling catheter: A type of catheter that remains in the bladder on a temporary or permanent basis. It's used only when intermittent catheterization isn't possible or is medically contraindicated. See *catheter*.

inflammation: A tissue's immunologic response to injury, characterized by mobilization of white blood cells and antibodies, swelling, and fluid accumulation.

intention tremor: Rhythmic shaking that occurs in the course of a purposeful movement, such as reaching to pick something up or bringing an outstretched finger in to touch one's nose.

interferon: A group of immune system proteins, produced and released by cells infected by a virus, which inhibit viral multiplication and modify the body's immune response.

intermittent self-catheterization (ISC): A procedure in which the person periodically inserts a catheter into the urinary opening to drain urine from the bladder. ISC is used in the management of bladder dysfunction to drain urine that remains after voiding, prevent bladder distention, prevent kidney damage, and restore bladder function.

intramuscular: Into the muscle. Used in the context of an injection of a medication directly into the muscle.

intrathecal space: The space surrounding the brain and spinal

534

cord that contains cerebrospinal fluid.

intravenous (IV): Within a vein. Often used in the context of an infusion (slow drip) of a liquid medication into a vein.

involuntary emotional expression disorder (IEED): A condition (also called pseudobulbar affect or pathological laughing and crying) in which episodes of laughing and/or crying occur with no apparent precipitating event. The person's actual mood may be unrelated to the emotion being expressed.

lesion: A wound to body tissue. A lesion that occurs in the myelin of the central nervous system because of MS is called a plaque. See *plaque.*

Lhermitte's sign: An abnormal sensation of electricity or "pins and needles" going down the spine into the arms and legs that occurs when the neck is bent forward so that the chin touches the chest.

living will: See *advance (medical) directive.*

Lofstrand crutch (also called a Canadian or forearm crutch): A type of crutch with an attached holder for the forearm that provides extra support.

lumbar puncture (also called a spinal tap): A diagnostic procedure that uses a hollow needle to penetrate the spinal canal to remove cerebrospinal fluid for analysis.

lymphocyte: A type of white blood cell that's part of the immune system.

macrophage: A white blood cell with scavenger characteristics that has the ability to ingest and destroy foreign substances, such as bacteria and cell debris.

magnetic resonance imaging (MRI): A diagnostic procedure that produces visual images of different body parts without the use of X-rays.

Minimal Record of Disability: A standardized method for quantifying the clinical status of a person with MS. See *Expanded Disability Status Scale (EDSS).*

monoclonal antibodies: Laboratory-produced antibodies, which can be programmed to react against a specific antigen in order to suppress the immune response.

Multiple Sclerosis Functional Composite (MSFC): A three-part, standardized, quantitative assessment instrument for use in clinical trials in MS.

myelin: A soft, white coating of nerve fibers in the central nervous system, composed of lipids (fats) and protein. Myelin serves as insulation and as an aid to efficient nerve fiber conduction.

myelin basic protein: One of several proteins associated with the myelin of the central nervous system, which may be found in higher than normal concentrations in the cerebrospinal fluid of individuals with MS and other diseases that damage myelin.

nerve: A bundle of nerve fibers (axons).

nervous system: Includes all of the neural structures in the body. The central nervous system consists of the brain, spinal cord, and optic nerves. The peripheral nervous system consists of the nerve roots, nerve plexi, and nerves throughout the body.

neurogenic: Related to activity of the nervous system.

neurogenic bladder: Bladder dysfunction associated with neurologic malfunction in the spinal cord and characterized by a failure to empty, failure to store, or a combination of the two.

neurologist: A physician who specializes in the diagnosis and treatment of conditions related to the nervous system.

neurology: The study of the central, peripheral, and autonomic nervous systems.

neuron: The basic nerve cell of the nervous system. A neuron consists of a nucleus within a cell body and one or more processes (extensions) called dendrites and axons.

neuropsychologist: A psychologist with specialized training in the evaluation of cognitive functions. See **cognition** and **cognitive impairment.**

nocturia: The need to urinate during the night.

nystagmus: Rapid, involuntary movements of the eyes horizontally or, occasionally, vertically.

occupational therapist (OT): A therapist who assesses functioning in activities of everyday living, including dressing, bathing,

536

grooming, meal preparation, writing, and driving, which are all essential for independent living.

oligoclonal bands: A diagnostic sign indicating abnormal types of antibodies in the cerebrospinal fluid. These bands are seen in approximately 79 to 90 percent of people with multiple sclerosis, but they aren't specific to MS.

oligodendrocyte: A type of cell in the central nervous system that's responsible for making and supporting myelin.

open-label study: A preliminary (Phase I) clinical trial in which all patients receive an experimental treatment and all participants in the trial (patients and physicians) know which drug is being given.

optic neuritis: Inflammation or demyelination of the optic (visual) nerve with transient or permanent impairment of vision and occasional pain.

orthotic (also called orthosis): A mechanical appliance, such as a leg brace or splint, that's specially designed to control, correct, or compensate for impaired limb function.

orthotist: A person skilled in making orthotics, such as leg braces or splints, that help support limb function.

oscillopsia: Continuous, involuntary, and chaotic eye movement that results in a visual disturbance in which objects appear to be jumping or bouncing.

osteoporosis: Decalcification of the bones, which can result from the lack of mobility experienced by wheelchair-bound individuals.

paresis: Weakness or partial paralysis.

paresthesia: A spontaneously occurring sensation of burning, prickling, tingling, or creeping on the skin that may or may not be associated with any physical findings on a neurologic examination.

paroxysmal spasm: A sudden, uncontrolled limb contraction that occurs intermittently, lasts for a few moments, and then subsides.

paroxysmal symptom: Any one of several symptoms that have sudden onset, apparently in response to some kind of movement or sensory stimulation, last for a few moments, and then subside.

periventricular region: The area surrounding the four fluid-filled cavities within the brain. MS lesions are commonly found in this region.

physiatrist: A physician who specializes in physical medicine and rehabilitation, including the diagnosis and management of musculoskeletal injuries and pain syndromes, electrodiagnostic medicine, and rehabilitation of severe impairments (including those caused by neurologic disease or injury).

physical therapist (PT): A therapist who's trained to evaluate and improve movement and function of the body, with particular attention paid to physical mobility, balance, posture, fatigue, and pain.

pilot study: In clinical trials, an early, small- to moderate-sized study (also known as Phase II) that follows Phase I (the "safety study") and is designed to begin determining the effectiveness of the experimental treatment.

placebo: An inactive, non-drug compound that's designed to look just like a test drug being used in a double-blind clinical trial.

placebo effect: An apparently beneficial result of therapy that occurs because of the patient's expectation that the therapy will help.

plaque: An area of inflamed or demyelinated central nervous system tissue. Also called a lesion.

plasma exchange (also called plasmapharesis): An exchange that involves removing blood from a person, mechanically separating the blood cells from the fluid plasma, mixing the blood cells with replacement plasma, and returning the blood mixture to the body.

post-void residual test (PVR): A test that involves passing a catheter into the bladder following urination to drain and measure any urine that's left in the bladder after urination is completed.

pressure ulcer: An ulcer of the skin (previously called a decubitis ulcer) resulting from pressure and lack of movement as would

538

occur when a person is bed- or wheelchair-bound. The ulcers occur most frequently in areas where the bone lies directly under the skin, such as elbow, hip, or over the coccyx (tailbone).

prevalence: The number of all new and old cases of a disease in a defined population at a particular point in time.

primary-progressive MS: A clinical course of MS characterized from the beginning by progressive disease, with no plateaus or remissions, or an occasional plateau and very short-lived, minor improvements.

prognosis: Prediction of the future course of the disease.

progressive-relapsing MS: A clinical course of MS that shows disease progression from the beginning, but with clear, acute relapses, with or without full recovery from those relapses along the way.

pseudobulbar affect: See *involuntary emotional expression disorder (IEED)*.

pseudoexacerbation: A temporary aggravation of disease symptoms, resulting from an elevation in body temperature or other stressor (for example, an infection, severe fatigue, or constipation), that disappears after the stressor is removed. See *relapse*.

quad cane: A cane that has a broad base on four short "feet," which provide extra stability.

quadriplegia: The paralysis of both arms and both legs.

randomized study: A clinical trial in which all patients are assigned randomly (by chance) to be in an experimental group (receiving the experimental treatment) or a control group (receiving the placebo or control substance).

recent memory: The ability to remember events, conversations, or content of reading material or television programs from a short time ago (for example, an hour or two ago or the previous night).

rehabilitation: A multidisciplinary process directed toward helping a person recover or maintain the highest possible level of functioning and realize his or her optimal physical, mental, and social potential given any limitations that exist.

relapse: The appearance of new symptoms or the aggravation of old ones, which lasts at least 24 hours. Usually associated with inflammation and demyelination in the brain or spinal cord. Also called an exacerbation, flare-up, attack, or episode.

relapsing-remitting MS: A clinical course of MS that's characterized by clearly defined, acute attacks with full or partial recovery and no disease progression between attacks.

remission: The complete or partial recovery that follows an MS relapse. See *relapse*.

remyelination: The repair of damaged myelin.

residual urine: Urine that remains in the bladder following urination.

retrobulbar neuritis: See *optic neuritis*.

sclerosis: Hardening of tissue. In MS, sclerosis is the body's replacement of lost myelin around central nervous system nerve cells with scar tissue.

scotoma: A gap or blind spot in the visual field.

secondary-progressive MS: A clinical course of MS that's initially relapsing-remitting and then becomes progressive at a variable rate, possibly with an occasional relapse and minor remission.

sign: An objective physical problem or abnormality identified by the physician during the neurologic examination. Neurologic signs may differ significantly from the symptoms reported by the patient because they're identifiable only with specific tests and may cause no overt symptoms.

single-blind clinical study: A study in which the experimental subjects don't know who is taking the test drug or the placebo (control), but the examining doctors, attending nurses, or other research staff do know.

spasm: A sudden involuntary muscle contraction or cramp.

spasticity: A change in the normal elasticity of the muscles (caused by altered nerve impulses), which results in tightness or stiffness.

speech/language pathologist: A physician who specializes in the diagnosis and treatment of speech and swallowing disorders. Be-

540

cause of their expertise with speech and language difficulties, these specialists also provide cognitive remediation for individuals with cognitive impairment.

sphincter: A circular band of muscle fibers that tightens or closes a natural opening of the body, such as the external anal sphincter, which closes the anus, and the internal and external urinary sphincters, which close the urinary canal. See **urinary sphincter.**

spinal tap: See **lumbar puncture.**

steroids: See **adrenocorticotropic hormone (ACTH), corticosteroid,** and **glucocorticoid hormones.**

subcutaneous: Under the skin. Used in connection with the shallow injection of a medication under the top layer of skin.

symptom: A subjectively perceived problem or complaint reported by the patient.

T-cell: A lymphocyte (white blood cell) that develops in the bone marrow, matures in the thymus, and works as part of the immune system in the body.

tandem gait: A test of balance and coordination that involves alternately placing the heel of one foot directly against the toes of the other foot.

trigeminal neuralgia: Lightning-like, acute pain in the face caused by demyelination of nerve fibers at the site where the sensory (trigeminal) nerve root for that part of the face enters the brainstem.

urethra: Duct or tube that drains the urinary bladder.

urinary frequency: Feeling the urge to urinate even when urination has occurred very recently.

urinary hesitancy: The inability to urinate spontaneously even though the urge to do so is present.

urinary incontinence: See **incontinence.**

urinary sphincter: The muscle closing the urethra, which in a state of flaccid paralysis causes urinary incontinence and in a state of spastic paralysis results in an inability to urinate.

urinary urgency: The inability to postpone urination after the need has been felt.

urine culture and sensitivity: A diagnostic procedure to test for urinary tract infection and identify the appropriate treatment.

urologist: A physician who specializes in the branch of medicine concerned with the anatomy, physiology, disorders, and care of the male and female urinary tract, as well as the male genital tract.

urology: A medical specialty that deals with disturbances of the urinary (male and female) and reproductive (male) organs.

vibration sense: The ability to feel vibrations against various parts of the body. Vibration sense is tested (with a tuning fork) as part of the sensory portion of the neurologic exam.

videofluoroscopy: A radiographic study of a person's swallowing mechanism that's recorded on videotape. Videofluoroscopy shows the physiology of the pharynx, the location of the swallowing difficulty, and confirms whether food particles or fluids are being aspirated into the airway.

visual acuity: Clarity of vision. Acuity is measured as a fraction of normal vision. For example, 20/20 vision indicates an eye that sees at 20 feet what a normal eye should see at 20 feet; 20/400 vision indicates an eye that sees at 20 feet what a normal eye sees at 400 feet.

visual evoked potential: A test in which the brain's electrical activity in response to visual stimuli (for example, a flashing checkerboard) is recorded by an electroencephalograph and analyzed by a computer.

vocational rehabilitation (VR): A program of services carried out by individually created state agencies designed to enable people with disabilities to become or remain employed.

white matter: The part of the brain that contains myelinated nerve fibers and appears white, in contrast to the cortex of the brain, which contains nerve cell bodies and appears gray.

Additional Resources

*E*ven though we've included in this book everything you need for the basics of living with multiple sclerosis (MS), you may want to delve deeper into a particular topic of interest. Luckily information about MS is now available from countless sources and in a variety of formats and languages. Your challenge is to zero in on the good stuff—the information that's accurate, up-to-date, and relevant. The books and Web sites listed here are only a limited sample of what's out there for you—but each is a resource that we recommend with confidence.

Reading Other Books about MS

All of the books in this list were written by specialists in the field of MS or chronic illness, or by people living with a chronic illness. So that you have a good idea of what you can expect, we give you a brief description of each book.

You'll notice that several titles are published by Demos Medical Publishing (www.demosmedpub.com). We're big fans of Demos Medical Publishing titles because they represent the work of respected colleagues who are dedicated to the care and quality of life of people with MS.

- *Alternative Medicine and Multiple Sclerosis*, 2nd edition, by Allen C. Bowling (Demos Medical Publishing, 2007). Lots of reliable, unbiased information on the relevance, safety, and effectiveness of various alternative therapies.

- *Barrier-Free Travel: A Nuts and Bolts Guide for Wheelers and Slow Walkers*, 2nd edition, by Candy Harrington (Demos Medical Publishing, 2005). An impressive collection of useful tips for safe and comfortable travel.

- *The Comfort of Home: A Step-by-Step Guide for Multiple Sclerosis Caregivers* by Maria M. Meyer and Paula Derr (Demos Medical Publishing, 2006). A helpful look at caregiving options and strategies that take into account the complex needs of both the person with MS and the caregiver.

- *Facing the Cognitive Challenges of MS* by Jeffrey N. Gingold (Demos Medical Publishing, 2006). A personal account of one man's struggle with the cognitive changes caused by MS.

- *Fall Down Laughing* by David L. Lander (Tarcher/Putnam, 2000). A poignant but humorous account of David "Squiggy" Lander's journey with MS and his efforts on behalf of others with the disease.

- *Health Insurance Resource Manual: Options for People with a Chronic Disease or Disability*, 2nd edition, by Dorothy E. Northrop, Stephen Cooper, and Kim Calder (Demos Medical Publishing, 2007). A must-read for anyone trying to navigate the world of insurance.

- *Managing the Symptoms of Multiple Sclerosis*, 4th edition, by Randall T. Schapiro (Demos Medical

Publishing, 2003). Comprehensive, easy-to-understand recommendations for managing the symptoms that MS can cause.

➤ *Meeting the Challenge of Progressive Multiple Sclerosis* by Patricia K. Coyle and June Halper (Demos Medical Publishing, 2001). A clear explanation of what progressive disease is all about, complete with suggestions regarding how to manage the symptoms and cope with potential life changes.

➤ *Multiple Sclerosis: 300 Tips for Making Life Easier*, 2nd edition, by Shelley Peterman Schwarz (Demos Medical Publishing, 2006). A wealth of practical and clever how-tos.

➤ *Multiple Sclerosis: A Guide for Families*, 3rd edition, by Rosalind Kalb (Demos Medical Publishing, 2006). A resource to help families make room for MS in their lives without giving it more time or attention than it needs.

➤ *Multiple Sclerosis: A Guide for the Newly Diagnosed*, 3rd edition, by Nancy Holland, T. Jock Murray, and Stephen C. Reingold (Demos Medical Publishing, 2007). A thorough yet readable introduction to MS for you and your family.

➤ *Multiple Sclerosis: A Self-Care Guide to Wellness*, 2nd edition, by Nancy Holland and June Halper (Demos Medical Publishing, 2005). Practical tips designed to promote wellness and independence for people who are old hands at MS.

➤ *Multiple Sclerosis: The Questions You Have; The Answers You Need*, 3rd edition, by Rosalind Kalb (Demos Medical Publishing, 2004). Information about virtually every aspect of the disease, in a readable question-and-answer format.

➤ *Multiple Sclerosis: Understanding the Cognitive Challenges* by Nicholas LaRocca and Rosalind Kalb (Demos Medical Publishing, 2006). The first comprehensive discussion of cognitive symptoms, including evaluation, treatment, and coping strategies.

➤ *One Particular Harbor: The Outrageous True Adventures of One Woman with Multiple Sclerosis Living in the Alaskan Wilderness* by Janet Lee James (iUniverse, 2000). A fun and fascinating memoir by a feisty woman with progressive MS.

➤ *Speedbumps* by Teri Garr and Henriette Mantel (Hudson Street Press, 2005). The whole truth and nothing but the truth—with humor and grace.

➤ *The Disabled Woman's Guide to Pregnancy and Birth* by Judith Rogers (Demos Medical Publishing, 2005). Helpful information straight from the mouths of women with disabilities.

➤ *The Winning Spirit: Lessons Learned in Last Place* by Zoe Koplowitz (Doubleday, 1997). The tales of a gutsy woman with MS who came in 28,657th at the New York City Marathon, 27 hours and 36 minutes after starting the race. Zoe describes herself as "the human post-it note you stick to your refrigerator to remind yourself, 'You can do this!'"

➤ *We are not Alone: Learning to Live with Chronic Illness* by Sefra Pitzele (Workman Publishing, 1986). A comforting, amusing, and endlessly helpful book from a woman who's been there.

➤ *Yoga and Multiple Sclerosis: A Journey to Health and Healing* by Loren M. Fishman, M.D. and Eric Small

(Demos Medical Publishing, 2007). A comprehensive guide to applying the principles of yoga to the management of some of your MS symptoms.

Finding Helpful Information Online

The Internet is a mixed bag of ever-changing information. The sites we've listed here are helpful starting points in your ongoing search for information. As you continue your search, remember that not all information is created equal. The bottom line is—you can't believe everything you read. If you see something on the Internet that seems too good to be true, it probably is. So, check things out with your healthcare team or the National MS Society, and don't make any big changes in your MS treatments without running them by your neurologist first.

General information sites

The sites listed here are great places to further explore the world of MS. Each one of these sites will add to your understanding of MS, its treatments, and the tools and resources available to help you.

✔ **Multiple Sclerosis Association of America** (www.msaa.com): Helpful information about MS and about the Association's valuable support services.

✔ **Multiple Sclerosis Foundation** (www.msfacts.org/index.php): Support groups, an MS cruise, and a multimedia library providing information in English and Spanish.

✔ **Multiple Sclerosis Society of Canada** (www.mssociety.ca): Useful information as well as opportunities to connect with others and ask questions of the experts online.

- **Multiple Sclerosis International Federation** (www.msif.org): Information about MS in English, German, Spanish, French, Italian, and Russian, and a listing of MS Societies around the world.

- **National Multiple Sclerosis Society** (www.nationalmssociety.org): Gobs of information about MS, including up-to-date research reports and Web-based programs on a variety of topics.

- **Disabled Online** (www.disabledonline.com): A world of resources for people with disabilities and their families.

- **Quackwatch** (www.quackwatch.org): A wealth of information about health-related frauds, myths, fads, fallacies, and misconduct. This site is a great place to check out those things that are too good to be true.

- **CenterWatch Clinical Trials Listing Service** (www.centerwatch.com): A listing of ongoing clinical research, including industry- and government-sponsored clinical trials.

Assistive technology sites

Take a look at these sites for a glimpse of all the tools, gadgets, and software that are out there to help you do whatever you want to do in the easiest possible way:

- **ABLEDATA** (www.abledata.com): A database of objective information about assistive technology products and rehabilitation equipment available from domestic and international sources.

✔ **AbilityHub** (www.abilityhub.com): Lots of good information and resources for people with disabilities who want to use computers.

Government sites

Here are just a few of our favorite government resources:

✔ **ADA home page** (www.usdoj.gov/crt/ada): Provides information and technical assistance concerning the Americans with Disabilities Act.

✔ **Department of Veterans Affairs** (www.va.gov): Provides benefits and services to veterans and their families.

✔ **Library of Congress—National Library Service for the Blind and Physically Handicapped** (www.loc.gov/nls): Administers a free library program of Braille and audio materials circulated by postage-free mail to eligible borrowers in the United States.

✔ **National Library of Medicine** (www.nlm.nih.gov): Provides information and research services in all areas of biomedicine and healthcare.

✔ **National Parks Service** (www.nps.gov): Provides information about the accessibility of each of the national parks in the country.

Organizations and services

Check out the information, products, and services offered by these groups to help you and your family live more comfortably with MS:

- **AARP** (www.aarp.org): Provides invaluable information and tips about health and quality of life even for youngsters under the age of 50.

- **Allsup, Inc.** (www.allsupinc.com): Provides assistance with Social Security applications.

- **The Heuga Center** (www.heuga.org): A nonprofit organization that offers multidisciplinary health and wellness programs for people with MS and their partners at locations around the country.

- **International Association of Medical Assistance to Travelers** (www.iamat.org): A nonprofit organization that makes competent medical care available to travelers, by western-trained, English-speaking physicians.

- **Lighthouse International** (www.lighthouse.org): A nonprofit organization providing information, resources, and referrals for people with visual limitations.

- **Medic Alert** (www.medicalert.org): A nonprofit organization that provides products and services built around your personalized and *private* electronic health record.

- **National Family Caregivers Association** (www.nfcacares.org): A nonprofit group that supports, empowers, educates, and advocates for the more than 50 million Americans who care for chronically ill, aged, or disabled loved ones.

- **Well Spouse Association** (www.wellspouse.org): A nonprofit organization that offers support for spouses and partners of people with a wide range of illnesses and disabilities. It also offers monthly meetings in many areas and a quarterly newsletter called *Mainstay*.

Chat rooms and bulletin boards

These sites offer you a variety of ways to communicate with others who have MS or care about someone who does:

✔ **CLAMS—Computer Literate Advocates for Multiple Sclerosis** (www.clams.org): A nonprofit organization that offers online bulletin board and chat room opportunities, as well as some fun and useful resources.

✔ **MS World Communications** (www.msworld.org): A great place to find chat rooms and message boards or to sign up for a pen pal or an e-mail group.

✔ **FaceofMS.org** (www.faceofms.org): A place to add your voice and story to hundreds of others.

Appendix C

Medications Commonly Used in MS

*T*he following table lists the medications commonly used in the management of multiple sclerosis (MS). For each product, the table gives the brand name, the chemical name, and the common usage in MS. Some of these medications are available under several different brand names. For the purposes of this table, we have included only the most commonly used brands.

You can use this table as a handy reference to help you sort out the various ways that different types of medications are used to treat MS and its symptoms. Products available without a prescription are so indicated (+).

Table C-1	Medications Used for MS Treatment	
Brand Name	**Chemical Name**	**Usage in MS**
No brand name formulation available	mineral oil+	Constipation
No brand name formulation available	papaverine	Erectile dysfunction
Antivert (U.S.)	meclizine	Nausea; vomiting; dizziness

Aricept	donepezil HCl	Memory problems
Atarax	hydroxyzine	Paroxysmal itching
Avonex	interferon beta-1a	Disease-modifying agent
Bactrim; Septra	sulfamethoxazole	Urinary tract infections
Betaseron	interferon beta-1b	Disease-modifying agent
Buspar	buspirone hydrochloride	Anxiety
Celexa	citalopram HBr	Depression; anxiety
Cialis	tadalafil	Erectile dysfunction
Cipro	ciprofloxacin	Urinary tract infections
Colace	docusate[+]	Constipation
Concerta	methylphenidate	Fatigue
Copaxone	glatiramer acetate	Disease-modifying agent
Cymbalta	duloxetine hydrochloride	Pain; depression
Dantrium	dantrolene	Spasticity
DDAVP Nasal Spray	desmopressin	Urinary frequency
DDAVP Tablets	desmopressin	Urinary frequency
Decadron	dexamethasone	Acute relapses
Deltasone	prednisone	Acute relapses
Detrol, Detrol LA	tolterodine	Bladder dysfunction

Dilantin	phenytoin	Pain (dyesthesias)
Ditropan	oxybutynin	Bladder dysfunction
Ditropan XL	oxybutynin (extended release formula)	Bladder dysfunction
Elavil	amitriptyline	Pain (paresthesias); depression
Effexor	venlafaxine	Depression
Dulcolax	Bisacodyl+	Constipation
Enablex	darifenacin	Bladder dysfunction
Enemeez Mini Enema	docusate stool softener laxative+	Constipation
Fleet Enema	sodium phosphate+	Constipation
H.P. Acthar Gel	adrenocorticotropic hormone (ACTH)	Acute relapses
Hiprex, Mandelaminetions	methenamine	Urinary tract infections (preventative)
Intrathecal Baclofen (ITB Therapy)	baclofen (intrathecal)	Spasticity
Klonopin (U.S.)	clonazepam	Tremor; pain; spasticity
Laniazid; Nydrazid	isoniazid	Tremor
Levitra	vardenafil	Erectile dysfunction
Lexapro	escitalopram oxalate	Depression; anxiety
Lidoderm patch	lidocaine	Localized pain

		Spasticity
Lioresal	baclofen	
LMX 4 cream	lidocaine	Localized pain
Macrodantin	nitrofurantoin	Urinary tract infections
Medrol	methylprednisolone	Acute relapses
Metamucil	psyllium hydrophilic mucilloid[+]	Constipation
MUSE	alprostadil	Erectile dysfunction
Neurontin	gabapentin	Pain (dysesthesias)
Novantrone	mitoxantrone	Disease-modifying agent
Oxytrol (Oxybutynin Transdermal System)	oxybutynin	Bladder dysfunction
Pamelor (U.S.)	nortriptyline	Pain (parasthesias); depression
Paxil	paroxetine	Depression
Phillips' Milk of Magnesia	magnesium hydroxide[+]	Constipation
Pro-Banthine	propantheline bromide	Bladder dysfunction
Prostin VR; Caverject	alprostadil	Erectile dysfunction
Provigil	modafinil	Fatigue
Prozac	fluoxetine	Depression; fatigue
Pyridium	phenazopyridine	Urinary tract infections (symptom relief)

555

Rebif	interferon beta-1a	Disease-modifying agent
Ritalin	methylphenidate	Fatigue
Sanctura	trospium chloride	Bladder dysfunction
Sani-Supp suppository	glycerin+	Constipation
Solu-Medrol	methylprednisolone	Acute relapses
Symmetrel	amantadine	Fatigue
Tegretol	carbamazepine	Pain (trigeminal neuralgia)
Tofranil	imipramine	Bladder dysfunction; pain
Tysabri	natalizumab	Disease-modifying agent
Valium	diazepam	Spasticity (muscle spasms)
Vesicare	solifenacin succinate	Bladder dysfunction
Viagra	sildenafil	Erectile dysfunction
Wellbutrin	bupropion	Depression
Zanaflex	tizanidine	Spasticity
Zoloft	sertraline	Depression

Index

559

560

561

562

566

572

574

575

577

581

582

Murray, T. Jock (*Multiple Sclerosis: A Guide for the Newly Diagnosed*), 92, 545
muscular dystrophy, 349
myelin, 47, 49, 536
Mysoline (medication), 201
myths, 513–518

N

NAb (neutralizing antibody), 149
naltrexone, 271
nap, 426
natalizumab, 154–156, 259, 405
National MS Society, 52, 91, 109, 141
Nelson, Jane (*Positive Discipline*), 433
nerve, 47, 536
nervous system
  definition, 47, 536
  effect of MS, 48–51
  function, 47–48
  MRI process, 77–79
neurogenic bladder, 536
neurologic exam, 73–76
neurologist
  action after diagnosis, 93–94
  decision-making tips, 107
  definition, 35, 536
  diagnosis criteria, 69–70
  diagnosis difficulties, 68
  MRI explanation, 77
  must-do's, 508
  rationale for use, 111
  routine care pattern, 115–116, 285–286
  second opinion, 85
  selection, 111–115

592

594

About the Authors

The authors' shared commitment to multiple sclerosis (MS) began more than 25 years ago at the MS Care Center at the Albert Einstein College of Medicine, under the direction of Labe Scheinberg, MD, who is considered by many to be the father of MS comprehensive care.

Rosalind Kalb, PhD, is Associate Vice President of the Professional Resource Center at the National Multiple Sclerosis Society in New York City. After receiving her doctorate in clinical psychology from Fordham University in 1977, Dr. Kalb began her career at the MS Care Center, providing individual, group, and family therapy for people living with MS. Dr. Kalb is the author of the National MS Society's *Knowledge Is Power* series for individuals newly diagnosed with MS and is an editor of *Keep S'myelin,* the newsletter for children who have a parent with MS. Dr. Kalb has edited two books on MS—*Multiple Sclerosis: The Questions You Have, The Answers You Need, 3rd Edition* (Demos Medical Publishing, 2004), and *Multiple Sclerosis: A Guide for Families, 3rd Edition* (Demos Medical Publishing, 2006). She is also coauthor, along with Nicholas LaRocca, PhD, of the book *Multiple Sclerosis: Understanding the Cognitive Challenges* (Demos Medical Publishing, 2006).

Nancy Holland, EdD, RN, is Vice President of Clinical Pro-

601

grams at the National Multiple Sclerosis Society in New York City. Prior to joining the Society, Dr. Holland served as the MS Care Center's Clinic Coordinator and Director of Training for 15 years. She is a founding director of the International Organization of MS Nurses. She is also author or editor of more than 60 MS-related articles, chapters, and books, including *Comprehensive Nursing Care in Multiple Sclerosis*, 2nd Edition (Demos Medical Publishing, 2002), *Multiple Sclerosis: A Self-Care Guide for Wellness*, 2nd Edition (Demos Medical Publishing, 2005), and *Multiple Sclerosis: A Guide for the Newly Diagnosed*, 3rd Edition (Demos Medical Publishing, 2007). Dr. Holland earned a doctorate in higher and adult education from Columbia University, and holds undergraduate and graduate degrees in nursing.

Barbara Giesser, MD, is an Associate Clinical Professor of Neurology and Clinical Director of the MS Program at the University of Los Angeles (UCLA) David Geffen School of Medicine. She also serves as the Medical Director of the UCLA Marilyn Hilton MS Achievement Center.

Dr. Giesser has specialized in the care of persons with MS since 1982, beginning with her training at the MS Care Center. She has been an invited lecturer to speak about MS in regional, national, and international venues, and has published research in the areas of cognition, gender issues, and rehabilitation strategies in persons with MS. Additionally, she has been active in developing educational materials about MS for medical students, residents, healthcare professionals, and people with MS for organizations including the NMSS and the American Academy of Neurology.

The employees of Thorndike Press hope you have enjoyed this Large Print book. All our Thorndike and Wheeler Large Print titles are designed for easy reading, and all our books are made to last. Other Thorndike Press Large Print books are available at your library, through selected bookstores, or directly from us.

For information about titles, please call:

(800) 223-1244

or visit our Web site at:

www.gale.com/thorndike
www.gale.com/wheeler

To share your comments, please write:

Publisher
Thorndike Press
295 Kennedy Memorial Drive
Waterville, ME 04901

603